Obesity Medicine
Board Review Questions

Obesity Medicine Board Review Questions

Kevin B. Smith, DO, FACP
ABOM Diplomate

225+ Board Style Review Questions to Prepare for the American Board of Obesity Medicine Certification

2023 Edition

ISBN: 9798373792769

Independently published

Disclaimer: All efforts have been made to ensure accuracy and that the most up-to-date information is provided. Information in this review book should be used for study, not as a reference for patient care. It is up to the provider to ensure all information is accurate, and the author will not be held liable for inadvertent errors.

The item domains and rubrics for the Certification Examination for Obesity Medicine Physicians are available without charge on the ABOM website to facilitate individual study as well as review course development. The author of this review book has not been provided information regarding examination questions, nor does the author have preferential knowledge regarding actual questions included in the examination.

Copy editing performed by Kelly Smith

For correspondence, including questions, concerns, or errata, please contact: obesitymedicinereview@gmail.com

Free weekly study blogs, book updates, and discounts can be found at obesitymedicinereview.com or by scanning QR code.

Need More Practice Questions?

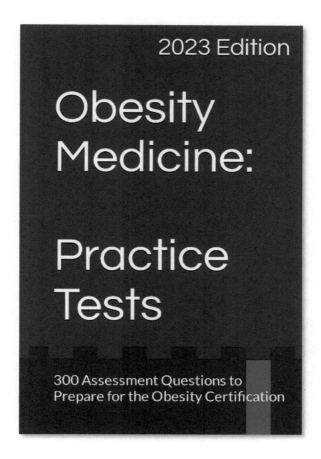

Obesity Medicine: Practice Tests (2023 Edition) provides 300 additional complementary questions to supplement studying for the American Board of Obesity Medicine (ABOM) examination.

I. Basic Concepts
Page 1

II. Diagnosis and Evaluation
Page 23

III. Treatment
Page 51

IV. Practice Management
Page 113

Answer Explanations
Page 121

Test Content Outline and
Answer List Summary
Page 351

I. Basic Concepts

1. A 41-year-old male is seen in the hospital on postoperative day one status post Roux-en-Y gastric bypass. Home medications include glargine 30 units nightly and aspart sliding scale with meals. Since surgery, he has not required any insulin to maintain normal glucose levels and has plans to be discharged on a low dose of immediate-release metformin. The increased endogenous hormone responsible for this diabetic medication adjustment

A. is only secreted in the small intestine
B. is secreted in response to fat and protein ingestion
C. reduces hepatic gluconeogenesis
D. has the same quantitative effects as seen after sleeve gastrectomy
E. causes gallbladder contraction

2. A 24-year-old female presents for genetic counseling regarding obesity. She is frustrated by the lack of ability to lose weight and being classified as "overweight" at a very young age despite her tall stature. She admits to wanting to give up regarding weight loss since obesity "is a family curse." She has diabetes and is on metformin. Previous testing indicated that she had significantly elevated circulating insulin levels. Which of the following genetic abnormalities is most likely present?

A. MC4R
B. POMC
C. FTO
D. PCSK1
E. LEPR

3. A 51-year-old female presents to the health clinic with questions about a diet she heard about through a health magazine. Although she cannot remember the name of the diet, it promoted a higher intake of omega fat than other diets she has researched. Benefits included lowering cardiovascular disease and preventing type 2 diabetes, both of which run in her family. In addition, she will still be able to consume seafood, an important component given her fishing hobby. What is the most likely diet that this patient is referencing?

A. Vegan
B. Pescatarian
C. Lacto-ovo
D. Mediterranean
E. Low carbohydrate

4. A 31-year-old female wants to know her total energy expenditure. She estimates her non-exercise activity thermogenesis to be 300 kcal/day, her thermic effect of meals to be 10% of her total expenditure, and her calories from exercise to be 400 kcal/day. What other testing is necessary to determine her total energy expenditure accurately?

A. Indirect calorimeter
B. Skinfold calipers
C. Duke's treadmill score
D. Bioelectric impedance analyses
E. Basal body temperature

5. A research team is developing a thesis regarding intrauterine predisposition to factors, such as how maternal obesity affects the developing fetus through adulthood. So far, the longitudinal study has shown that a mother's body mass index correlates with comorbidities of cognitive deficits and autism spectrum disorders. This type of research is best associated with which of the following?

A. Neurohormonal physiology
B. Epigenetics and environment
C. Behavioral determinants
D. Mutations of genetic DNA
E. Socioeconomic and culture

6. A longitudinal study was completed looking at the effects of sleep on weight. Both weight and the time of quality sleep, measured through a smartwatch device, were documented over 10 years. At the end of the study, what hormones or receptor levels would be expected to be increased in those who received 5 hours of sleep compared to those that received 8 hours?

A. Leptin and neuropeptide Y
B. α-MSH and peptide YY
C. POMC receptors and ghrelin
D. Cortisol and leptin
E. Ghrelin and orexin A

7. A 65-year-old male is following up with his dietician after starting a low-fat diet six weeks ago. He has increased his exercise to 250 minutes/week and has noticed a 1% total body weight loss since initiating these lifestyle changes. He comments that he has always had to work hard to maintain or lose weight, and it seems that if he stops dieting for a few weeks, he regains weight rapidly. In contrast, he states that his wife can eat whatever she likes, has always remained thin, and seldomly exercises. Compared to his wife, this patient most likely has which of the following?

A. Decreased energy harvest from food
B. Higher fasting-induced adipose factor expression
C. Increased levels of Firmicutes in his gut
D. Higher AMPK

8. A research study is underway in which patients fast for 8 hours, followed by consuming a meal of 500 kcal. Several hormones are monitored every 2 hours during the fasting and postprandial period for 12 hours. Six hours into the fast, ghrelin hormone levels are at their peak. What other finding would most likely be present during this time?

A. Y1 and Y5 receptor stimulation
B. Leptin hormone elevation
C. Suppressed agouti-related peptide hormone levels
D. Activation of the POMC/CART pathway
E. Orexin A and B hormone suppression

9. A 31-year-old female presents to her primary care physician for follow-up regarding weight-gain. Over the past three months, she has noticed a weight gain of approximately 10 pounds (4.5 kg), which is discouraging because she has been trying to get healthy and lose weight before her wedding in 2 months. She quit smoking with the help of bupropion and has been walking daily. She had a copper intrauterine device inserted four months ago. Although she goes to bed later due to wedding planning, she states she still sleeps 8 hours nightly. Which of the following is most likely playing a role in her weight gain?

A. Bupropion
B. Intrauterine device
C. Decreased tobacco
D. Sleep habits

10. Several medical students are trying to create a project to determine the best way to impact childhood obesity rates, as this rate has nearly tripled in the past 30 years. They begin to review epidemiologic data on a national level to see who is most affected by obesity prevalence, focusing on children 2-19 years old. They compare age, race, gender, and financial status. During their research, what are they most likely to find?

A. The highest prevalence of obesity is in Hispanic female children
B. Class 3 obesity in children has declined over the past decade
C. Asian adolescents had higher obesity rates than Hispanics
D. The highest income class had the lowest obesity rates
E. The prevalence of obesity was nearly 40% in all children

11. A 19-year-old female presents to her family practice practitioner and requests a referral to a lymphedema clinic. She states that since she was 15 years old, she has gained excessive weight, predominantly in her lower extremities. She says her grandmother had similar findings on her upper extremities after undergoing a mastectomy, and she was treated at a lymphedema clinic with good results. She has a normal waist circumference and a BMI of 26 kg/m². Her lower extremities have a sensation of round peas when the fatty tissue is palpated. What other findings would be expected in this patient?

A. Decreased lymphatic flow
B. Positive cuff sign
C. Marked pitting edema
D. Eventual progression to arms
E. Positive Stemmer's sign

12. A 33-year-old female recently underwent a sleeve gastrectomy and is losing weight appropriately. She is most impressed by her decreased appetite, irrespective of meals, which has helped maintain a significant calorie deficit. The hormone most likely responsible for her decreased appetite initially acts on what area of the brain?

A. Dorsal vagal complex
B. Amygdala
C. Nucleus of the tractus solitarius
D. Arcuate nucleus
E. Lateral hypothalamus

13. A dietician is reviewing terminology with one of her students. She discusses a term that describes the value of the amount of a nutrient estimated to meet the requirement of half of all healthy individuals in a population. What term is she defining?

A. Estimated average requirement
B. Adequate intake
C. Recommended daily allowance
D. Tolerable upper intake level
E. Daily value

14. A human research study is ongoing and is recruiting patients with a body mass index > 30 kg/m² who have not previously been diagnosed with thyroid disease and do not have symptoms of overt hypothyroidism. Inclusion criteria requires a thyroid-stimulating hormone (TSH) level > 5 mcU/mL (reference range 0.4-4.2 mcU/mL). At the end of the study, 130 patients met the above criteria. The patients were then provided resources to assist in losing 5% of their total body weight. Which lab finding would be expected after they achieved their weight-loss goal?

A. Increased thyroid-releasing hormone
B. Increased T₄ (thyroxine) levels
C. Decreased T₃ (triiodothyronine) levels
D. Unchanged thyroid level changes

15. A 49-year-old male presents to the office to discuss weight-related complications. He states he was recently promoted to chief operating officer of a Fortune 500 company and the fear of messing up and losing the associated lifestyle, prestige, and salary is "driving me mad." Per chart review, it is noted that since starting this new position, he has gained nearly 45 lbs (20.4 kg). Compared to before the promotion and now, which hormonal change is most likely?

A. Insulin sensitivity increase with glucagon suppression
B. Activation of α-MSH and increased levels of leptin
C. Poor quality of sleeping activating the POMC/CART pathway
D. NPY activation related to excess cortisol section
E. Suppressed ghrelin levels due to vagal nerve suppression

16. A researcher is looking to evaluate different climates' effects on obesity rates. He believes warmer temperatures should allow more outdoor activity, thus lowering obesity rates. He wants to begin his research in the state with the lowest obesity rates. Which state should he start his research?

A. Colorado
B. Mississippi
C. Oklahoma
D. Florida
E. West Virginia

17. An endocrinologist is discussing with a medical student the vast number of hormones that play a role in obesity and satiety. In particular, one hormone is an insulin sensitizer, in which levels are inversely related to body fat mass. In addition, the endogenous levels of this hormone decrease in the setting of type 2 diabetes. The hormone described above most likely originates from which of the following structures?

A. Adipose tissue
B. Gastric fundus
C. Duodenum
D. Beta cells of the pancreas
E. Alpha cells of the pancreas

18. A 44-year-old male with a past medical history of insomnia presents for an annual wellness exam. He denies any current complaints but does admit to right knee pain that is worsened with prolonged walking. He has a moderate score on the Epworth sleepiness scale. His body mass index is 31 kg/m², his waist circumference is 81.3 cm (32 inches), and his body fat composition is 24%. Laboratory work, including a hemoglobin A1c, complete metabolic panel, and lipid panel, is unremarkable. An x-ray of his right knee shows moderate osteophytes and joint space narrowing. Which of the following best describes his condition?

A. Sick fat disease
B. Obesity class II
C. Obesity based on % body fat
D. Fat mass disease
E. Abdominal obesity

19. A 6-year-old male is being seen by a pediatric endocrinologist subspecialist for severe obesity. The mother states that the patient had a normal birth weight and even required nutrient supplementation due to failure to thrive early on. However, since age three, he has had extreme hunger, which has led to progressive weight gain. The child currently weighs 178 lbs (80.7 kg). A genetic mutation is discovered, and subsequent treatment with hormone replacement is initiated with impressive results. Which of the following neuromodulators was most likely activated with the hormone replacement?

A. Orexin A and B
B. Alpha melanocyte-stimulating hormone
C. Agouti-related peptide
D. Melanin-concentrating hormone

20. Researchers are looking at potential intravenous medications to assist in weight loss. One treatment that has shown promise is a synthetic form of a gastrointestinal hormone produced in both the large and small intestines and is found to be elevated within 1 hour after meals. Its contributions to weight loss are due to its potent appetite suppressant and ability to delay gastric emptying and intestinal transit time. The hormone level increases irrespective of macronutrient intake. What is the hormone most likely being studied?

A. Ghrelin
B. Cholecystokinin
C. Glucagon-like peptide 1
D. Oxyntomodulin
E. Peptide YY

21. A previously healthy 9-year-old female presents to her pediatrician for a well-child check. Her growth chart is shown below. Her percentile BMI has steadily increased over the last four visits despite lifestyle changes incorporated within her family. She has breast bud development. Which of the following conditions may be contributing to these findings?

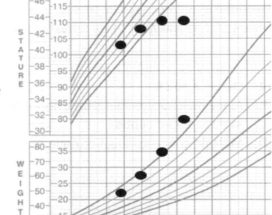

A. Excessive caloric intake
B. Precocious puberty
C. Bulimia
D. Achondroplasia
E. Hypothyroidism

22. A 7-year-old female presents with her mother for a dietician evaluation and education session. The family drinks a lot of sweetened tea in the home and inquires about changing from sugar to nonnutritive sweeteners (NNS). The best response to her inquiry would be that NNS:

A. are a preferred alternative to sucrose
B. increase the risk of ADHD in children
C. may help with weight loss, as they are calorie-neutral
D. can cause a dysregulation in appetite
E. are regarded as "not safe for children" by the FDA

12

23. A 5-year-old male with the disease of obesity is seen in the pediatric clinic for follow-up after meeting with a childhood obesity specialist. This patient has had many difficulties, including significant intellectual disability, retinal dystrophy, and polydactyly. Renal malformations have led to polyuria and polydipsia, requiring a percutaneous endoscopy gastrostomy tube to be placed to keep up with fluid replenishment. Given these findings, the patient most likely carries which of the following diagnoses?

A. Prader-Willi syndrome
B. Cohen syndrome
C. Borjeson-Forssman-Lehmann syndrome
D. Albright hereditary osteodystrophy
E. Bardet-Biedl syndrome

24. A previously healthy 29-year-old male with a diagnosis of obesity presents to the clinic for a physical examination. He is an accountant and thus is relatively inactive during the day. Vital signs are within normal limits. His BMI is 35 kg/m². He is frustrated that despite exercising and eating similarly to his identical twin brother, he is nearly 40 lbs (18.1 kg) heavier than his brother, who is a mail carrier. Which of the following best explains the weight difference between him and his twin brother?

A. Basal metabolic rate
B. Non-exercise activity thermogenesis
C. Intentional exercise
D. Resting energy expenditure
E. Dietary thermogenesis

25. On a medical mission trip, a 7-year-old patient is being seen in the clinic. He appears very malnourished, but he seems unphased by his lack of nutrition. His abdomen is distended, and anasarca is present. He is supplemented with low doses of protein in incremental amounts to prevent refeeding syndrome. Which of the following must be consumed in his diet, as his body cannot produce it?

A. Alanine
B. Aspartate
C. Glycine
D. Leucine
E. Proline

26. A researcher is trying to create a calculator that will take into account epigenetic factors contributing to childhood obesity rates to predict which children are most prone to obesity. He plans to have a smartphone application that contains a checklist of risk factors for childhood obesity, thus providing a percent risk of obesity based on current risk factors. Practitioners would then be able to discuss with the parents how reducing certain risk factors could improve the odds of a healthy-weight in their children. Which of the following should be taken into account for his predictive calculator?

A. Kids have similar obesity rates whether one/both parents have obesity
B. Cesarean-section babies are more likely to be affected by obesity
C. Maternal smoking leads to decreased childhood obesity rates
D. Breastfed infants have fewer infections but increased obesity rates
E. Insufficient gestational weight gain is protective against obesity

27. A 36-year-old female status post sleeve gastrectomy six years prior presents to her primary care physician complaining of numbness to her lower extremities. She has lost 120 lbs (54.4 kg) postoperatively. She is currently taking prenatal vitamins. Physical examination reveals diminished vibratory sense bilaterally in her lower extremities and a positive Romberg test. What is the most likely underlying cause of this patient's clinical presentation?

A. Decreased intrinsic factor production
B. Anti-parietal antibodies
C. Tissue transglutaminase antibodies
D. Impaired terminal ileum absorption
E. Decreased dietary intake

28. A 31-year-old female presents to her dietician's office five months after undergoing a sleeve gastrectomy. During this period, she has lost 43 lbs (19.5 kg) and is encouraged and motivated to continue working toward weight loss. She has followed all dietary recommendations and vitamin replacement. What is the most accurate statement regarding the hormone most affected by this surgery, contributing to her weight loss?

A. Patients with Prader-Willi syndrome have normal levels
B. Those with a vagotomy would have similar qualitative levels
C. Glucose suppresses the hormone for extended periods
D. Sleep deprivation reduces this hormone, while stress increases it
E. Leptin levels are directly proportionate to this hormone

29. A pathophysiologist is lecturing medical students on the hormones secreted by adipose tissue. In particular, one of these hormones plays a role in energy balance and is directly proportionate to the amount of adipose tissue in the body. As adipose increases, this hormone increases, signaling satiety and increasing the rate of energy expenditure. Patients with a deficiency of this hormone have obesity at an early age. Which of the following is most similar to the described hormone in both duration of action, and effects on satiety?

A. Pancreatic polypeptide
B. Cholecystokinin
C. Insulin
D. Glucagon-like peptide 1
E. Ghrelin

30. A 33-year-old female presents to her primary care physician for follow-up regarding her polysomnography results. Her results reveal her apnea-hypopnea index was > 30, indicating severe obstructive sleep apnea; the test was split with continuous positive airway pressure (CPAP) titration. She has a prescription for a CPAP machine but has not picked it up yet. Given these findings, which neurohumoral hormone would be expected to be decreased?

A. Ghrelin
B. Orexin
C. Leptin
D. Neuropeptide Y

31. A physician is discussing with a medical student the ethnic disparities within obesity. Of the following ethnicity and gender combinations in adults, which would likely have the most significant disparity of increased obesity (based on percentage)?

A. Asian males
B. Hispanic males
C. White females
D. Black females

32. A patient is presenting to discuss weight loss options. He has tried several dietary plans without success and has trouble maintaining a persistent exercise schedule. Which of the following statements would be most accurate?

A. If you consume less calories than what you use, you will lose weight
B. For every 3500 kcal you decrease in your diet, you will lose 1 lb
C. Losing weight is all about willpower and motivation
D. It is easier to maintain weight loss, rather than lose it
E. Subcutaneous fat can affect health similarly to visceral fat

33. A 46-year-old female presents for an annual follow-up with her obesity medicine specialist. She underwent a successful biliopancreatic diversion and duodenal switch seven years ago. She has been adherent with all nutritional visits and supplemental vitamin intake. She had lost 162 lbs (73.5 kg), but has regained 10 lbs (4.5 kg) in the past year. She denies any new symptoms. Laboratory work reveals a microcytic anemia with a decreased ferritin level. Which gastrointestinal area is most likely responsible for this patient's laboratory abnormalities?

A. Stomach
B. Duodenum
C. Jejunum
D. Ileum
E. Colon

34. A nutritionist is discussing how energy relates to food intake and nutrition labels. How much energy would it take to raise 1 kilogram of water by 1 °C?

A. 1 Calorie
B. 10 kilocalories
C. 100 Calories
D. 1,000 Calories
E. 10,000 calories

35. A 23-year-old male presents to his family practice physician after he read an article on high-dose calcium intake related to weight loss. He is currently taking twice the recommended daily allowance, but hasn't noticed a significant weight loss at this point. He asks if this is an effective obesity treatment. His current BMI is 27 kg/m². His only complaint is constipation. Given his current status, which of the following is most likely increased in this patient?

    A. Parathyroid hormone activity
    B. Vitamin D levels
    C. Lipogenesis
    D. Lipolysis
    E. Fat storage levels

36. A group of physicians are developing a program to address patients with coronary artery disease who are at the highest risk of mortality within the next five years. To simplify the program, they only evaluate the body mass index and waist circumference. Those with the highest mortality risk will be entered into an intensive physical, dietary, and behavioral modification program. Which of the following parameters of patients should receive priority entrance into this class?

    A. BMI 22 kg/m²; Waist circumference 85 cm
    B. BMI 22 kg/m²; Waist circumference 101 cm
    C. BMI 26 kg/m²; Waist circumference 85 cm
    D. BMI 30 kg/m²; Waist circumference 85 cm
    E. BMI 30 kg/m²; Waist circumference 101 cm

37. A 49-year-old female is discussing a recent incident with her health coach. She states that she recently dropped off her only child at college. A week later, she walked by a bakery and the smell brought back memories of her and her child baking bread on the weekends. Despite recently finishing up lunch and not being hungry, she indulged in two large pieces of bread. Which area of activation played the largest role in this incident?

A. Amygdala
B. Hippocampus
C. Pre-frontal cortex
D. Hypothalamus
E. Occipital lobe

38. A 4-year-old male with weight and height consistently in the 95th percentile presents to his pediatrician for follow-up regarding tumor surveillance. He recently underwent an abdominal ultrasound showing hepatosplenomegaly without concerning findings for malignancy. What genetic characteristic is most likely associated with this condition?

A. Autosomal recessive inheritance
B. Chromosome 15q deletion
C. Chromosome 8q22 mutation
D. Chromosome 11p15.5 dysregulation
E. ALMS 1 mutation

39. A 32-year-old pregnant female presents for education regarding her recent diagnosis of gestational diabetes mellitus (GDM). In particular, she wants to know the risk factors for her infant developing the disease of childhood obesity in order to make appropriate changes. Which would be the most accurate information to provide to this patient?

A. High protein intake early in life increases BMI at age 2
B. Breastfeeding only for the first week of life reduces toddler weight
C. Gestational diabetes does not influence childhood obesity rates
D. Early complementary feedings result in reduced caloric intake at 12 months
E. A cesarean section reduces unfavorable microbiota leading to reduced childhood weight

40. A 37-year-old female presents to her surgeon for a 12-month follow-up after a successful sleeve gastrectomy. She has followed all diet and exercise regimens as prescribed by her dietician and electrophysiologist. However, she has noticed that even though she has increased her exercise time to 220 minutes weekly, she has not seen a significant decrease in weight as expected. She has lost 95 lbs (43 kg) postoperatively but has plateaued. Which of the following most likely explains this plateau effect?

A. Increased total energy expenditure
B. Increased muscle efficiency
C. Adaptive thermogenesis
D. Modified set-point
E. Increased leptin levels

41. A 29-year-old male plans to run a marathon in the next four months. He has been training daily and can run nearly 18 miles without stopping. What is true of the muscle fibers he predominantly utilizes to prepare for this marathon?

A. Energy is from glycolysis
B. Creates forceful contractions
C. Fatigue susceptible
D. Increased mitochondria are present

42. A 66-year-old female presents to the clinic for worsening vision. She states that this has been progressing for the past six months, but recently nearly caused a car accident. She has also had daily headaches, which she attributes to the vision changes, and reports she always feels hungry. Her vital signs are normal except for her BMI, which has increased from 31 to 33 kg/m² since last year. Physical exam reveals bilateral loss of the lower peripheral visual fields. Laboratory work reveals a TSH is 0.1 µU/mL (reference range: 0.5–5.0 µU/mL) and a T₄ is 2 µg/dL (reference range: 5–12 µg/dL). Prolactin levels are normal. Which of the following is the most appropriate next step?

A. Brain imaging
B. Levothyroxine replacement
C. Ophthalmology referral
D. Radioactive iodine scan of the thyroid
E. Growth hormone and ACTH levels

43. A double-blinded study is performed with patients who have a body mass index between 25-30 kg/m². They receive either a placebo or an intravenous medication theorized to increase brown adipose tissue (BAT) activation. At the end of the infusion, patients undergo a positron emission tomography (PET) scan to evaluate the presence of BAT. After the trial, there was an 11% increased tracer uptake, as evidenced by the PET scan, in those receiving the medication compared to the placebo group. Which of the following most accurately describes the studied adipose tissue?

A. Its brown color is due to increased lysosomes
B. It couples oxidative phosphorylation, increasing ATP production
C. It is stimulated by acetylcholine of the parasympathetic system
D. Resting metabolic rate is inversely proportional to BAT levels
E. It utilizes glucose and free fatty acids to increase lipolysis

44. A 29-year-old health-conscious female is discussing her diet with a nutritionist. Although not focused on weight loss, she is interested to see if her diet matches the recommendations based on the acceptable macronutrient distribution range, as set forth by the United States Department of Agriculture (USDA). Which of the following would meet that criteria if the macronutrient was listed as a percentage of her total calories?

A. Protein 45%
B. Carbohydrate 60%
C. Fat 40%
D. Linoleic acid (Ω -6 fatty acid) 15%
E. α-Linolenic acid (Ω-3 fatty acid) 5%

45. A 29-year-old female presents for a follow-up appointment with her primary care physician. Over the past year, she has lost 40 lbs (18.1 kg), which she attributes to meal replacements and an effective exercise regimen. A recent body composition scan revealed a 3% reduction in adipose tissue. However, over the past two months, she has regained 5 lbs (2.3 kg). She denies a change in her diet or exercise regimen but does admit to "sneaking a few extra snacks here and there," as she states her hunger has increased. Which of the following neurohormonal changes is most likely contributing to her increased weight gain?

A. Increased leptin levels
B. Loss of inhibition of the NPY/AgRP pathway
C. Melanocortin 4 receptor activation
D. Orexin A and B hormone suppression
E. Inhibition of neurotrophic factor

II. Diagnosis and Evaluation

46. A 34-year-old female with a BMI of 29 kg/m^2 presents to her primary care physician with overeating concerns. She states that she often eats a large amount of food, lacking control while eating during these episodes. She hides this behavior from her roommate as she feels intense embarrassment and guilt. Given the most likely diagnosis, what other finding would most likely be expected?

A. Eating more rapidly than normal
B. Compensatory purging
C. Consuming > 25% of calories after dinner
D. Repetitive behaviors
E. Eating small, unplanned amounts of food

47. A 43-year-old female is presenting with increased thirst and urination. She states that over the past 2-3 months, she has woken up multiple times in the night to urinate and feels like she cannot "drink enough water". She has a past medical history of autoimmune hemolytic anemia and obesity class II. In addition to other age-appropriate screenings, which laboratory test is most sensitive to diagnose her with the most likely condition?

A. Hemoglobin A1c
B. Fasting glucose levels
C. HOMA-IR levels
D. Oral glucose tolerance test
E. Fructosamine levels

48. A 3-year-old male is brought into the pediatric office, as the mother has recently noticed increased weight gain and an insatiable appetite that was not previously present. After reviewing the growth chart, it is noted that his height has maintained the 60th percentile. However, his weight has increased from the 50th percentile to the 90th percentile in the past 1.5 years. A speech therapist has seen him for delayed speech, and he is scheduled to see a therapist for late motor development. Which of the following would most likely be seen on physical examination?

A. Short 4th and 5th metacarpals
B. Hepatosplenomegaly
C. Polydactyly
D. Macroglossia
E. Almond-shaped eyes

49. A 33-year-old Caucasian female is presenting to her primary care physician for an annual exam. She is up to date on her preventative screenings and immunizations. Although she exercises and avoids eating at fast-food restaurants, she is concerned about her cardiovascular risk, as her father had a heart attack at age 42. In this patient, at which body mass index would a waist circumference provide the most useful information regarding cardiovascular risk?

A. 18 kg/m²
B. 24 kg/m²
C. 33 kg/m²
D. 40 kg/m²

50. Researchers are performing a study on obesity and the effects on the associated comorbidities as weight fluctuates over two years. They desire the most accurate fat composition measurements at a molecular level, regardless of cost. Which of the following measurement modalities would meet these criteria?

A. Skinfold calipers
B. Deuterium dilution hydrometry
C. Bioelectric impedance analyses
D. Dual-energy x-ray absorptiometry
E. Body mass index

51. A 23-year-old healthy female presents for an annual examination at her family practice physician's clinic. She has decided to pursue a vegan diet in place of the pescatarian diet she had previously consumed. She wants to ensure she does not become malnourished and asks about vitamin supplementation. What deficiency will most likely be present if supplementation is not initiated within the next year?

A. Vitamin C
B. Cyanocobalamin
C. Vitamin D
D. Folate
E. Vitamin K

52. A 61-year-old male diagnosed with hypertension and obesity class II presents to his sleep specialist to discuss his overnight polysomnography results. His primary care physician referred him after he was experiencing unrefreshing sleep and waking up holding his breath. His spouse also had concerns about loud snoring with pauses in his breathing. Given this patient's history, what is the minimal apnea-hypopnea index (AHI) needed to diagnose obstructive sleep apnea?

A. 5 per hour
B. 15 per hour
C. 30 per hour
D. 60 per hour

53. A physician is working in a weight loss clinic and seeing a patient with inadequate insurance coverage. The patient meets criteria for pharmacologic therapy and is interested, but cannot afford name-brand combination medications. Therefore, the physician discusses the off-label use of medications, including emulating the newer combination medications by prescribing the two medications separately. The patient comes back one month later with no weight loss. He explains that he lost one of the two prescriptions. Which medications did he most likely take for the past month?

A. Topiramate
B. Phentermine
C. Bupropion
D. Liraglutide
E. Naltrexone

54. A 9-year-old female is brought to her pediatrician for a well-child check. A few years ago, she was diagnosed with depression. Although the medications prescribed have helped with her mood symptoms, her appetite has significantly increased. She eats approximately 3500 kcal/day and admits to playing on the computer and watching more television than previously. Lab work including thyroid hormone levels are normal. Her weight is displayed on the growth chart below. Which stature curve would best correlate with her height?

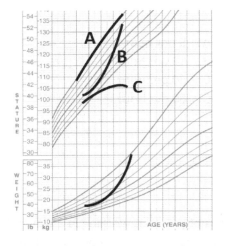

A. Line A
B. Line B
C. Line C

55. A 27-year-old female with a history of hypertension and recently diagnosed obstructive sleep apnea (OSA) presents for evaluation after having failed many name-brand diets. She states she has always been "on the heavier side," but needing a CPAP machine for OSA motivated her to lose weight. Physical examination reveals a rounded face and truncal obesity with widened abdominal striae. Laboratory work reveals a hemoglobin A1c in the pre-diabetes range. What other findings would most likely be present on physical exam?

A. Scalloped tongue
B. Hirsutism
C. Decreased deep tendon reflexes
D. Periumbilical hernia
E. Superficial ecchymosis

56. A female sprinter undergoes indirect calorimetry to determine her respiratory quotient (RQ), which is obtained by measuring carbon dioxide eliminated divided by oxygen consumed. It is determined that when the athlete is slowly jogging, she mostly consumes lipids. However, during sustained sprinting, her RQ would be expected to be near which of the following values?

A. 0.5
B. 0.7
C. 1.0
D. 1.3

57. A 44-year-old female presents for a follow-up three years after undergoing a Roux-en-Y gastric bypass. She is pleased with her results, having lost nearly 55% of her total body weight loss and she states she continues to lose weight despite no longer following the dietician's recommendations or exercising. She denies depression and says she feels well but admits to diarrhea. Preoperative BMI was 47.3 kg/m^2, and today it is 22.7 kg/m^2. Physical exam is normal except for some excess skin in the abdomen and arms. She has not followed up with her surgeon after the first year. Which of the following may explain her weight loss?

A. Vitamin deficiency
B. Anastomotic stricture
C. Small intestinal bowel overgrowth
D. A shorter common intestinal channel
E. Expected post-surgical weight loss

58. A 14-year-old female with a BMI of 39 kg/m² presents to her family practitioner for recurrent headaches. She states the headaches are pulsatile and occasionally cause loss of appetite. In addition, she now has difficulty seeing the board during school and must sit toward the front of her class. She has intermittent loss of vision and diplopia when standing up. Which of the following would be the best test to determine her cause of headaches?

A. Orthostatic vital signs
B. Overnight sleep study
C. Ophthalmologic evaluation
D. Brain imaging
E. Cerebral spinal fluid studies

59. A mother brings her 9-year-old son to his pediatrician for evaluation, as is concerned that his height and weight are increased in comparison to his peers. The mother states that her son does tend to watch 4-5 hours of television daily and is "constantly snacking." The son has no known health concerns, and overall appears happy. Physical examination reveals a BMI of 19.75 kg/m², which is the 86th percentile for his age and gender. Which of the following most accurately describes his weight categorization?

A. Underweight
B. Healthy weight
C. Overweight
D. Class 1 obesity
E. Class 2 obesity

60. A 19-year-old male presents to his primary care physician for an annual physical evaluation. He admits to eating significantly more since he started college. He relates this to stress and a change in sleep habits since moving to the dormitories. He states he has gained approximately 20 lbs (9.1 kg) over the past five months. His BMI is 29 kg/m². Laboratory findings include a hemoglobin A1c of 5.9% (reference range: < 5.7%), and his fasting cholesterol panel is consistent with dyslipidemia. To diagnose him with metabolic syndrome, what additional finding is necessary?

A. Abdominal circumference of 100 cm (39 inches)
B. Diagnosis of obstructive sleep apnea
C. Diastolic blood pressure of 82 mmHg
D. Being treated with amlodipine

61. A 14-year-old female presents to her pediatrician's office for an annual examination. She denies any concerns but appears withdrawn. She states school is "going okay." When asked about diet, she says she hardly eats because she is "fat and ugly." Physical examination reveals a BMI of 17 kg/m², with a global cachectic appearance. Which of the following is most associated with her underlying condition?

A. Tachycardia
B. Urinary phosphate wasting
C. Increased osteoblast activity
D. Decreased luteinizing hormone
E. Respiratory alkalosis

62. A sports medicine physician is working with athletes to optimize their performance. He has them undergo testing to determine the VO_2 maximum, in order to calculate their cardiorespiratory fitness level. Which of the following statements is most accurate regarding VO_2 max?

A. VO_2 max increases with age
B. Professional athletes have low levels of VO_2 max
C. Decreasing body fat percentage improves VO_2 max
D. VO_2 max is similar among genders

63. A 34-year-old male presents to the clinic after attending a bariatric seminar. He is interested in weight loss surgery. He takes amlodipine for hypertension and is adherent with continuous positive airway pressure (CPAP) for his obstructive sleep apnea. He denies any tobacco or alcohol history. Which of the following would be the most appropriate initial screening test for metabolic-associated fatty liver disease at this time?

A. History
B. Physical exam findings
C. Laboratory work
D. Right upper quadrant ultrasound
E. Liver biopsy

64. A 22-year-old male is frustrated by his recent diagnosis of "overweight," which was made at an insurance screening exam. He weight-lifts for 3-4 hours daily and competes at the state and national level for body-building. Prior testing reveals an 18% body fat composition. What other condition would act similarly to this patient in terms of an increased BMI with a discordant obesity-related risk association?

A. Congestive heart failure
B. Increased age
C. Southeast Asian ethnicity
D. Sarcopenia
E. Osteoporosis

65. A 63-year-old female presents to her primary care physician's office for follow-up after starting methotrexate with complaints of a sore tongue and irritability. She was diagnosed with polymyalgia rheumatic two years ago and was placed on 15 mg of prednisone daily. However, she had gained nearly 60 lbs (27.2 kg) while on prednisone. Eight months ago, she was transitioned to methotrexate for glucocorticoid-sparing therapy. Her BMI is 35 kg/m². Which of the following is most responsible for her current condition?

A. Vitamin B_1
B. Vitamin B_2
C. Vitamin B_3
D. Vitamin B_9
E. Vitamin B_{12}

66. A 14-year-old male presents to his family practice physician for his annual physical examination. He is in the 105th percentile for weight and the 65th percentile for height. His upper arm circumference is 37 cm. Which of the following would likely cause an inaccurately elevated systolic blood pressure?

A. Using a large adult-sized cuff (16x36 cm)
B. Sitting in a chair with back support
C. Having the patient rest his arm by his side
D. Telling the patient not to talk during inflation
E. Deflating the cuff at 5-10 mmHg per second

67. A 44-year-old female presents to the office with concerns about weight-gain. She rarely eats breakfast but instead eats from the time she gets home from work until bedtime. She occasionally awakens and consumes calories at night. The only medication she takes is zolpidem for insomnia. Which of the following questions would be most helpful to determine if the nocturnal caloric intake is caused by zolpidem versus night eating syndrome?

A. Are you aware during your nocturnal eating episodes?
B. What is the dose of your zolpidem?
C. Do you have a prior history of sleep walking?
D. Do you take any other over-the-counter medications?
E. Are you drowsy in the mornings after taking zolpidem?

68. A university hospital is working with the Centers for Medicare and Medicaid Services (CMS) regarding billing and repayments. The current system allows for an increased hospital length of stay based on body mass index alone. The new proposal is to establish repayments and recommended appropriate length of stay on comorbidities and functional limitations. Which of the following would be the best categorization method to initiate?

A. New York Heart Association Classification
B. Edmonton Obesity Staging System
C. Epworth Sleepiness Score
D. World Health Organization Obesity Classification
E. King's Obesity Staging Criteria

69. A physician is discussing the different terminology used in body composition to a rotating internal medicine resident. She describes a term that encompasses muscles, organs, water, bones, ligaments, tendons, and essential fat, but does not include nonessential or storage adipose tissue. Which of the following terms is she most likely describing?

A. Fat mass
B. Fat-free mass
C. Lean body mass
D. Total body mass
E. Percent body fat

70. A 37-year-old mother of two presents to her primary care physician's office for follow-up after recently being diagnosed with binge-eating disorder (BED). She has started cognitive behavioral therapy and has noticed improvements. She states that upon researching BED, she has seen a lot of the same tendencies and characteristics of her condition in her 11-year-old daughter. Her daughter is scheduled to meet with her pediatrician and will likely be diagnosed with which of the following?

A. Grazing
B. Anorexia nervosa
C. Loss of control eating disorder
D. Night eating syndrome
E. Bulimia nervosa

71. A patient is discussing with a physician a news story that was heard earlier in the day. The report stated patients who have a BMI ≥ 25 kg/m^2 have a longer life expectancy than those with a BMI < 25 kg/m^2. The patient now questions the utility of obtaining a BMI at each visit. Which is a true statement regarding the correlation between BMI and obesity-related comorbidities?

A. A BMI of 35 kg/m^2 decreases life expectancy the same as smoking
B. BMI is the best indicator of cardiovascular disease
C. 50% of type 2 diabetes is directly related to obesity-range BMI
D. A 5-unit increase in BMI increases ischemic stroke risk by 20%

72. A 3-year-old female is referred to a geneticist for evaluation after persistent milestone delays and a recent seizure. The child appears very happy, smiling, and frequently laughing during the examination. Her movements are spastic and she is only able to pull herself up to a seated position and stand with assistance. She does not talk and only babbles intermittently. What would the genetic workup most likely reveal?

A. Angelman syndrome
B. Turner syndrome
C. Borjeson-Forssman-Lehmann syndrome
D. Albright hereditary osteodystrophy
E. Fragile-X syndrome

73. A 68-year-old female with a history of type 2 diabetes presents to the clinic following a bariatric seminar. Although she understands there is no definitive age limit to surgery, she elects to undergo medical management. Her current diabetic medication regimen includes a maximum dose of metformin. Her hemoglobin A1c is 9.6%. The risks and benefits of a daily FDA-approved injectable, anti-obesity medication for long-term use is discussed. What medical history would be necessary for the physician to inquire about before starting this medication?

A. Papillary thyroid carcinoma
B. Suicidal ideation
C. History of cholelithiasis
D. Diabetic gastroparesis

74. An 11-year-old male presents to his pediatrician for complaints of right lower extremity pain. He states the pain has worsened over the past month, describing it as a dull ache. There was no preceding trauma. His mother brought him in after she noticed him walking with a limp. His BMI is in the 120th percentile for his age and gender. Physical examination reveals limited internal rotation of his right hip and an antalgic gait. Which of the following is most likely the culprit of his presenting condition?

A. Blount disease
B. Slipped capital femoral epiphysis
C. Osgood-Schlatter disease
D. Legg-Calve-Perthes disease
E. Aseptic necrosis

75. A mother of three children presents to her family practitioner for well-child examinations. Two of the children have been diagnosed with obesity. The mother has not followed up with the dietician as recommended, and the children are still consuming high-caloric density packaged food. Which of the following would be the most appropriate question to ask now?

A. Do you run out of food towards the end of the month?
B. Is your transportation adequate for making appointments?
C. Do you feel like you are suited to take care of your children?
D. What sweets could be eliminated from your children's diets?
E. How can we incorporate physical activity?

76. A 25-year-old male presents to his primary care physician's office with the complaint of weight gain. Over the past two years, he has gained nearly 35 lbs (15.9 kg). He states that he first noticed the weight gain once he began to work the night shift. He says he still exercises 30 minutes daily before work but does admit to increased hunger and snacking throughout his shift. Compared to 4 years ago, which of the following would most likely be observed in the patient at this visit?

A. Decreased orexin
B. Increased cortisol
C. Suppressed ghrelin
D. Increased melatonin
E. Increased adiponectin

77. A 31-year-old male presents as a 2-week follow-up to his weight-loss clinic. Since being seen previously, he has decreased his soda consumption and has reduced the number of times he eats fast food from three times weekly to once. Also, he has started to briskly walk around his neighborhood for approximately 30 minutes three times weekly. He has lost 4 lbs (1.8 kg) since his last appointment. According to current minimum recommendations, what goal should be set regarding his 30-minute exercise sessions?

A. Increase to daily sessions
B. Increase to 5 sessions weekly
C. Change from walking to jogging
D. Set a goal in terms of miles, not minutes
E. No changes necessary

78. A 16-year-old female presents to her family practitioner at the request of her mother after being found to be self-inducing vomiting. The patient states this is something she has done for the past few months, most often after she eats more than she intends to, saying it helps with the guilt. She is active in sports, has several close friends, and is getting good grades. Given the underlying diagnosis, which of the following abnormalities is most likely to develop in this patient if left untreated?

A. Anion gap metabolic acidosis
B. Shortened corrected QT interval
C. Mallory-Weiss tear
D. Melanosis coli
E. Keratoconjunctivitis sicca

79. A 26-year-old female is presenting to her family practitioner for an infertility evaluation. She states that although she has unprotected sex approximately three times weekly, she has not become pregnant for the past two years. She says she averages one heavy menstrual cycle every three months. Her BMI is 34 kg/m². Physical examination reveals facial hair stubble. Pelvic examination is unremarkable; however, clitoromegaly is noted. An ovarian ultrasound is unrevealing. Given these findings, which lab test would most likely be present?

A. Increased luteinizing hormone
B. Decreased free thyroxine levels
C. Decreased androgen levels
D. Elevated cortisol levels
E. Elevated vitamin D (25-OH) levels

80. A 45-year-old female presents to her internist with concerns of bleeding within her mouth. She states that she has been utterly frustrated with her weight and has decided to go on an "extreme diet" for the past three months. She has been consuming water and only small amounts of protein and carbohydrates. She lost nearly 45 lbs (20.4 kg) during this time. A physical exam shows dried blood on her gums and spiral hair on her arms. Given her most likely deficiency, which of the following is a potential complication?

A. Peripheral neuropathy
B. Hallucinations
C. High-output cardiac failure
D. Dermatitis
E. Poor wound healing

81. A 63-year-old female presents to her primary care office for a routine evaluation. Her lab results reveal a TSH level of 11.1 mU/L (reference range: 0.4-4.5 mU/L) with a normal T₄ level. She had similar lab values two months prior, completed for insurance screening purposes. She feels well overall and denies fatigue, constipation, or cold intolerance. Which of the following would be the next best step?

A. Start levothyroxine if the patient begins having symptoms
B. Order thyroid peroxidase antibodies levels
C. Initiate weight-based synthetic thyroxine replacement
D. Repeat TSH, T₃, and T₄ levels in 3 months
E. Discuss desiccated thyroid replacement therapy

82. A 27-year-old male presents to a new primary care physician's office for evaluation of fatigue. He has not been seen by a physician "since high school," as he has felt well and has not been seriously ill. He denies alcohol or tobacco use and states that he tries to avoid fast-food. Vital signs are within normal limits, besides a BMI of 28 kg/m². Physical examination reveals hyperpigmented skin in his axillary folds and the nape of his neck. Other physical exam findings are unremarkable. A cholesterol panel reveals total cholesterol to be 220 mg/dL (reference range < 200 mg/dL), and an HbA1c of 6.0% (reference range: < 5.7%). What other physical examination finding is most likely present?

A. Xanthoma
B. Easy bruising
C. Acrochordons
D. Dry skin
E. Corkscrew hairs

83. A mother brings her child to the pediatrician for his 18-month well-child exam. He has met all of his age-appropriate milestones, including starting to walk at 12 months old. She states that he has gained more "rolls" in the arms and legs and seems to be gaining weight faster than she recalls of her other children. Which would be the most accurate way to track this patient's weight parameters?

A. Weight-for-height
B. Body mass index
C. Age-adjusted growth
D. Weight-for-length
E. CDC growth charts

84. A 46-year-old male with a BMI of 38 kg/m² presents for follow-up regarding his diabetes. He is being treated with metformin and empagliflozin; his last HbA1c was 6.8%. He has mild knee pain with prolonged exercise but otherwise feels well. According to the Edmonton Obesity Staging System, he would be classified as which of the following?

A. Stage 0
B. Stage 1
C. Stage 2
D. Stage 3
E. Stage 4

85. A 21-year-old male with a past medical history of depression and obesity presents to a dietician for a nutrition evaluation. He states that he has overeaten at night for as long as he can remember. He admits to craving sweets and even sometimes wakes up throughout the night to get a snack. Given his most likely underlying diagnosis, which of the following findings is likely to be seen in this patient?

A. Daytime fatigue
B. Excessive daily protein intake
C. Pica
D. Frequent daytime grazing
E. Morning anorexia

86. An electrophysiology study is being performed, which evaluates the resting metabolic rate of individual organs in an average person without excess body weight. A radiotracer is injected into a patient who is lying still, and a subsequent body scan is performed. The tissue with the highest metabolic rate displays the brightest on body scan imaging, with quantitative data extrapolated. Based on this scan, which of the following tissue would most likely display the brightest on imaging?

A. Kidneys
B. Heart
C. Digestive system
D. Liver
E. Fat

87. A 33-year-old male presents to his family practice physician at his wife's request for "sleep-eating." He states that his wife has caught him multiple times in the middle of the night eating large amounts of food before returning to bed. He has no recollection of this in the morning but has noticed that he has consistently been gaining weight, despite a relatively healthy diet and exercise. He does admit to working rotating shifts. Given this history, which medication is this patient most likely taking?

A. Diphenhydramine
B. Eszopiclone
C. Ramelteon
D. Trazodone
E. Ginkgo biloba

88. A 51-year-old female is undergoing a preoperative evaluation for a planned Roux-en-Y gastric bypass. She admits to often feeling tired during the day, occasionally falling asleep during conversations. Her spouse has told her that she snores very loudly, sometimes requiring him to sleep in another bedroom. Vital signs are within normal limits. BMI is 39 kg/m^2, and her neck circumference is 17 inches (43.2 cm). What is the next best step in evaluating for obstructive sleep apnea?

A. Inquire if she has stopped breathing during sleep
B. Place a referral for an overnight pulse-oximetry test
C. Place a referral for polysomnography
D. Perform a physical exam, focusing on the oral exam
E. Order a daytime arterial blood gas

89. A 17-year-old female presents to her family medicine doctor for a sports physical. She has no prior medical history, although she feels more fatigued than average. Vital signs reveal a heart rate of 60 BPM and a BMI of 22 kg/m^2. A physical exam reveals parotid gland enlargement and scrapes over the dorsum of her second metacarpal phalangeal joint. She is elusive when asked questions about her eating habits. Which medication is contraindicated given her underlying diagnosis?

A. Trazodone
B. Bupropion
C. Topiramate
D. Sertraline
E. Buspirone

90. A 29-year-old male presents to an internist to establish care. His chief concern is related to his lack of upper body strength, in particular the muscle size. He states despite working out his arms for nearly 3 hours daily, his arms still appear smaller than he would like. He has difficulty focusing on his work as a car salesman, as he feels people notice his arms and admits to being very self-conscious. A physical exam reveals a healthy, muscular-appearing male in no distress. If inquired, the patient most likely would admit to experiencing which of the following?

A. Compulsive behaviors
B. Anxiety attacks
C. Severe calorie restriction
D. Nocturnal eating
E. Delayed sleep onset

91. A university is conducting a research study. The primary objective is to correlate quantitative sex hormone binding globulin (SHBG) levels with different patient characteristics. In particular, age, weight, and comorbid conditions such as polycystic ovarian syndrome (PCOS) are analyzed. Which of the following patients would have an increased SHBG level compared to their comparative matched cohort?

A. A patient with a BMI of 45 kg/m²
B. A female with a diagnosis of PCOS
C. A younger individual
D. A male with decreased total testosterone
E. A patient six months status post gastric bypass

92. A pediatrician is evaluating a young patient in the office and determines that the body mass index charts utilized for most children in her practice is inadequate for this patient, and a specialized BMI chart is utilized. The patient most likely has which of the following findings on physical examination?

    A. Bicuspid aorta
    B. Macrocephaly
    C. Macroglossia
    D. Ovarian agenesis
    E. Upslanting palpebral fissures

93. A 41-year-old Caucasian male presents to his primary care physician for an annual health screen. His immunizations are up to date. A recent diabetes and hypertension screening completed through work were within normal limits. His height is 70 inches (178 cm), and his weight is 260 lbs (117 kg). By utilizing the chart below, his weight would best be described as being in which of the following categories?

BMI	28	29	30	31	32	33	34	35	36	37	38	39	40	41	42	43	44	45	46
5'4"	163	169	174	180	186	192	197	204	209	215	221	227	232	238	244	250	256	262	267
5'5"	168	174	180	186	192	198	204	210	216	222	228	234	240	246	252	258	264	270	276
5'6"	173	179	186	192	198	204	210	216	223	229	235	241	247	253	260	266	272	278	284
5'7"	178	185	191	198	204	211	217	223	230	236	242	249	255	261	268	274	280	287	293
5'8"	184	190	197	203	210	216	223	230	236	243	249	256	262	269	276	282	289	295	302
5'9"	189	196	203	209	216	223	230	236	243	250	257	263	270	277	284	291	297	304	311
5'10"	195	202	209	216	222	229	236	243	250	257	264	271	278	285	292	299	306	313	320
5'11"	200	208	215	222	229	236	243	250	257	265	272	279	286	293	301	308	315	322	329

(Note: Weight is in pounds)

    A. Normal weight
    B. Overweight
    C. Class I obesity
    D. Class II obesity
    E. Class III obesity

94. A 49-year-old female with a history of severe obesity is following-up with her pulmonologist regarding her pulmonary hypertension, confirmed with a right-heart catheterization. She has no prior tobacco or occupational exposures, and her polysomnography test was negative. Given this information, which of the following would most likely be seen in this patient?

A. Class 4 Mallampati score
B. Increased Epworth sleepiness scale
C. $FVC/FEV_1 < 0.70$
D. Increased respiratory disturbance index
E. Arterial blood gas $PaCO_2 > 45$ mmHg

95. A mother brings her previously healthy 10-year-old daughter to her family medicine physician for an annual examination. The patient has been spending more time on the computer and watching television, with decreased physical activity. Her weight has steadily increased. Her body mass index is in the 86th percentile for age and gender. The patient denies any symptoms or concerns, including fatigue, polyuria, or hirsutism. Given this, which test should be ordered for screening purposes?

A. Fasting lipid profile
B. Aspartate aminotransferase
C. Fasting glucose
D. Creatinine
E. Thyroid-stimulating hormone

96. After injuring his finger, a 6-year-old male with class III obesity presents to the emergency department. The mother states that the child was trying to swing at a local park when his finger became stuck in the chain. The patient has full range of motion but increased swelling of his third digit. An x-ray is shown below. Which other finding is most likely?

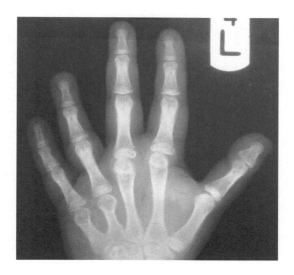

A. Pseudohypoparathyroidism
B. History of seizures
C. Almond-shaped eyes
D. Microorchidism

III. Treatment

97. A 44-year-old female presents to her primary care physician with dysuria and malodorous urine. She denies abdominal pain. She has type 2 diabetes and was recently started on a medication to help with weight loss and diabetes control. In addition, she initiated a new diet this week. Her urinalysis dipstick results are below. Given these findings, the diet she has started most likely encourages which of the following components?

Leukocyte	1+	Specific gravity	1.011
Nitrite	2+	Ketone	2+
Protein	Trace	Bilirubin	Not detected
Blood	1+	Glucose	3+

A. Significant carbohydrate restriction
B. Avoiding foods with a glycemic index > 70
C. Increasing omega-3 intake with extra virgin vegetable oil
D. Limiting fat intake to 20-25% of daily calories
E. Intake of 5 servings of fruit minimum

98. A 14-year-old male presents for his annual checkup at his pediatrician's clinic. He has no prior medical history. His BMI is 31 kg/m². The pediatrician discusses healthy eating choices, exercise, and lifestyle changes to prevent weight-related complications. This discussion is an example of which of the following phases of prevention in chronic obesity?

A. Primary prevention
B. Secondary prevention
C. Tertiary prevention

99. A patient had a previous bariatric procedure performed ten years ago in which a band was placed around the top of the stomach, creating a small pouch. Although adjustable, the patient has had difficulty following up and thus is interested in a surgical revision. The patient has had three adjustments during the past decade, initially losing 32 lbs (14.5 kg), but has since regained this weight. Which is true of this bariatric procedure?

A. It is considered a malabsorptive procedure
B. The minimum BMI required for placement is 30 kg/m²
C. The mortality rate is similar to other bariatric procedures
D. Adjustment requires conscious sedation
E. It is the most common weight loss procedure worldwide

100. A healthy 6-year-old female presents with her father to her primary care physician for an annual exam. She has no prior medical conditions and is up to date on immunizations. Her father has no concerns about her current health but is concerned about preventing weight gain, as her sibling has excess weight. The patient's BMI is in the 50th percentile, with consistent height and weight in the 55th and 60th percentile, respectively. Which of the following is the most appropriate recommendation for this child?

A. Consume 3 or more fruits and vegetables daily
B. Minimize screen time to < 3 hours daily
C. Allow the child to self-regulate meals
D. Encourage at least 8 hours of sleep nightly
E. Eat as a family at least 3 times weekly

101. A 53-year-old male is presenting for evaluation for weight loss. He has started the bridge-to-transplant program, which requires a BMI of 35 kg/m² or less in order to be listed on the kidney transplant list. His current BMI is 44 kg/m². Both medication and surgical options are discussed. He prefers to undergo bariatric and metabolic surgery. Which of the following surgical options is most preferred?

A. Single anastomosis duodeno-ileal bypass
B. Roux-en-Y gastric bypass
C. Vertical sleeve gastrectomy
D. Gastric balloon
E. Aspiration device

102. A 34-year-old male with a past medical history of hypothyroidism presents for an initial evaluation regarding weight-loss surgical options. In particular, he is interested in an aspiration device. He affirms this would work well with his lifestyle, as he works remotely at home. He has good family support and performs daily aerobic physical activity for 30 minutes. He has already begun behavioral therapy, including chewing his food slowly and thoroughly. Which of the following would be a contraindication to this device?

A. Night eating syndrome
B. Prior hemicolectomy
C. Gastroesophageal reflux disease
D. Diastolic heart failure
E. Zenker diverticulum

103. A mother brings her 6-year-old daughter, who is in the 95th percentile for weight based on her BMI, to her pediatrician's office due to persistent constipation despite increased water intake. They have been using over-the-counter stool softeners without relief. The mother states that the child is not picky regarding food and eats "whatever is available." The physician recommends increasing whole grains. What effect will this indirectly have on the child?

A. Reduce HDL and triglyceride levels
B. Increase risk of irritable bowel syndrome
C. Increase nutrient-rich food intake
D. Increase saturated fat consumption
E. Diarrhea and potential fecal incontinence

104. A 57-year-old male presents to the emergency department two weeks after a Roux-en-Y gastric bypass for dehydration, nausea, and vomiting. His spouse has also noted some confusion recently. Vital signs reveal a heart rate of 110/min and a blood pressure of 89/58 mmHg. Physical exam reveals dry mucus membranes, nystagmus, and difficulty walking. He is alert and oriented x 1. Given his most likely nutritional deficiency, what other clinical sequelae may be seen if left untreated?

A. Macrocytic anemia
B. Dermatitis (pellagra)
C. Seizure disorder
D. Glossitis and cheilitis
E. Peripheral neuropathy

105. A 59-year-old male presents to his internist with the desire to start pharmacotherapy for weight loss. The physician is interested in starting a particular combination medication but first inquires about a history of calcium oxalate stones, as this medication should be avoided in those with a history of renal nephrolithiasis. Given the most likely medication eluded to, what is a contraindication of this medicine?

A. Chronic malabsorption syndrome
B. Family history of medullary thyroid cancer
C. Concurrent history of glaucoma
D. History of epilepsy or risk of seizures
E. Uncontrolled hypertension

106. A 36-year-old female with diabetes mellitus type 2 presents to her primary care physician's clinic for a bariatric surgery evaluation. Her diabetes has been poorly controlled despite being on metformin, semaglutide, empagliflozin, and high-dose insulin. She exercises 250 minutes weekly and has been on a low glycemic index dietary plan for the past nine months. Despite this, her hemoglobin A1c is 8.9% (reference range: 4.2-5.7%). Her body mass index is 32 kg/m². Regarding her bariatric surgery eligibility question, would she be a good candidate?

A. No: Her body mass index is not in an appropriate range
B. No: She only has one obesity-related comorbidity
C. No: She should pursue an insulin pump instead
D. Yes: Her diabetes is difficult to control
E. Yes: She meets the criteria for Roux-en-Y gastric bypass only

107. A 52-year-old male presents to his primary care physician with concerns of decreased libido. He states he has no current sexual desire, and does not wake up with a morning erection. Physical exam reveals small testicles, gynecomastia, and a BMI of 52 kg/m². Morning testosterone levels are low on two occasions, while a prostate-specific antigen is within normal limits. Starting testosterone in this patient would likely have what effect?

A. Increase HbA1c
B. Decrease fertility
C. Increase weight
D. Worsening lipid panel
E. Increasing blood pressure

108. A 47-year-old male with end-stage renal disease is presenting to his primary care physician's office with the desire to lose weight. To be considered for a renal transplant, he must lose an additional 22 lbs (10 kg). Although he has incorporated lifestyle modifications, he has failed to meet his weight loss goals. He is interested in bariatric medications. Which of the following would be the most appropriate medication to prescribe?

A. Phentermine/topiramate ER
B. Naltrexone/bupropion ER
C. Liraglutide
D. Phentermine monotherapy
E. Metformin

109. A patient presents to her internist with concerns about supplements she has been taking. She was started on L-carnitine and green tea extract at the recommendation of an herbalist. However, since starting, she has noticed increased anxiety, palpitations, and a slight tremor. Both of these supplements theoretically work by which mechanism?

A. Energy expenditure
B. Satiety
C. Carbohydrate metabolism
D. Blocking fat absorption
E. Increase in fat oxidation

110. A 52-year-old female has presented for a follow-up visit to the bariatric clinic. A rotating resident is interviewing the patient and is asking questions such as "What weight-loss techniques have worked for you in the past?" and "So, swimming was an exercise you could do long-term?" After further discussions, the resident expresses hope stating, "It sounds like you are ready to pursue and maintain weight loss." He summarizes the visit, and the patient leaves the office. Which skill did this resident utilize?

A. OARS
B. FRAMES
C. SMART goals
D. RULE

111. An obesity medicine specialist is working with an internal medicine resident and discusses ways to improve surgical outcomes, including decreased hospitalization and recovery times. Which of the following should routinely be performed to improve outcomes?

A. Preoperative carbohydrate loading
B. Intraoperative low-molecular-weight heparin
C. Nasogastric nutritional supplementation
D. Intraoperative high ventilator tidal volumes
E. Postoperative intravenous opioid administration

112. A surgeon consults an obesity medicine specialist after a 39-year-old female develops a provoked lower extremity deep venous thrombosis (DVT) extending to the femoral artery on post-operative day three from a Roux-en-Y gastric bypass. Post-op complications included persistent nausea and vomiting, which have now subsided. The surgeon requests assistance with anticoagulation therapy. What is the most appropriate recommendation to provide?

A. Initiate rivaroxaban and check anti-Xa levels in 3 days
B. Bridge anticoagulation with fondaparinux and warfarin
C. Start an unfractionated heparin drip and place an IVC filter
D. Consult vascular surgery for mechanical thrombectomy
E. Discharge patient with weight-based enoxaparin

113. A recently published study has shown weight-loss success and diabetes improvement with a subcutaneous injectable medication undergoing continued clinical testing. The medication contains GLP-1 and another hormone that is endogenously secreted by the K cells in the proximal small intestines. This dual medication has been shown to have more significant effects on diabetes and weight than with a GLP-1 alone due to its dual incretin effect. The described medication combined with a GLP-1 is

A. Amylin
B. Oxyntomodulin
C. Glucagon
D. Gastric inhibitory peptide
E. Peptide YY

114. A 44-year-old female with a history of ovarian cancer recently completed chemotherapy. During cancer treatment, she lost substantial weight and currently has a BMI of 20 kg/m². She states she does not have a significant appetite and must force herself to remember to drink protein shakes, although she has no nausea. Her diabetes mellitus type 2 initially had improved with the unintended weight loss and she quit all of her medications during treatment. Her most recent hemoglobin A1c is 7.4% (reference range: ≤5.7%). Which is the most appropriate medication to initiate at this time?

A. Semaglutide
B. Sitagliptin
C. Tirzepatide
D. Insulin
E. Dapagliflozin

115. A 26-year-old male is presenting for psychiatric evaluation as part of a multi-disciplinary team approach before bariatric surgery. He admits that he eats until he feels uncomfortably full, even eating large amounts when he doesn't feel hungry. This is something that has caused significant guilt and depression. He eats much more over a short period compared to his friends. He states it feels "like I lose control when food is around." Which of the following classes of medications is FDA approved to treat his underlying condition?

A. Central nervous system stimulant
B. Anticonvulsant
C. Atypical antipsychotic
D. Selective serotonin neuromodulator
E. Glucagon-like peptide analog

116. A 14-year-old male presents for a sports physical for the upcoming football season. He has always been at the 95th-100th percentile of his weight compared to his peers. His weight today is 204 lbs (92.5 kg). He has unhealthy eating habits and consumes multiple sodas daily. The concern about his weight is discussed, including the health risks. He seems perplexed by this, as he feels he is at a good weight for football. After further discussion, he agrees to a focused follow-up visit regarding dietary modifications. Which of the following stages of change is this patient experiencing?

A. Pre-contemplation
B. Contemplation
C. Preparation
D. Action
E. Maintenance

117. A 57-year-old business executive returns to his primary care physician for follow-up regarding his exercise prescription. Although the prescription clearly states 300 minutes of exercise weekly in the form of brisk walking, he does not have that amount of time to devote to exercise and did not fulfill his prescription. His current BMI is 31 kg/m². What would be the most appropriate modification to his exercise prescription?

A. Change to water walking
B. Increase exercise intensity
C. Change to resistance training
D. Focus on dietary components instead
E. Confront him on his priorities

118. A general surgeon is discussing one potential bariatric surgical option with a patient in which 80% of the greater curvature of the stomach is resected laparoscopically, allowing for 2-3 ounces (60-90 mL) of volume intake. Which of the following is true regarding the described procedure?

A. Dumping syndrome is a common complaint
B. It is the second most common bariatric procedure
C. The procedure does not affect hunger hormones
D. Patients are prone to experience vitamin B_{12} deficiency
E. This surgery is most effective for treating diabetes

119. A 39-year-old female with a history of type 2 diabetes and sleep apnea is presenting to her general surgeon after undergoing a Roux-en-Y gastric bypass six months ago. She has noted a weight loss of 47 lbs (21.3 kg) and is happy with the results. She regularly meets with her dietician and the weight loss clinic. Her only complaint is that after she eats certain meals, she experiences facial flushing and lightheadedness. Given the most likely etiology of these symptoms, what other associated finding is she likely to encounter?

A. Intermittent constipation
B. Excessive belching
C. Wheezing
D. Reactive hypoglycemia
E. Bacterial overgrowth

120. A rapid response is called on a 33-year-old female 12 hours after undergoing a Roux-en-Y gastric bypass. She complains of progressively worsening mid-epigastric pain with radiation to her left chest and mild dyspnea. Vital signs reveal a heart rate of 120 BPM, respirations 24/min, and oxygen saturation of 99% on room air. A portable chest x-ray shows a new left-sided pleural effusion. A complete blood count reveals a white blood cell count of 13.4 x 10^3/mcL (reference range: 4.8-10.8 x 10^3/mcL). What is the next best step in management?

A. Start empiric ceftriaxone and azithromycin
B. Order a stat CTA of the chest
C. Administer 1 mg/kg low molecular weight heparin
D. Contact the attending surgeon
E. Order an electrocardiogram

121. A 39-year-old female presents to the clinic due to nausea, vomiting, and increased fatigue over the past three weeks. Past medical history includes class II obesity, migraines, and polycystic ovarian syndrome (PCOS). She is on oral combined birth control and phentermine/topiramate ER. She has lost 19 lbs (8.6 kg) over the past 4 months but has recently started to regain some weight over the past month. Which of the following could have prevented the underlying cause of her symptoms?

A. Adhering to the Risk Evaluation and Mitigation Strategy program
B. Referral to a dietician to discuss a low-carbohydrate diet
C. Prophylactic ondansetron to take before anti-obesity medication
D. Cognitive behavioral therapy to prevent anxiety from phentermine
E. Adding metformin to treat the current PCOS symptoms

122. A 39-year-old male presents to the obesity clinic for a 2- month follow-up appointment. He was started on semaglutide six months ago and has maintained exercise of 200 minutes weekly. He states he feels well and plans to continue his current treatment regimen. Vital signs are within normal limits. Over the past year, he has lost 34 lbs (15.4 kg), accounting for an 8% total body weight loss. He is now at his lowest weight since being seen at the clinic. If he maintains his current regimen, what can you predict about his weight loss in the future?

A. He will continue to lose weight but at a slower pace
B. Eventually he will plateau and regain weight
C. He will lose weight until he plateaus at his ideal body weight
D. Eventually he will relapse to his previous weight

123. A 44-year-old male is being evaluated in the intensive care unit after a biliopancreatic diversion with duodenal switch. The surgery was particularly time-consuming due to anatomic variation and significant scar tissue from prior abdominal surgeries. The nurse is concerned as his urine has darkened, and the urine output has decreased to < 40 mL per hour despite adequate fluid hydration. His abdomen is soft, with no bowel sounds appreciated. Which of the following tests will most likely be abnormal?

A. Urinalysis hemoglobin
B. Renal parenchymal ultrasound
C. Renal vasculature doppler
D. Urine eosinophil count
E. Urine microscopy

124. A 62-year-old female is presenting to her primary care physician's office to discuss semaglutide (Wegovy®) for weight loss. Her medical comorbidities include diabetes type II and hypertension. She is currently taking metformin, rosuvastatin, sitagliptin, and chlorthalidone. She drinks two alcoholic beverages nightly and quit tobacco products six years ago. Which of the following is the most appropriate action before starting semaglutide?

A. Obtain baseline lipase levels
B. Discontinue one of her current medications
C. Inquire about a family history of MEN 1 syndrome
D. Require alcohol cessation due to interactions
E. Obtain triglyceride levels

125. A 42-year-old female presents with chronic diarrhea, abdominal pain, and bloating for six months. She underwent a duodenal switch approximately eight years ago and has had minimal follow-up due to losing insurance. She admits to now feeling weak and lightheaded with exertion. Laboratory examination reveals macrocytic anemia with increased folate levels. Which of the following tests is most appropriate at this time?

A. Urea breath test
B. Carbohydrate breath test
C. Hydrogen breath test
D. Stool cultures
E. Endoscopic evaluation

126. A 37-year-old male with type 1 diabetes presents to his primary care practitioner to discuss anti-obesity medication. In particular, he would like to start semaglutide. His last HbA1c was 7.4% (reference range: < 5.7%) and he is on 18 units of glargine nightly and dosing the aspart based on carbohydrate counting. His current BMI is 31 kg/m², which has increased from 27 kg/m² since last year. Which of the following is the most accurate statement regarding his inquiry?

A. Semaglutide is contraindicated in patients with type 1 diabetes
B. I will discuss this with your endocrinologist
C. You do not meet the criteria for anti-obesity medications
D. Tirzepatide would be a safer alternative
E. I would like to discuss intermittent fasting or a ketogenic diet today

127. A 9-year-old female presents to her pediatrician's office after her mother has concerns about her weight. Her mother states that the patient snores loudly and has episodes where she appears to hold her breath. Compared to other kids her age, the mother states her daughter seems much larger. She is at the 100th percentile for her weight and 56th percentile for height. Her weight is 174 pounds (78.9 kg). Which of the following is the recommended initial course of action for this patient?

A. Monitor dietary intake
B. Perform overnight pulse-oximetry
C. Discuss pharmacologic therapy
D. Initiate meal replacement
E. Provide reassurance

128. A geriatrician notices that many of his patients have lost muscle mass with debility or reduced physical activity, but continue to gain excess fat mass. Although some of these patients have certain conditions predisposing them to muscle wasting, including malignancy, fractures, and neurodegenerative conditions, the majority experience frailty independent of any underlying diseases. Which of the following would be an important part of the multidisciplinary treatment plan in regard to preventing sarcopenia and subsequent frailty?

A. Prescribe megestrol acetate
B. Encourage resistance training
C. Target protein intake of 0.8 g/kg/day
D. Consider testosterone supplements (males)
E. Encourage water aerobics

129. A 26-year-old female presents to the emergency department with a laceration above her right eye from a fall. She underwent a single anastomosis duodeno-ileal bypass with sleeve gastrectomy (SADI-S) six months prior and has not followed up with any providers since the surgery. She states she felt light-headed when getting up to go to the restroom and "passed-out" in the bathroom. Her skin turgor is normal. Which of the following questions will assist in preventing future similar hospital admissions?

A. Have you been drinking sufficient fluids?
B. Are you taking your daily vitamins?
C. Have you discontinued your sitagliptin post-operatively?
D. Did you have any alcohol before the fall?
E. Are you still taking blood pressure medication?

130. A 9-year-old male is presenting for follow-up regarding elevated blood pressures. Both of his parents have concerns about his sedentary lifestyle and picky eating habits that often cause him to snack throughout the day. His BMI is in the 80th percentile for age and gender, and his height has maintained the 60-65th percentile. He undergoes 24-hour ambulatory blood pressure monitoring, which shows normal blood pressure levels. Which is the most appropriate treatment modality for his current weight?

A. Prevention
B. Stage 1: Prevention plus
C. Stage 2: Structured weight management
D. Stage 3: Comprehensive multidisciplinary intervention
E. Stage 4: Tertiary care intervention

131. A patient presents to her nutritionist to discuss an article she read on the internet. It discussed making dietary changes by adding nutrients that have potentially favorable effects beyond basic nutrition. She most likely read an article on which of the following topics?

A. Supplements
B. Over-the-counter medications
C. Functional foods
D. Prescription medications
E. Herbal remedies

132. A 28-year-old healthy male presents to his primary care physician frustration with his inability to lose a significant amount of weight. For the past six months, he has changed to a vegan diet and exercises 30 minutes daily. Although he has lost 8 lbs (3.6 kg), he feels he should have lost more. His current BMI is 31 kg/m². After reviewing the side-effects of medications, he chooses one that he feels will be a safe option. After two months, he returns with no significant weight loss. Which of the following anti-obesity medication was he most likely prescribed?

A. Phentermine/topiramate ER
B. Orlistat
C. Naltrexone/bupropion ER
D. Liraglutide

133. A 24-year-old male is discussing his concerns about blood clots after his planned sleeve gastrectomy surgery next month. His father died from a pulmonary embolism (PE) one week after undergoing a total hip arthroplasty. The patient has no history of deep venous thrombosis, and besides his father, he knows of no other family history. He denies smoking. Which of the following would be the most appropriate statement regarding venous thromboembolism (VTE) in this patient?

A. Start VTE prophylaxis at least 24 hours after surgery
B. Low-molecular-weight heparin 40 mg twice daily is considered standard
C. Failure to wean from ventilator support may indicate VTE
D. He should be on extended chemoprophylaxis upon discharge
E. Given his family history, an IVC filter should be discussed

134. A psychiatrist is evaluating a patient in a psychiatric hospital for a recent episode of mania. The patient has a diagnosis of bipolar type I. The patient states that she has stopped her lithium due to excessive weight gain, leading to this current episode. The patient would like to discuss alternative options that would not cause this adverse effect. Which option should be discussed with the patient?

A. Valproate
B. Sertraline
C. Divalproex
D. Gabapentin
E. Lamotrigine

135. A 48-year-old male presents for follow-up with the dietician. He has been doing research and wants to discuss some dietary plans. He has obesity class I without other obesity-related comorbidities and is currently taking no medications besides a daily multivitamin. He asks for an opinion related to frequently used dietary plans. Which of the following recommendations is most accurate?

A. Intermittent fasting allows for a time of restricted eating followed by unregulated calorie consumption
B. The Dietary Approach to Stopping Hypertension (DASH) diet plan provides significant weight loss with cardiovascular benefits
C. Low carbohydrate diets are more effective long-term for weight loss compared to low-fat dietary plans
D. Eating low-density foods increases the sensation of fullness and thus promotes weight loss in comparison to high-density foods

136. A patient is meeting with a bariatric surgeon to discuss potential surgical options. Although she has done a lot of research, she still has not committed to one surgery. She asks about the estimated number of bariatric surgeries performed, including which are popular and which are becoming obsolete. Which of the following statements is accurate regarding bariatric surgery statistics over the past ten years?

A. The number of bariatric surgeries have declined in the past five years
B. Gastric banding has persistently made up 5% of bariatric surgeries
C. Roux-en-Y gastric bypass remains the most common surgery
D. Sleeve gastrectomy surgeries have nearly doubled in number
E. Intragastric balloons have been available since 2012

137. A 29-year-old female with a past medical history of migraine headaches and pre-diabetes is presenting to a local weight-loss clinic frustrated about her lack of weight loss. She currently exercises 300 minutes/week, restricts her calories to 1200 kcal/day, and takes no medications. She has been working with a weight-loss coach for the past six months. She is interested in weight-loss surgery. Her BMI is 29 kg/m², and her vital signs and physical exam are otherwise unremarkable. Which of the following would be the most appropriate action to take now?

A. Further intensify lifestyle modifications
B. Begin weight-loss pharmacotherapy
C. Referral for bariatric surgery
D. Referral for dietician
E. Provide reassurance

138. You are discussing with a patient their interest in physical activity. After asking the patient to grade their motivation in readiness to initiate a workout plan, the patient states they are at a 6 out of 10. What is the most appropriate reply to their assessment?

A. Why did you not select a number higher than that?
B. Great- it seems like you are motivated
C. Why did you not select a 3?
D. What can I do to convince you to get it to a 10?
E. It doesn't seem like you are quite ready yet

139. A patient is six months post biliopancreatic diversion with duodenal switch and has been happy with her weight loss thus far. However, she has noticed that her hair has grown slower and started to fall out. This is very concerning to her. She admits to taking one prenatal vitamin daily and following all food restrictions. Recent thyroid levels and complete metabolic panel were normal. Given these findings, what micro deficiency is the most likely explanation for her symptoms?

A. Selenium
B. Zinc
C. Copper
D. Vitamin K
E. Vitamin A

140. A family practice physician sees multiple patients during her dedicated bariatric clinic session. A number of them have approached her regarding evaluation for bariatric surgery. Which of the following patients would be the best current candidate for weight-loss surgery?

A. 29-year-old male (BMI 36 kg/m²) who is a current tobacco user with a history of hypertension and obstructive sleep apnea
B. 34-year-old female (BMI 41 kg/m²) with a history of cervical cancer status post hysterectomy with clean margins
C. 52-year-old female (BMI 55 kg/m²) with a history of hypertension, refusing to undergo mammography and colonoscopy
D. 60-year-old male (BMI 34 kg/m²) with a history of osteoarthritis, hyperlipidemia, diabetes type 2, and chronic kidney disease stage 2

141. A 48-year-old female with the disease of obesity presents as a follow-up appointment regarding increased liver enzymes. She recently completed a right upper quadrant ultrasound that revealed fatty liver infiltration. She denies any significant alcohol use. Which of the following diets should be recommended to her at this time?

A. Mediterranean-style
B. DASH diet
C. Low glycemic index
D. Low fat
E. High protein

142. A 42-year-old male presents to a dietary clinic for his initial consultation. He admits that his work schedule is hectic, requiring him to travel frequently, and thus, he feels his weight gain is most likely due to his fast-food intake. He is not interested in calorie counting. His weight loss goals include losing approximately 10% of his weight within the next year, based on mostly diet changes, as he already exercises every morning. His BMI is 37 kg/m^2, and he has no prior medical history. Given these preferences, which would be the best fit regarding weight-loss management?

A. Mediterranean diet
B. Paleo diet
C. Bariatric surgery
D. Meal replacement
E. Pharmacotherapy

143. A 52-year-old male presents for follow-up at the transplant center. He was diagnosed with cirrhosis secondary to long-standing metabolic-associated fatty liver disease. He has minimal ascites and his last hospitalization was three months ago for hepatic encephalopathy. His BMI is currently 38 kg/m^2, and he must lose 25 lbs (11.3 kg) before being placed on the liver transplant list. Which of the following anti-obesity medications is contraindicated in this patient?

A. Setmelanotide
B. Naltrexone/ bupropion ER
C. Semaglutide
D. Orlistat
E. Cellulose and citric acid hydrogel

144. A patient returns to the office extremely concerned because she recently found out her grandfather had medullary thyroid carcinoma (MTC). She started on semaglutide at her prior appointment to help with weight loss. Which of the following is the best advice to provide the patient?

A. "It is fine to continue the medication, as MTC is not associated with this class of medications."
B. "The associated risk of MTC has only been shown in animal studies, not in human trials."
C. "We must monitor calcitonin levels and order a RET oncogene test while on this medication."
D. "Unfortunately, the risk of developing MTC has increased significantly, given your family history."

145. A 37-year-old male presents to discuss bariatric surgical options. He had a friend that underwent a single anastomosis duodeno-ileostomy with sleeve gastrectomy (SADI-S) and has done well. He is wondering about the benefits and risks of this procedure compared to a Roux-en-Y gastric bypass. What is the best advice to provide?

A. The SADI-S has more anastomotic sites than the RYGB
B. The SADI-S reduces ghrelin significantly more than RYGB
C. A RYGB requires more frequent monitoring of vitamin levels
D. The RYGB leads to increased remission rates of diabetes mellitus
E. The SADI-S is done through an open abdominal procedure

146. A recently graduated advanced practice nurse is prescribing pharmacologic therapy in the clinic. Although she has received her national provider identifier (NPI) number, she currently does not have her drug enforcement agency (DEA) license. Because of this limitation, which of the following medications is she able to prescribe?

A. Diethylpropion
B. Phentermine/topiramate ER
C. Phendimetrazine
D. Naltrexone/bupropion ER

147. A 29-year-old female affected by obesity is presenting for help with losing and maintaining weight. During discussions, the importance of losing 5-10% of her baseline weight related to her health is reiterated, specifically related to improving current medical conditions and preventing future issues. This discussion falls into which of the following categories of the "5 A's of obesity management"?

A. Ask
B. Assess
C. Advise
D. Agree
E. Arrange/assist

148. A 67-year-old male presents for lifestyle modification education after recently having a cardiac stent placed for unstable angina. In particular, he is wondering about "good fats" that his wife has talked about. Which of the following is the most accurate statement?

A. Saturated fats are unlikely to be absorbed and thus preferred
B. Trans fats should only be consumed in moderation
C. Increasing polyunsaturated fats reduces cardiac risk factors
D. Coconut oil is preferred instead of vegetable oil
E. Tilapia is a cheaper alternative to salmon with similar benefits

149. A 52-year-old female presents to the emergency room by ambulance after a witnessed seizure. The patient is not on any current medications. She underwent a successful Roux-en-Y gastric bypass nearly two years ago, with hypertension currently in remission. Her husband states she has complained of lightheadedness and fatigue 1-2 hours after meals for the past few months. However, this is the first time she has had a seizure. Point of care glucose on arrival is 23 mg/dL (reference range: 74-106 mg/dL). Which of the following daily medications may have prevented her seizure?

A. Semaglutide
B. Metformin
C. Metoprolol
D. Acabrose
E. Sitagliptan

150. A 28-year-old female with a history of rheumatoid arthritis and epilepsy presents to a multidisciplinary weight loss clinic after not meeting weight loss goals with lifestyle modifications. Her BMI is 36.2 kg/m². She is interested in long-term weight loss options in combination with behavioral therapy. Which of the following would be the most appropriate option for her?

A. Gastric balloon
B. Naltrexone/bupropion ER
C. Open sleeve gastrectomy
D. Aspiration device
E. TransPyloric shuttle

151. An 8-year-old male with excess weight presents to his pediatrician, accompanied by his mother. The patient appears happy and has no other medical conditions and takes no medications. The mother states the school year has been busy with music lessons and chess tournaments, which he prefers over sports. She says he is physically inactive but has eliminated soda from his diet. Given the mother's work schedule, they often pick up food from restaurants in the evening. Which of the following would be the most effective method to promote weight loss in this patient?

A. Initiate pharmacotherapy
B. Wake patient up early to exercise
C. Restrict dinner portion sizes
D. Sign the patient up for soccer
E. Involve the family in weight loss

152. A 31-year-old female with a body mass index of 36 kg/m² presents to her primary care physician after discussing weight loss medications with her friend. She is interested in starting a medication but is unsure of the best option. She denies any tobacco or alcohol abuse. Past medical history reveals a history of recurrent nephrolithiasis and epilepsy. Physical exam reveals truncal obesity with a small and reducible umbilical hernia with minimal abdominal striae. Of the options below, which would be her best long-term option?

A. Phentermine/topiramate ER
B. Phentermine monotherapy
C. Liraglutide
D. Naltrexone/bupropion ER
E. Orlistat

153. A 59-year-old female presents to an obesity medicine specialist. She has tried numerous dietary plans and becomes frustrated with the associated restrictions and rules. Since the beginning of the covid pandemic, she has worked from home, exercises 200-300 minutes weekly, and does resistance training twice weekly. She is interested in anti-obesity medications but also wants to continue working on lifestyle modifications. Which of the following recommendations would be most useful for her?

A. Recommend increasing her weekly physical activity
B. Provide resources on mindful eating
C. Discuss phone-based applications to count calories and macronutrients
D. Initiate medications and put lifestyle changes on hold
E. Begin sertraline to help with depression and improve motivation

154. A 37-year-old female is following up with her bariatric surgeon after undergoing a successful Roux-en-Y gastric bypass procedure three weeks prior. Overall she is doing well, however, she points to her mid-epigastric region as having increased constant pain, which is not relieved with famotidine. Also, yesterday she noticed nausea, and today she has had two bouts of emesis. She does admit to starting smoking again, but only 4-5 cigarettes daily. Her last bowel movement was three days ago. Which of the following is the most likely diagnosis?

A. Internal hernia
B. Gastric outlet obstruction
C. Mesenteric ischemia
D. Anastomotic stricture
E. Marginal ulcer

155. A 31-year-old previously healthy male presents to his family care physician for evaluation of his chronic condition of obesity. He started seeing a dietician and is very happy with his progress regarding dietary changes and calorie counting. He has not begun to exercise but is interested. A history and physical is performed, with no limitations to exercise perceived. An exercise prescription is being written. Which of the following is directly part of this prescription?

A. Patient safety
B. Barriers to exercise
C. Motivational interviewing
D. Enjoyment of activity
E. Physical limitations

156. A 49-year-old female presents to her family practitioner with a complaint of weight gain. She was on fenfluramine in combination with phentermine in the distant past and would like to start on something similar, as it was very effective. She is started on phentermine 15 mg in the morning. What is the most common side effect this patient will likely experience?

A. Xerostomia
B. Nausea and vomiting
C. Diarrhea
D. Dysgeusia
E. Headaches

157. A 42-year-old female with a medical history of difficult to control diabetes mellitus type 2 and obesity class III presents for a bariatric seminar to learn more about surgical options. She is particularly interested in a more recently endorsed malabsorptive procedure. It is described as having a high diabetes remission rate and causing a significant reduction in hunger due to the removal of a portion of the stomach. Which surgical procedure is she referring to?

A. Single anastomosis duodeno-ileostomy with sleeve gastrectomy
B. Vertical sleeve gastrectomy
C. Roux-en-Y gastric bypass
D. Biliopancreatic diversion with a duodenal switch
E. One anastomosis gastric bypass

158. A 27-year-old female with a history of epilepsy is returning for a one month-follow up to her primary care physician's office. Three months ago, she was started on phentermine/topiramate ER after lifestyle changes failed to achieve her weight loss goals. Her current dose is 7.5/46 mg phentermine/topiramate ER daily. She is tolerating the medication well, but is unsure of its effectiveness. During the past three months, her weight has decreased from 220 lbs (100 kg) to 216 lbs (98 kg). Which option would be the most appropriate to initiate at this time?

A. Monitor for weight loss for an additional month
B. Take an additional phentermine/topiramate ER 3.75/23 mg tab at night
C. Change the medication to naltrexone/bupropion ER
D. Titrate up to phentermine/topiramate ER 15/92 mg daily
E. Titrate off medication, then start liraglutide

159. A 31-year-old male presents for his initial 1-week post-bariatric surgery (sleeve gastrectomy) follow-up appointment with his dietician. He has continued on a liquid diet and has been taking crushed vitamin supplementation. His current vitamin intake includes the following:

- Two adult multivitamins
- Elemental calcium of 1200 mg daily
- 1000 international units of vitamin D
- 65 mg of iron taken on an empty stomach

Which of the following recommendations should be made to this patient?

A. Take iron with calcium for increased absorption
B. Avoid concentrated carbohydrates to prevent dumping syndrome
C. Double the amount of vitamin D intake
D. Decrease the multivitamin to one tablet daily
E. Ensure the multivitamins contain vitamin K

160. A 31-year-old female status post Roux-en-Y gastric bypass is being seen 4 hours postoperatively on the general medical floor by the hospitalist. There were no immediate surgical complications. The patient has type 2 diabetes mellitus and was previously on empagliflozin, tirzepatide, and metformin. She has tolerated a small amount of oral liquid intake. Point-of-care glucose testing reveals a current glucose level of 150 mg/dL. Of the following options, what is the most appropriate management of this patient's diabetes?

A. Decrease empagliflozin by 50%
B. Continue to monitor glucose levels
C. Initiate semaglutide
D. Change metformin to extended-release
E. Start insulin drip to maintain glucose levels of 140-180 mg/dL

161. A 34-year-old male is presenting for a 2-week follow-up with his health coach. He had lost 3 lbs (1.4 kg) the first week but has regained that back. He states that work is busy, and he has difficulty avoiding eating fast food, which is convenient. The health coach agrees that losing weight does take effort and then states, "You are showing motivation to lose weight by coming to the office, but yet you continue to eat fast food frequently. How do those two go together?" What motivation interview principle did the coach display?

A. Empathy
B. Avoiding arguments
C. Developing discrepancy
D. Resolving ambivalence
E. Supporting self-efficacy

162. A 24-year-old female presents for smoking cessation counseling. She has mild depression symptoms and increased weight gain since starting the night shift. The clinician starts her on a single medication that can treat all of these components. Which of the following parameters may increase once starting this medication?

A. LDL
B. Triglycerides
C. Glucose levels
D. Blood pressure
E. Heart rate

163. A 35-year-old female is following up with her primary care physician two years after undergoing a Roux-en-Y gastric bypass. She has lost and maintained 65% of her excess body weight. Today, her vitamin D (OH-25) is 8 ng/mL (reference range > 30 ng/ml), her parathyroid hormone is slightly elevated, and her corrected calcium levels are normal. She undergoes a bone density scan, which is consistent with osteopenia. Which of the following is the most appropriate treatment at this time?

A. Calcitriol
B. Ergocalciferol
C. Calcium oxalate
D. Oral alendronate
E. Intravenous zoledronic acid

164. A 41-year-old male with a body mass index of 61 kg/m² presents for a surgery consultation regarding bariatric surgical options. Comorbidities include well-controlled obstructive sleep apnea, hypertension, and right knee osteoarthritis. Upon discussing goals, he states his primary goal is maximum weight loss. Given his prior medical history and weight loss goals, which of the following would be the most appropriate surgical option for him?

A. Laparoscopic adjustable gastric banding (LAGB)
B. Sleeve gastrectomy (SG)
C. Roux-en-Y gastric bypass (RYGB)
D. Biliopancreatic diversion with duodenal switch (BPD/DS)

165. A 43-year-old female presents to the office for increased weight since her last appointment. She was started on amlodipine for blood pressure and has noted a 2.2 lb (1 kg) weight gain despite no other changes to physical activity. What is the most likely explanation for this?

A. Increased interstitial edema
B. Increased appetite
C. Decreased energy expenditure
D. Activation of POMC/CART pathway
E. Placebo effect

166. A 52-year-old female presents to her primary care physician with intermittent post-prandial fullness, nausea, and occasional vomiting. She underwent a laparoscopic Roux-en-Y gastric bypass two years prior and has been very happy with her weight loss. A barium swallow and subsequent EGD fail to explain her findings. The following week she goes to the emergency department for biliary emesis. The most likely cause of her symptoms is a(n)

A. mesenteric defect
B. small intestinal bowel overgrowth
C. H. pylori infection
D. marginal ulcer
E. anastomotic stricture

167. A 41-year-old female presents to her primary care physician for concerns of diaphoresis, weakness, and tunnel vision approximately 2 hours after meals. She underwent a Roux-en-Y gastric bypass (RYGB) 3 years ago and subsequently lost 103 lbs (46.7 kg) with a current BMI of 26.1 kg/m². She denies ever having similar symptoms. She has decreased her carbohydrate intake, which helped minimally. Which of the following conditions most accurately describes her symptoms?

A. Dumping syndrome
B. Insulinoma
C. Post-gastric bypass hypoglycemia
D. Nesidioblastosis
E. Noninsulinoma pancreatogenous hypoglycemia syndrome

168. A 39-year-old Caucasian female with a past medical history of obstructive sleep apnea adherent with CPAP and gout presents to her primary care office for follow-up regarding elevated blood pressures. Over the last three months, home and in-office blood pressures have ranged from 150-170/90-105 mmHg. Today her blood pressure is 164/98 mmHg with a BMI of 34 kg/m². Which of the following is the most appropriate medication to prescribe now?

A. Losartan
B. Naltrexone/bupropion ER
C. Chlorthalidone
D. Metoprolol

169. An 8-year-old female affected by obesity is returning for a follow-up visit regarding weight. Over the past five months, she has met biweekly with either a dietician, physician, or psychiatrist for behavioral therapy to address her weight. During this time, she has continued to gain weight despite following recommendations. She has increased from the 97th percentile for BMI to the 99th percentile. Which of the following is the most appropriate recommendation at this time?

A. Send the patient to a tertiary weight loss center
B. Maintain current weight with continued growth
C. Initiate pharmacotherapy
D. Target a 2-pound weekly weight loss
E. Limit screen time to 2 hours daily

170. A 51-year-old female is presenting to her primary care physician with plans to undergo a sleeve gastrectomy. She has a prior diagnosis of polycystic ovarian syndrome and hypertension, for which she is taking metformin and lisinopril. Overall she states she feels well. Her physical activity consists of briskly walking (5 metabolic equivalents) for 45 minutes daily. Physical examination is unrevealing. Her STOP-BANG score is 1. Which would be the most appropriate test to perform before surgery?

A. Pharmacologic stress test
B. Fasting lipid panel
C. Thyroid-stimulating hormone
D. Dexamethasone suppression test
E. Overnight polysomnography

171. A patient is researching different bariatric procedures and is considering a duodenal switch. In discussing this procedure with the patient, which of the following most accurately describes this procedure?

A. It is preferred in those with a BMI < 45 kg/m²
B. The common channel is less than 20 cm in length
C. Digestive enzymes enter the digestive loop
D. A portion of the stomach is removed

172. A clinical trial is evaluating an oxyntomodulin analog, which is a potential investigational obesity therapy that has shown promising effects in animal studies. It is theorized that this medication will increase satiety, decrease food intake, and potentially have beneficial glucose effects in patients with type 2 diabetes mellitus. The beneficial effects of this intravenous peptide most likely occur as a result of which of the following mechanisms?

A. GLP-1 receptor agonist
B. Glucagon receptor antagonism
C. NPY/AgRP direct antagonist
D. Increase in central serotonin levels
E. Ghrelin binding and inactivation

173. A 52-year-old male presents to a gastroenterologist for evaluation of esophageal dysphagia. He underwent an open Roux-en-Y gastric bypass 15 years prior. Although he has maintained significant weight loss, he has not been adherent to physical activity or taking vitamins. An image from the upper gastrointestinal series is shown below. Given this finding, which other feature is likely found on physical examination?

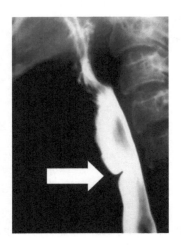

A. Koilonychia
B. Hepatomegaly
C. Dermatitis
D. External hemorrhoids
E. Actinic cheilitis

174. A 29-year-old female presents to the clinic with concerns about an abnormal fasting lipid panel on screening blood work for life insurance.

Test	Value	Reference Range
Total cholesterol	287 mg/dL	< 200 mg/dL
LDL	188 mg/dL	< 130 mg/dL
HDL	31 mg/dL	> 40 mg/dL
Triglycerides (TG)	388 mg/dL	< 150 mg/dL

In discussing a carbohydrate versus fat-restricted diet, which of the following would be an accurate statement to provide to this patient?

A. A ketogenic diet is preferred to improve the LDL value
B. A diet consisting of < 30% fats will preferentially improve HDL
C. Genetic hypercholesterolemia responds to carbohydrate restriction
D. Low-fat diets do not affect insulin resistance or glucose levels
E. Carbohydrate-restricted diets would have a greater effect on TG

175. A 42-year-old female presents for her 3-month follow-up appointment with her diabetes specialist. The patient has noticed increased polyuria over the past month and admits to having some "slip-ups" following her carbohydrate-restricted diet. Medical history includes type 2 diabetes, heart failure with preserved ejection fraction, and mild diabetic nephropathy. Medications include metformin 2000 mg daily, lisinopril 10 mg daily, and hydrochlorothiazide 25 mg. Body mass index is 34 kg/m², whereas vital signs and physical examination are otherwise normal. Her most recent HbA1c is 8.6% (reference range: < 5.7%), an increase of 0.5% since her prior appointment. Which of the following is the most appropriate management change at this time?

A. Increase metformin
B. Initiate basal insulin
C. Start a DPP-4 inhibitor
D. Prescribe an SGLT-2 inhibitor
E. Lifestyle changes only

176. A patient presents to a bariatric seminar, as he is interested in undergoing surgery for weight loss. He has struggled with weight his entire life, and despite recommended dietary and physical activity changes, his body mass index is still > 60 kg/m². At the end of the seminar, he discusses with the surgeon an option that he has read about, but was not presented by the surgeon, which included placing a balloon into the stomach for weight loss. Which of the following is a true statement regarding this procedure for weight loss?

A. This device is not FDA-approved for use in the United States
B. Intragastric balloons account for 10% of bariatric procedures
C. Indications include a BMI between > 30-40 kg/m² with comorbidities
D. Intragastric balloons have been proven ineffective for weight loss
E. The balloons are placed for 12 months, then removed

177. A 61-year-old male presents to his primary care office with a desire to start a newer medication to treat his diabetes and help with weight loss. The medication discussed has two mechanisms of action. Which of the following is a contraindication to this medication?

A. History of prior alcohol-induced pancreatitis
B. End-stage renal disease
C. Suicidal ideation
D. Family history of medullary thyroid carcinoma
E. History of nephrolithiasis

178. A 26-year-old female with severe obesity presents to a bariatric surgery consultation. Her prior medical history includes gastroesophageal reflux and obstructive sleep apnea. She takes prenatal vitamins and famotidine and admits adherence regarding her continuous positive airway pressure machine. Physical examination reveals acanthosis nigricans on the back of her neck and narrow striae on her abdomen. A recent complete metabolic panel and thyroid-stimulating hormone level were normal. Which of the following must be completed before this patient undergoes bariatric surgery?

A. Preoperative *Helicobacter pylori* testing
B. Right upper quadrant ultrasound
C. Serum dehydroepiandrosterone-sulfate (DHEA-S)
D. Psychosocial-behavioral evaluation
E. 5% mandatory weight loss preoperatively

179. A 29-year-old female who is one month postpartum is being evaluated for weight management. She is currently breastfeeding, and her BMI is 36 kg/m². She states her BMI has never been below 30 kg/m² during her adult life. She would like to start treatment to help with returning to her pre-conception weight. Which option would be most appropriate to initiate at this time?

A. Semaglutide
B. Phentermine/topiramate ER
C. Naltrexone/bupropion SR
D. Cellulose and citric acid hydrogel
E. Metformin

180. A 39-year-old female is presenting to her general surgeon, who performed her gastric bypass four months prior. She is having vague episodes of sharp mid- to upper abdominal pain that lasts 2-3 hours and then resolves. During these episodes, she feels nauseated but denies emesis. These occur 2 hours after eating, but she is unsure of the correlation to certain foods. She does admit to taking naproxen occasionally for a headache but is on concurrent omeprazole. A right upper quadrant ultrasound reveals cholelithiasis without cholecystitis. In working up her abdominal pain, which of the following statements is true?

A. She should be given a trial of rifaximin
B. NSAIDs should never be used after bariatric surgery
C. Endoscopic evaluation is high-risk after bariatric surgery
D. Traditional ERCP is preferred for choledocholithiasis evaluation
E. Ursodeoxycholic acid may have prevented her symptoms

181. A 22-year-old female is presenting to the weight-loss clinic to discuss the FDA-approved, long-term use anti-obesity medications. She denies any prior eating disorders, including bulimia and anorexia nervosa, which you state are contraindications to the combination oral medication that you want to prescribe. In addition, this medication carries a black box warning for which of the following conditions?

A. Congenital defects
B. Suicidal ideation
C. Medullary thyroid carcinoma
D. Pancreatitis
E. Ventricular arrhythmia

182. A female patient meets with her dietician one final time before undergoing a Roux-en-Y gastric bypass. The dietician discusses starting a high-protein, liquid diet 2 weeks before the surgery. What is the reasoning behind this?

A. Develop good dietary habits for the post-operative period
B. To prevent surgical complications from organ injury
C. Reduce inflammation in the stomach and proximal intestines
D. Decrease colonic stool burden and risk of an intestinal leak
E. Increase the total percentage of post-operative weight loss

183. A 47-year-old female presents for a comprehensive metabolic and bariatric surgery consultation. Her BMI has consistently been over 50 kg/m² for the past ten years, which she attributes to pregnancies and genetics. She has a family history of endometrial cancer in her mother and prostate cancer in her father. Per the Centers for Disease Control and Prevention (CDC), aggressive weight loss will likely reduce the risk of malignancy affecting which of the following areas?

A. Thyroid
B. Lymph nodes
C. Lung
D. Skin
E. Oral

184. A 6-year-old male presents to a geneticist after he is found to have hyperphagia. Testing reveals that pro-insulin levels are increased. The child's BMI is 150% of the 95th percentile. Genetic testing returns positive for a variant of the proprotein convertase subtilisin/Kexin type 1 (PCSK1) gene. Which of the following should be administered to this child?

A. Amylin analogs
B. Metreleptin
C. Semaglutide
D. Setmelanotide
E. Gastric inhibitory polypeptide

185. A 33-year-old female presents for a pre-operative consultation with a desire to undergo a Roux-en-Y gastric bypass. She is concerned as she states that she has been on buprenorphine-naloxone for the past five years due to a history of intravenous heroin use. Since stopping heroin, she has had a steady increase in weight, and her current BMI is 41 kg/m². She has an accountability partner, has been sober for the past 5 years, and is now counseling others on the effects of substance use. Which of the following statements is accurate to present?

A. A history of substance use is a contraindication to surgery
B. Buprenorphine-naloxone must be stopped prior to surgery
C. The risk of alcohol use disorder is increased after surgery
D. An underlying eating disorder will improve after surgery
E. Weekly urine drug screens will ensure adherence after surgery

186. A 32-year-old female is being evaluated by psychiatry before bariatric surgery. During the interview, the patient understands the risks and benefits of the planned gastric sleeve but shows a lack of motivation to maintain the dietary and exercise changes. The patient is asked to write a list of potential pitfalls or concerns the patient has regarding maintaining weight postoperatively. What key process of motivational interviewing is being displayed?

A. Engagement
B. Focusing
C. Evoking
D. Planning

187. A multi-disciplinary weight management center has recently added the TransPyloric Shuttle (TPS)® to its list of options for weight loss. What is true regarding this device?

A. It is best for those with significant BMI levels as a bridge to surgery
B. It can only be kept in place for six months maximum
C. It is safe in pregnancy, although it must be removed before birth
D. Patients must be on chronic acid suppression while device is in place
E. Bowel obstruction is the most common adverse side effect

188. A 29-year-old female presents for a two-month follow-up appointment after her initial obesity medicine consultation. At the prior appointment, her medroxyprogesterone injection was discussed as being weight positive. She was started on tirzepatide to assist in weight loss and treat her diabetes mellitus type 2. She has since changed to an oral estrogen-progesterone contraceptive pill and is tolerating the tirzepatide well. Which lab finding may occur within the next year if her current medications are not addressed?

A. Increased renin levels
B. Hypokalemia
C. Increased urine anion gap
D. Hypoglycemia
E. Positive urine HCG

189. A 21-year-old female is having frequent migraines leading to missed days of work. Most headaches last up to two days and she has approximately eight debilitating headaches per month. She has tried NSAIDs and sumatriptan for abortive therapy and topiramate and propranolol for prevention. None of these have been effective. Recent head imaging was normal. She does not want to start on medications that will cause weight gain. Which is the best pharmacologic treatment for this patient?

A. Atenolol
B. Amitriptyline
C. Acetazolamide
D. Erenumab
E. Valproic acid

190. A 34-year-old male with a past medical history of anxiety and diabetes presents to his primary care physician two years after undergoing a sleeve gastrectomy. He initially lost 60 lbs (27.2 kg) within the first year, but then over this past year, he has slowly regained approximately 30 lbs (13.6 kg). Medications include metformin, detemir, and fluoxetine. He does admit nonadherence with his recommended daily vitamins but continues to exercise three times weekly. Given these findings, which of the following most likely explains his postoperative weight regain?

A. Dilated gastric pouch
B. Excess insulin administration
C. Dietary indiscretion
D. Psychologic issues
E. Vitamin deficiencies

191. A 49-year-old female who was recently widowed after her husband had complications from obesity presents to her family medicine physician for weight loss counseling. Her BMI is 42 kg/m^2, and she has a past medical history of hypertension, diabetes, and asthma. Comprehensive lifestyle changes are discussed. What is a reasonable weight loss goal, in terms of total body loss, for this patient within the next six months, according to the "2013 ACC/AHA/TOS Guidelines for the Management of Overweight and Obesity in Adults"?

A. 0-5%
B. 5-10%
C. 10-15%
D. 15-20%

192. A 33-year-old female with a past medical history of class III obesity, diabetes type 2, tobacco abuse, and polycystic ovarian syndrome presents for a bariatric evaluation. She is interested in a "gastric bypass." Her medications include metformin, oral contraceptive birth control, and a prenatal vitamin. After a thorough history and physical examination, you discuss preoperative recommendations, including a physical activity plan and healthy dietary patterns. What other perioperative education would be necessary for this patient?

A. Avoid becoming pregnant for at least 6 months after surgery
B. Birth control must be discontinued 1 week before surgery
C. Her hemoglobin A1c should be less than 9% preoperatively
D. Metformin is contraindicated after Roux-en-Y gastric bypass
E. Tobacco products must be stopped 6 weeks before surgery

193. A 24-year-old female presents to her primary care physician's office for an evaluation regarding weight gain. She states she has been exercising five times weekly for approximately 30 minutes during her sessions. She has decreased her calories to 1200 kcal daily, focusing on a low-fat diet, but still has noticed a 10 lb (4.5 kg) weight gain in the past year. Medical history includes bipolar disease, which is well-controlled on aripiprazole. Previous laboratory work was within normal limits, including HbA1c, TSH, and CMP. Which would be the most effective in treating her weight gain?

A. Prescribe metformin
B. Prescribe orlistat
C. Intensify calorie restrictions
D. Change aripiprazole to olanzapine
E. Intensify exercise regimen

194. A 12-year-old female who has struggled with obesity for the past five years is presenting to a bariatric tertiary center for a vertical sleeve gastrectomy evaluation. She has hypertension and severe obstructive sleep apnea that did not respond to tonsillectomy. She is sexually active and developmentally is at a Tanner Stage 3. Her BMI is currently 37 kg/m². Psychiatry evaluation reveals mild depression and a lack of understanding of the risks regarding the surgical procedure. Which of the following is a contraindication for this adolescent to undergo bariatric surgery?

A. Tanner Stage 3
B. Body mass index
C. Sexual activity
D. Depression
E. Risk appreciation

195. A 28-year-old female is presenting to her primary care physician's office six months after undergoing a laparoscopic adjustable gastric banding (LAGB). She states two weeks ago, she had eaten too quickly, with subsequent nausea and vomiting. Since then, she has been unable to keep solids down and will regurgitate undigested food after small meals. In addition, her acid reflux has significantly worsened during this time. Which of the following is the next best step in management?

A. CT of the abdomen
B. Remove fluid from the band
C. Surgical revision
D. Diet changes
E. Start omeprazole

196. A 35-year-old female presents as a follow-up three years after undergoing a sleeve gastrectomy. She states she had significant weight loss within the first year post-operatively but has since plateaued in her weight, approximately 30 lbs (13.6 kg) short of her goal. She has followed all recommendations but admits to an increased appetite. She would like to discuss anti-obesity medications to assist in helping with reaching her goals. Which of the following is the most appropriate recommendation to provide?

A. Weight-loss medications are contraindicated after bariatric surgery
B. Cellulose and citric acid hydrogel is preferred post-operatively
C. Revision surgery is most appropriate to reach your target weight
D. Body contouring surgery will likely allow you to reach your goal
E. Starting semaglutide and phentermine will reduce weight

197. A 14-year-old female is being evaluated for a sleeve gastrectomy given her body mass index and comorbidities. Where should this evaluation be completed?

A. Primary care physician's office
B. Pediatric weight management center
C. Tertiary care center
D. Pediatric general surgery office

198. A 59-year-old male is interested in initiating the exchange diet into his daily routine. He is currently planning on eliminating one of his snacks daily and substituting two servings of vegetables for 2 starches.

American Diabetes Association Exchange Servings				
1 Serving	Protein	Carbohydrate	Fat	Calories
Starches	3 g	15 g	<1 g	80 kcal
Vegetables	2 g	5 g	0 g	25 kcal
Fat	0 g	0 g	0 g	45 kcal
Fruit	0 g	15 g	0 g	60 kcal
Dairy	8 g	15 g	0-8 g	90-150 kcal
Protein	7 g	0 g	2-5 g	55-75 kcal
Snacks	3 g	15 g	0-1 g	80 kcal

How many daily calories will he reduce by making these changes?

A. 80 kcal/day
B. 130 kcal/day
C. 190 kcal/day
D. 240 kcal/day
E. 270 kcal/day

199. A 19-year-old female presents to her obstetrician to discuss options for birth control. She wants to maintain a healthy weight, given her family history of diabetes and early-onset coronary artery disease. She is sexually active and does not want to become pregnant. Which of the following is associated with the most weight gain?

A. Intrauterine device
B. Barrier method
C. Progesterone-only pill
D. Etonogestrel implant
E. Progesterone depo injections

200. A 32-year-old male presents to his primary care physician for yellowing of his eyes and noticing increased fatigue. He takes no prescribed medication, but does admit to taking a combination herbal supplement for weight loss. Although it is recommended to take twice daily, he has been taking approximately ten daily, and has noticed a 14 lb (6.4 kg) weight loss. AST, ALT, bilirubin, and INR are markedly elevated. Which of the following ingredients in his supplement is most likely contributing to his current condition?

A. Chitosan
B. Ephedra
C. Glucosinolates
D. Green tea extract
E. Raspberry ketone

201. A 29-year-old male presents to his dietician after starting a very low-calorie diet. He has done some research and determined that he would like to maintain less than 800 kcal/day and eliminate all fat from his diet. Currently, he is consuming 1300 kcal/day without significant weight loss. The dietician discusses the importance of close monitoring and recommends adding some fat to his diet instead of eliminating it altogether. Without this recommendation, what possible complications could arise?

A. Electrolyte imbalance
B. Gout flares
C. Cholelithiasis
D. Electrolyte derangements
E. Cold intolerance

202. A 26-year-old female underwent a one-anastomosis gastric bypass and has since had a persistent burning sensation in her mid-epigastric region. She states that proton pump inhibitors have not helped and sucralfate provided no relief. She denies any other symptoms, including fever, nausea, or vomiting. Endoscopic evaluation reveals no strictures or anastomotic ulcers, and a histologic sample shows mild stomach inflammation. A CT of the abdomen is unremarkable. Which of the following is the most likely cause of her symptoms?

A. Cardiac ischemia
B. Bile acid gastritis
C. *H. pylori* infection
D. Recalcitrant acid reflux
E. Esophageal spasm

203. A 44-year-old male presents to his primary care clinician for a three-month follow-up appointment. He has a history of obesity class II, hypertension, obstructive sleep apnea, and hyperlipidemia. He started an off-label medication for weight loss at his prior appointment and is tolerating it well. His lab work before and after initiating the anti-obesity medication, is shown below. Which of the following medications was likely started?

Test	Initial	Today	Reference Range
Sodium	138 mEq/L	136 mEq/L	136–145 mEq/L
Potassium	3.8 mEq/L	4.1 mEq/L	3.5-5.0 mEq/L
Chloride	99 mEq/L	107 mEq/L	95-105 mEq/L
Bicarbonate	24 mEq/L	18 mEq/L	22–28 mEq/L
BUN	16 mg/dL	18 mg/dL	6-20 mg/dL
Creatinine	0.8 mg/dL	0.9 mg/dL	0.6–1.2 mg/dL
Glucose	88 mg/dL	83 mg/dL	70–110 mg/dL

A. Phentermine
B. Metformin
C. Bupropion
D. Topiramate
E. Tirzepatide

204. A 31-year-old female presents to her primary care physician's office with complaints of significant anxiety. She has tried counseling and has noted slight improvements, but the anxiety still interferes with her life. She denies depression. She is concerned that initiating pharmacotherapy for anxiety could cause her to gain weight. Vital signs are normal. BMI is 32 kg/m². If pharmacotherapy is started, which would be the most appropriate?

A. Bupropion
B. Fluoxetine
C. Duloxetine
D. Aripiprazole
E. Propranolol

205. A 38-year-old male with a history of obesity presents to his internist's office for an annual exam. The patient denies any new symptoms since his last appointment but has noticed some weight gain, especially around his waist. His current weight is 241 lbs (109.3 kg), which is an increase of 14 lbs (6.4 kg) since last year, placing his BMI at 39 kg/m². His lipid panel is within normal limits, however, his HbA1c is currently 5.9% (reference range: < 5.7%), and his fasting glucose level is 119 mg/dL (reference range: < 100 mg/dL). Which of the following would be the most appropriate recommendation at this time?

A. Initiate metformin therapy
B. Obtain C-peptide levels
C. Recheck HbA1c levels in 3 months
D. Recommend resistance training
E. Initiate an SGLT-2 inhibitor

206. A 52-year-old male presents for a follow-up for weight loss. He was started on phentermine 15 mg in the morning and states it works well, but he notices the effects wear off by midafternoon. He wants to avoid increasing the morning dose of phentermine due to some tremors he noticed on the higher dose. He has a history of nephrolithiasis and cannot afford GLP-1 medications due to a lack of insurance coverage. Which of the following would be a potential treatment option?

A. Initiate tirzepatide
B. Add diethylpropion in the afternoon
C. Add topiramate
D. Continue current regimen
E. Add metformin

207. A previously healthy 28-year-old female with a current BMI of 28 kg/m^2 presents for a follow-up appointment with her primary care. Over the past six months, she has intensified her exercise regimen to 200 minutes/week, restricted her diet to 1300 kcal/day, and eliminated fast food and soda. However, she is frustrated that she has not met her weight loss goals and is interested in pharmacotherapy. If prescribed, which would most likely help her accomplish her 10% weight loss goal if titrated to maximum recommended strength?

A. Phentermine/topiramate ER
B. Phentermine monotherapy
C. Liraglutide
D. Naltrexone/bupropion ER

208. A 17-year-old female who has struggled with the disease of obesity since childhood is meeting with a dietician to discuss weight loss goals. In addition to keeping a food diary, the patient downloads an application on her smartphone that keeps track of calories. Upon a follow-up visit, she is averaging 1900 kcal/day. She should be counseled to reduce her calories by a minimum of what additional amount?

A. 300 kcal/d
B. 600 kcal/d
C. 900 kcal/d
D. 1200 kcal/d

209. A 67-year-old male presents with concerns of uncontrolled diabetes and increased weight gain. He is petrified of needles and refuses medications that require administration through needles, including insulin. Medications include metformin ER and dapagliflozin. He exercises 30 minutes daily and follows recommendations from his dietician. Which of the following is the next best step in management?

A. Initiate oral semaglutide
B. Discuss tirzepatide
C. Start pioglitazone
D. Intensify exercise routine
E. Prescribe continuous glucose monitoring

210. A 59-year-old female presents to her bariatric surgeon's office one week before undergoing a Roux-en-Y gastric bypass. Her current comorbidities include hyperlipidemia, hypothyroidism, obstructive sleep apnea, osteoarthritis, hypertension, and type 2 diabetes. She is hopeful of decreasing or discontinuing some of her medications after surgery. Despite improvements in many obesity-related comorbidities, which of the following conditions may likely need to have medications increased after her bariatric surgery?

A. Hyperlipidemia
B. Diabetes
C. Hypertension
D. Hypothyroidism
E. Osteoarthritis

211. A medical student is rotating with a surgeon who is about to perform a Roux-en-Y gastric bypass. He describes the procedure as one in which he will create a gastric pouch, then connect this new pouch to the jejunum, bypassing the duodenum. He describes a potentially severe complication that may follow the procedure, associated with high morbidity and prolonged hospital stays. What is true of this potential complication?

A. Barium studies are the preferred imaging
B. Failure to extubate may be the presenting sign
C. Procalcitonin has no role in evaluation
D. It is more frequently seen in a sleeve gastrectomy

212. A patient with type 1 diabetes and obesity class I presents to the clinic to discuss an indicated medication to help reduce appetite and insulin intake. A subcutaneous medication is initiated after a thorough discussion, including hypoglycemia symptoms. Which mechanism or class of medication is associated with the initiated medication?

A. Amylin analog
B. Biguinide
C. GLP-1 receptor agonist
D. GLP-1 and GIP agonist
E. Sympathetic amine

213. A 37-year-old male with a past medical history of chronic migraines and well-controlled hypertension is presenting to his primary care physician for evaluation of weight management. He has lost 9 lbs (4 kg) with lifestyle modifications but has plateaued and wants to start pharmacotherapy. His current BMI is 32 kg/m². Insurance denies the use of combination weight loss pills. Which of the following, if used off-label, would be the most appropriate medication to start now?

A. Topiramate
B. Phentermine
C. Bupropion
D. Naltrexone
E. Metformin

214. A 29-year-old female, two months post-partum who is currently breastfeeding, presents to her family practitioner to jump-start weight-loss. She states her goals are to lose weight healthily and not disrupt milk production. She is up multiple times nightly with her infant and always feels tired. She walks for 15 minutes daily and drinks 1-2 sodas daily. Her pre-pregnancy weight was 178 lbs (80.7 kg). Currently, she is at 212 lbs (96.2 kg). Which of the following would be an example of a SMART goal to set for this patient while utilizing shared-decision making?

A. Decrease calories to < 1000 kcal/day
B. Increase exercise as much as tolerated
C. Lose 5 lbs (2.3 kg) weekly until at pre-pregnancy weight
D. Decrease soda intake by 3 cans weekly until discontinued
E. Start and titrate liraglutide to a goal of 3 mg daily

215. A neurologist calls to discuss a mutual patient who needs treatments for partial seizures. The neurologist offers a few options listed below but would like your feedback based on the patient's comorbidities. The patient has diabetes mellitus type II with retinopathy, obesity class I, and hypertension. Which of the following options is most appropriate to recommend?

A. Carbamazepine
B. Gabapentin
C. Valproate
D. Zonisamide
E. Pregabalin

216. A 45-year-old male with a past medical history of acid reflux, class III obesity, hypertension, and osteoarthritis presents for a bariatric surgery evaluation. He takes a proton pump inhibitor twice daily but admits that he still has gastroesophageal symptoms regularly. A barium swallow evaluation is performed, as shown below. If bariatric surgery is pursued, which of the following should be recommended?

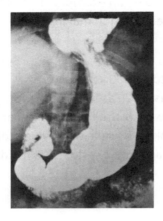

A. Sleeve gastrectomy
B. Biliopancreatic diversion with a duodenal switch
C. Adjustable gastric banding
D. Intra-gastric balloon
E. Roux-en-Y gastric bypass

IV. Practice Management

217. A 45-year-old male reluctantly presents to a bariatric seminar. He has wanted to attend for the past few years, but always cancels due to concerns of what others may think. In particular, his coworkers have already verbalized that he is less valuable compared to more active and fit employees. Thus, if he takes 2-3 weeks off from work for surgery, he feels this may exacerbate their views. What is the term that describes this labeling of decreased value that his coworkers have imparted on him?

A. Bias
B. Self-efficacy
C. Implicit bias
D. Prejudice
E. Stigma

218. A primary care physician is treating a patient who is interested in bariatric surgery. She wants to understand the potential mortality, morbidity, and predicted amount of weight loss she could experience, given her comorbidities. More specifically, she wants to compare and contrast these parameters between a sleeve gastrectomy and a Roux-en-Y gastric bypass to help her decide the best option for her. In addition to referring her to a bariatric surgeon, what resource will likely be able to assist in providing her with the information she is looking for?

A. American College of Sports Medicine
B. Metabolic and Bariatric Surgery Accreditation Quality Improvement
C. Obesity Medicine Association
D. The Obesity Society
E. United States Preventive Services Task Force

219. A cardiologist is teaming up with a bariatric clinic to provide multidisciplinary expertise regarding exercise safety. They have created an algorithm to screen asymptomatic individuals who would benefit from performing an exercise electrocardiogram stress test before engaging in a robust exercise program. Which patient would most likely fall into a moderate-risk category for suffering a cardiac event during exercise and, therefore, should be recommended for an exercise stress test before beginning aerobic exercise?

A. 52-year-old male starting moderate-intensity exercise
B. 49-year-old female initiating vigorous-intensity exercise
C. 61-year-old male starting water-walking
D. 41-year-old male beginning vigorous-intensity workouts

220. A mother of a 12-year-old son with cognitive delays and class III obesity has brought a formal complaint to the medical board regarding the denial of a metabolic bariatric surgery evaluation. The surgeon states that although the patient meets criteria for surgery based on body mass index and comorbidities, he is concerned that the cognitive disability would make post-operative follow-up more difficult. Thus, he denied the adolescent entrance into the comprehensive bariatric program. This physician may be found in violation of which of the following principles?

A. Respect for autonomy
B. Beneficence
C. Nonmaleficence
D. Justice
E. American disability act

221. A Master of Public Health candidate is interviewing clinicians for her dissertation focused on the biased treatment of those living with obesity. In particular, she wants to understand the clinician-patient relationship, including support staff, regarding the perception of those with obesity in the medical setting. Which of the following is the most accurate statement regarding this topic?

    A. Patients with obesity seek out medical care as a safe haven for bias
    B. The FDA treats medications for obesity similarly to other medications
    C. Clinicians with a normal BMI are more comfortable discussing weight
    D. Physicians self-report that obesity is a disease similar to diabetes
    E. Patients with obesity tend to receive longer office visits

222. An employer of a mid-level business is evaluating ways to improve productivity while decreasing costs. He would like to implement a physical activity initiative in which his employees would reap the cost-savings of an overall healthier workforce. Which of the following has the highest cost for an employer of workers affected by obesity compared to workers with a healthy weight?

    A. Absenteeism
    B. Health insurance premiums
    C. Presenteeism
    D. Retirement plans
    E. Accidental death insurance

223. A 19-year-old female presents to her primary care physician. She has a diagnosis of systemic lupus erythematosus with nephritis, and she has gained nearly 50 lbs (22.7 kg) since starting treatment. Her current BMI is 33 kg/m². Which of the following is the best primary diagnosis code used for billing in this patient?

A. E66.01: Severe obesity due to excess calories
B. E66.1: Drug-induced obesity
C. E66.9: Obesity, unspecified
D. Z68.33: Body mass index (BMI) 33.0-33.9, adult
E. Z68.53: BMI pediatric, 85% to less than 95th percentile for age

224. A primary care physician will start to see bariatric patients in his clinic as part of a multi-disciplinary approach to treating patients that are planning to undergo bariatric surgery. He plans to perform a preoperative screening, education, and postoperative follow-up visits. In preparing his office for this influx of patients with obesity, what would be recommended to make the patients feel more comfortable when presenting to his office?

A. Ensure his scales can weigh up to 300 lbs (136 kg)
B. Ensure standard chairs have handrails on either side
C. Order additional medium and large blood pressure cuffs
D. Ensure reading material in the waiting room is obesity-sensitive
E. Provide additional obesity-culture training only to the nursing staff

225. A physician is meeting with a United States senator regarding reimbursement for obesity therapy, including pharmacotherapy. The senator discusses the cost burden associated with obesity and his concerns that additional finances for coverage of extra office visits, bariatric surgery, and pharmacotherapy would ultimately not be worth the extra cost. Which of the following statements is true regarding the value of obesity therapy?

A. A patient with a BMI of 35 kg/m^2 infers an additional annual average medical cost of $500 compared to someone with a BMI of 25 kg/m^2
B. Nationally, the burden of obesity accounts for $50 billion in additional healthcare costs
C. Anti-obesity interventions cumulatively could generate $20 billion in savings for Medicare within ten years
D. Although bariatric surgery provides decreased morbidity, no studies have confirmed improved mortality rates
E. Physicians should only use FDA-approved anti-obesity medications despite the cost, as off-label medications have little evidence.

226. A school counselor is evaluating a 9-year-old male. The child states that two other boys in his class relentlessly tease him about his weight during recess. This has caused the student to withdraw from friends and academically decline. He is very conscious of what he eats now and states, "I wish they would just leave me alone!" The counselor calls the parents to discuss the situation. Which of the following would be the most constructive advice to provide to the parents?

A. Encourage them to seek medical care for the child's weight
B. Reassure the parents this will likely resolve with disciplinary action against the students initiating the bullying
C. Recommend scheduled counseling for the child
D. Encourage parents to teach the child to stand up for himself
E. Inform the parents that ignoring bullying is an effective technique

227. A 14-year-old male with Down syndrome and class II obesity with obstructive sleep apnea, hyperlipidemia, and prediabetes presents for follow-up at a bariatric center. The patient has been evaluated for bariatric surgery and was started on lifestyle modifications. His mother states he eats what he is given and rarely snacks. The patient and his family have been walking together every night for 1 hour. However, he has not lost any weight despite these measures. When discussing the procedure, the patient does not show an understanding of the procedure but states, "I want to be skinny." What is the most appropriate surgical management?

A. Obtain surgical consent from the parents
B. Continue to educate the patient and only perform the surgery when he can understand and provide consent
C. Two physicians that agree that surgery is appropriate, along with the parent's consent, is sufficient for pre-operative consent
D. Do not perform surgery due to a lack of understanding
E. Intensify lifestyle modifications

228. An obesity clinic is trying to determine the best way to reach different ethnicities by utilizing cultural-specific resources effectively. Given the clinic's central location, its patient population consists of many minority groups. Generally speaking, which strategy would be the most effective therapeutic addition for a culturally tailored approach to weight-loss?

A. Provide a heart disease class for American Indians
B. Have Caucasians teach weight-loss strategies to Chinese Americans
C. Discuss alcohol avoidance within the Muslim population
D. Utilize a faith-based setting for African Americans

229. A 27-year-old male with a body mass index of 34 kg/m² presents to his primary care physician for follow-up from an emergency department visit for intractable nausea that has since resolved. He is very disappointed with his experience, as he requested hospital records and found in the emergency room notes that the physician used wording that he felt was hurtful and counterproductive. Which of the following statements would be an appropriate opening identifying statement regarding his weight?

A. A 27-year-old morbidly obese male
B. A 27-year-old individual affected by obesity
C. A 27-year-old obese patient
D. A class 1 obese 27-year-old male

Answer Explanations

1. (Content: I-B-7) A 41-year-old male is seen in the hospital on postoperative day one status post Roux-en-Y gastric bypass. Home medications include glargine 30 units nightly and aspart sliding scale with meals. Since surgery, he has not required any insulin to maintain normal glucose levels and has plans to be discharged on a low dose of immediate-release metformin. The increased endogenous hormone responsible for this diabetic medication adjustment

   A. is only secreted in the small intestine
   B. is secreted in response to fat and protein ingestion
   C. reduces hepatic gluconeogenesis
   D. has the same quantitative effects as seen after sleeve gastrectomy
   E. causes gallbladder contraction

(C) Glucagon-like peptide 1 is secreted in the distal small bowel and colon. This hormone has an incretin effect in response to carbohydrate ingestion, including glucose-dependent insulin secretion, **reduction of hepatic gluconeogenesis via glucagon suppression**, and delays in gastric emptying leading to increased satiety and reduced appetite. This hormone is responsible for the weight-independent, immediate improvements in diabetes after gastric bypass, as levels significantly increase after bypassing the proximal intestines.

Anorexigenic (Meal-Terminating) Intestinal Hormones		
Hormonal	Secretion Site	Action
Cholecystokinin (CCK)[1]	Duodenum and jejunum (I-cells)	Stimulates gallbladder contraction, slows gastric emptying, and reduces appetite
Glucose-dependent insulinotropic peptide (GIP) [3]	Duodenum and jejunum (K-cells)	Insulin incretin effect and slows gastric emptying
Glucagon-like peptide 1 (GLP-1)[2]	Distal small bowel and colon (L-cells)	**See paragraph above**
Oxyntomodulin (OXM)[3]	Distal small bowel and colon (L-cells)	Decrease appetite and increase energy expenditure
Peptide YY (PYY)[3]	Distal small bowel, colon, and rectum (L-cells)	Appetite suppression and delays gastric and intestinal emptying

[1]Secreted in response to fat/protein ingestion and gastric distention
[2]Secreted in response to carbohydrate ingestion. Reduced in obesity and type II diabetes
[3]Secreted in response to feeding

Reference: Miller GD. Appetite Regulation: Hormones, Peptides, and Neurotransmitters and Their Role in Obesity. Am J Lifestyle Med. 2017;13(6):586-601. Published 2017 Jun 23. doi:10.1177/1559827617716376

2. (Content: I-A-3) A 24-year-old female presents for genetic counseling regarding obesity. She is frustrated by the lack of ability to lose weight and being classified as "overweight" at a very young age despite her tall stature. She admits to wanting to give up regarding weight loss since obesity "is a family curse." She has diabetes and is on metformin. Previous testing indicated that she had significantly elevated circulating insulin levels. Which of the following genetic abnormalities is most likely present?

A. **MC4R**
B. POMC
C. FTO
D. PCSK1
E. LEPR

(A) Many of the above genes are involved in early-onset and often severe levels of obesity. **Melanocortin 4 receptor deficiency (MC4R)** is the most common monogenetic defect predisposing to obesity, shared within families. It is characterized by tall stature, increased bone mineral density ("big-boned"), and high insulin levels with insulin resistance.

MC4R mediates most of the anorectic effects of leptin; therefore, a deficiency leads to early-onset obesity via leptin resistance. Interestingly, leptin is also independently involved in linear bone growth, with increased levels causing tall stature, as seen in MC4R deficiency.

Other genetic abnormalities leading to early-onset obesity are listed below.

- **POMC:** Proopiomelanocortin gene mutations lead to an adrenal crisis in neonates due to ACTH deficiency, which is produced from POMC (hypothalamus) as well as alpha-melanocyte-stimulating hormone, which is involved in reducing food intake.
- **LEPR:** Leptin receptor gene defects (or those who have leptin deficiency) have difficulty suppressing their appetites and insulin resistance, but do not have tall stature.

Importantly, diagnosis allows for treatment options. Setmelanotide is approved for POMC and LEPR deficiency and Bardet-Biedl syndrome; leptin replacement (metreleptin) is approved for congenital leptin deficiency with lipodystrophy.

Reference: Up To Date: "Genetic contribution and pathophysiology of obesity"

3. (Content: I-D-4) A 51-year-old female presents to the health clinic with questions about a diet she heard about through a health magazine. Although she cannot remember the name of the diet, it promoted a higher intake of omega fat than other diets she has researched. Benefits included lowering cardiovascular disease and preventing type 2 diabetes, both of which run in her family. In addition, she will still be able to consume seafood, an important component given her fishing hobby. What is the most likely diet that this patient is referencing?

A. Vegan
B. Pescatarian
C. Lacto-ovo
D. Mediterranean
E. Low carbohydrate

(D) **A Mediterranean diet** (meal pattern) differs from other diets as it allows moderate fats (35-40% consumption), with extra virgin olive oil being the primary source of omega-3 fat. Fruits, vegetables, nuts, legumes, avocados, and whole grains are staples of the diet, which also allows moderate alcohol intake. Although limited amounts of poultry, dairy, and red meat intake is allowed, fish and seafood can be consumed in moderation.

Several studies have shown improvements in primary cardiovascular disease prevention and associated risk factors with a Mediterranean diet. Also, the Lyon Heart Study displayed secondary cardiovascular disease benefits.

Note: Although the Primary Prevention of Cardiovascular Disease with a Mediterranean Diet (PRIDIMED) has been retracted due to randomization errors, recalculation still displays a cardiac benefit from this diet.

Reference: Lyon Diet Heart Study: Benefits of a Mediterranean-Style, National Cholesterol Education Program/American Heart Association Step I Dietary Pattern on Cardiovascular Disease. Penny Kris-Etherton , Robert H. Eckel , Barbara V. Howard , Sachiko St. Jeor , Terry L. Bazzarre

4. (Content: I-B-5) A 31-year-old female wants to know her total energy expenditure. She estimates her non-exercise activity thermogenesis to be 300 kcal/day, her thermic effect of meals to be 10% of her total expenditure, and her calories from exercise to be 400 kcal/day. What other testing is necessary to determine her total energy expenditure accurately?

A. **Indirect calorimeter**
B. Skinfold calipers
C. Duke's treadmill score
D. Bioelectric impedance analyses
E. Basal body temperature

(A) **Indirect calorimetry** can determine the resting metabolic rate, as it is used as a proxy for resting energy expenditure, the last component needed in this patient to determine her total energy expenditure.

Indirect calorimetry estimates energy expenditure by measuring carbon dioxide production and oxygen consumption. Patients must wear a sealed mask, with gas exchange monitored through an electronic device. Testing can be done in the office. It is inexpensive, non-invasive, and reimbursable (CPT code: 94690).

Direct calorimetry: In contrast to indirect, direct calorimetry measures the heat generated by an organism via an enclosed chamber. Water circulates the chamber, and the incoming and outgoing water temperature differences are measured, which can then be used to calculate total energy expenditure.

The formula below calculates total energy expenditure (TEE) and approximate percentages of each component.

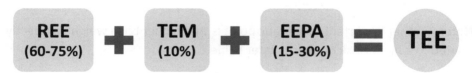

REE: Resting energy expenditure (basal metabolic rate)
TEM: Thermic effect of meals
EEPA: Energy expenditure from physical activity (exercise and non-exercise activity thermogenesis)

Note: Resting energy expenditure can also be estimated by the Mifflin St. Jeor (preferred in those with obesity) and Harris-Benedict equations.

Reference: Obesity medicine association: Obesity Algorithm (2021)

5. (Content: I-A-5) A research team is developing a thesis regarding intrauterine predisposition to factors, such as how maternal obesity affects the developing fetus through adulthood. So far, the longitudinal study has shown that a mother's body mass index correlates with comorbidities of cognitive deficits and autism spectrum disorders. This type of research is best associated with which of the following?

    A. Neurohormonal physiology
    B. Epigenetics and environment
    C. Behavioral determinants
    D. Mutations of genetic DNA
    E. Socioeconomic and culture

(B) The term **epigenetics** refers to the modification of genetic <u>expression</u> (not genetic mutations), often in the setting of inheritable changes. It is essential to understand that these effects do not modify the DNA sequence, only their expression.

The consequences of maternal obesity and the intrauterine environment affect the brain of the developing fetus. Studies have shown that increased maternal inflammatory markers, glucose, and lipids affect postnatal neurodevelopment and metabolism.

In addition to metabolism, the following increased risks were appreciated when maternal BMI was > 30 kg/m^2.

- Attention deficit disorders
- Autism spectrum disorder
- Cognitive deficits
- Impaired stress response

Note: Another important epigenetic point is that higher birth weight is directly related to a higher risk of obesity later in life.

In addition to the above, adverse childhood events (ACE) have been associated with an increased risk of obesity in children, adolescents, and even adults. Abuse, violence, incarceration or death of parents, divorce, etc. are all considered ACE, and cumulatively increase the risk of obesity later in life.

Reference: Assessing the fetal effects of maternal obesity via transcriptomic analysis of cord blood: a prospective case–control study. AG Edlow L Hui HC Wick I Fried DW Bianchi. First published: 29 December 2015

6. (Content: I-B-4) A longitudinal study was completed looking at the effects of sleep on weight. Both weight and the time of quality sleep, measured through a smartwatch device, were documented over 10 years. At the end of the study, what hormones or receptor levels would be expected to be increased in those who received 5 hours of sleep compared to those that received 8 hours?

    A. Leptin and neuropeptide Y
    B. α-MSH and peptide YY
    C. POMC receptors and ghrelin
    D. Cortisol and leptin
    E. **Ghrelin and orexin A**

(E) Long-term studies have been completed that have shown a progressive decrease in the duration of sleep for most Americans. There was a correlation between those that received fewer hours of sleep with increased weight compared to those that slept for longer periods of time, indicating sleep deprivation and subsequently increased hunger hormones lead to increased weight. These patients with decreased amounts of sleep would likely have **increased ghrelin from the stomach and increased release of orexin from the NPY/AgRP pathway,** with subsequent decreased leptin, leading to increased appetite and decreased energy expenditure.

Short amounts of sleep (approximately 5-6 hours) were correlated with a 60% increased rate of obesity and 20% with overweight. Shockingly, there was a 200% increased prevalence of obesity among those who slept <5 hours nightly.

Overall, the trend of sleep patterns indicates more people receiving < 6 hours of sleep and a decrease in those that received ideal sleep (7-8 hours) in the United States from 1977 → 2009 when this study was conducted.

Not only does sleep length play a role, but also interruptions of sleep that may occur from restless leg syndrome, obstructive sleep apnea, bed partner movements (including pets), circadian misalignment, and sleep-maintenance insomnia.

Reference: Jean-Louis G, Williams NJ, Sarpong D, Pandey A, Youngstedt S, Zizi F, Ogedegbe G. Associations between inadequate sleep and obesity in the US adult population: analysis of the national health interview survey (1977-2009). BMC Public Health. 2014 Mar 29;14:290. doi: 10.1186/1471-2458-14-290. PMID: 24678583; PMCID: PMC3999886.

7. (Content: I-B-2) A 65-year-old male is following up with his dietician after starting a low-fat diet six weeks ago. He has increased his exercise to 250 minutes/week and has noticed a 1% total body weight loss since initiating these lifestyle changes. He comments that he has always had to work hard to maintain or lose weight, and it seems that if he stops dieting for a few weeks, he regains weight rapidly. In contrast, he states that his wife can eat whatever she likes, has always remained thin, and seldomly exercises. Compared to his wife, this patient most likely has which of the following?

    A. Decreased energy harvest from food
    B. Higher fasting-induced adipose factor expression
    C. Increased levels of Firmicutes in his gut
    D. Higher AMPK

(C) The gut microbiome has been studied as it relates to obesity and the effects of dieting. The two most common gut bacteria are Firmicutes and Bacteroides, comprising 92% of gut flora. In general, those who are leaner, such as his wife, have higher levels of Bacteroides and decreased levels of Firmicutes compared to someone affected by obesity. Interestingly, with weight loss, gut bacteria will alter (Firmicutes will decrease, while Bacteroides increases). These levels will also eventually resemble lean individuals in those who undergo gastric bypass. Compared to his lean wife, this patient likely **has higher Firmicutes levels.**

Note: In rat studies, increased calories were found in stool samples of lean rats, indicating that rats with obesity had increased calorie absorption (i.e., energy harvesting and complex carbohydrate absorption) compared to lean rats.

Gut bacteria outnumber the number of human cells; therefore, the gut microbiome is an intriguing research area related to obesity. Ongoing studies include the effects of fecal transplants, probiotics (active, good bacteria), and prebiotics (sugars that serve as food for good bacteria).

Reference: Clarke SF, Murphy EF, Nilaweera K, et al. The gut microbiota and its relationship to diet and obesity: new insights. Gut Microbes. 2012;3(3):186-202. doi:10.4161/gmic.20168

8. (Content: I-B-8) A research study is underway in which patients fast for 8 hours, followed by consuming a meal of 500 kcal. Several hormones are monitored every 2 hours during the fasting and postprandial period for 12 hours. Six hours into the fast, ghrelin hormone levels are at their peak. What other finding would most likely be present during this time?

A. **Y1 and Y5 receptor stimulation**
B. Leptin hormone elevation
C. Suppressed agouti-related peptide hormone levels
D. Activation of the POMC/CART pathway
E. Orexin A and B hormone suppression

(A) In periods of fasting, ghrelin levels increase, which activates the orexigenic pathway, with subsequent **Y1 and Y5 receptor stimulation** on the orexin/melanin-concentrating hormone second-order neuron. These second-order neurons signal other brain regions, leading to decreased energy expenditure and increased hunger.

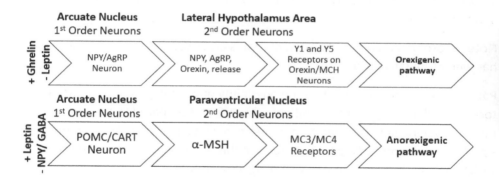

Note: AgRP inhibits melanocortin (MC4) receptors
POMC: Proopiomelanocortin; **CART:** Cocaine and amphetamine-regulated transcript; **α-MSH:** α melanocyte-stimulating hormone; **MC3R/MC4R:** Melanocortin 3 and 4 receptors; **NPY:** Neuropeptide Y; **AgRP:** Agouti-related peptide; **MCH:** Melanin-concentrating hormone

Reference: Varela L, Horvath TL. Leptin and insulin pathways in POMC and AgRP neurons that modulate energy balance and glucose homeostasis. EMBO Rep. 2012;13(12):1079-1086. doi:10.1038/embor.2012.174

9. (Content: I-A-4) A 31-year-old female presents to her primary care physician for follow-up regarding weight-gain. Over the past three months, she has noticed a weight gain of approximately 10 pounds (4.5 kg), which is discouraging because she has been trying to get healthy and lose weight before her wedding in 2 months. She quit smoking with the help of bupropion and has been walking daily. She had a copper intrauterine device inserted four months ago. Although she goes to bed later due to wedding planning, she states she still sleeps 8 hours nightly. Which of the following is most likely playing a role in her weight gain?

A. Bupropion
B. Intrauterine device
C. **Decreased tobacco**
D. Sleep habits

(C) **Tobacco cessation** is a common cause for patients to gain weight. It is likely related to decreased metabolic rate, increased caloric intake, change in food preference, and increased lipoprotein lipase activity. The average weight gain is 4-5 kg, although nearly 10% gain over 13 kg after cessation. These effects are more common in women, nonwhites, and heavier smokers.

Note: Bupropion is an anti-depressant that is also used in smoking cessation. It has weight-negative properties.

Patients should be counseled on the possibility of weight gain while quitting tobacco and develop habits to mitigate this effect. Compared to the often minimal weight gain, the long-term benefits of smoking cessation are more significant. Patients should be reminded of this and encouraged not to use weight gain as an excuse to delay smoking cessation.

Reference: Smoking cessation and weight gain. Filozof C, Fernández Pinilla MC, Fernández-Cruz A. Obes Rev. 2004;5(2):95
Reference: Smoking cessation, lung function, and weight gain: a follow-up study. Chinn S, Jarvis D, Melotti R, Luczynska C, Ackermann-Liebrich U, AntóJM, Cerveri I, de Marco R, Gislason T, Heinrich J, Janson C, Künzli N, Leynaert B, Neukirch F, Schouten J, Sunyer J, Svanes C, Vermeire P, Wjst M, Burney P Lancet. 2005;365(9471):1629.

10. (Content: I-C-2) Several medical students are trying to create a project to determine the best way to impact childhood obesity rates, as this rate has nearly tripled in the past 30 years. They begin to review epidemiologic data on a national level to see who is most affected by obesity prevalence, focusing on children 2-19 years old. They compare age, race, gender, and financial status. During their research, what are they most likely to find?

A. The highest prevalence of obesity is in Hispanic female children
B. Class 3 obesity in children has declined over the past decade
C. Asian adolescents had higher obesity rates than Hispanics
D. **The highest income class had the lowest obesity rates**
E. The prevalence of obesity was nearly 40% in all children

(D) Obesity affects nearly 20% of all children 2-19 years old. The prevalence is highest in those in the lowest (18.9%) and middle (19.9%) income levels, likely explained by the increased cost of healthy food and the lack of grocery stores in lower-income neighborhoods. In contrast, the **highest-income households had the lowest obesity rates (10.9%).**

The obesity epidemic disproportionately affects ethnic minorities, with African American girls and Hispanic boys having the highest prevalence. Class 3 obesity (140% of the 95th percentile BMI range) is growing most rapidly. Besides socioeconomic status and race, other risk factors are:

- Sedentary lifestyle and increased screen time
- Poorly balanced diet (sugary drinks, processed foods, etc.)
- Family history

The consequences of obesity are significant, ranging from psychiatric (depression, eating disorders), obstructive sleep apnea, gallstones, acid reflux, kidney stones, slipped capital femoral epiphysis, pseudotumor cerebri, hypertension, dyslipidemia, diabetes/insulin resistance, polycystic ovarian syndrome, metabolic syndrome, and intertrigo to name a few.

Reference: CDC: https://www.cdc.gov/obesity/data/childhood.html#Prevalence

11. (Content: I-B-4) A 19-year-old female presents to her family practice practitioner and requests a referral to a lymphedema clinic. She states that since she was 15 years old, she has gained excessive weight, predominantly in her lower extremities. She says her grandmother had similar findings on her upper extremities after undergoing a mastectomy, and she was treated at a lymphedema clinic with good results. She has a normal waist circumference and a BMI of 26 kg/m². Her lower extremities have a sensation of round peas when the fatty tissue is palpated. What other findings would be expected in this patient?

A. Decreased lymphatic flow
B. **Positive cuff sign**
C. Marked pitting edema
D. Eventual progression to arms
E. Positive Stemmer's sign

(B) This patient's presentation is classic for lipedema, which is abnormal subcutaneous fat deposition affecting the lower extremities; this is in contrast to lymphedema, which is a pathology of the lymphatic system (fluid), as seen in her grandmother. One differentiating physical exam finding is a **"cuff sign,"** **which occurs due to fat tissue overhanging the minimally involved feet.**

Lipedema treatment includes decongestive lymphatic therapy, exercise (aqua therapy), pain control, and potentially even surgery (liposuction).

Lymphedema versus Lipedema		
Condition	Lymphedema	Lipedema
Pathophysiology	Lymphatic pathology	Lipodystrophy
Demographics	Men and women, affecting any age	Women, between the ages of 15-30
Family history	Not common	Common
Physical findings	-Firm, with marked pitting edema -Stemmer's sign[1] -Foot involvement	Soft and minimally pitting, with a "round pea" sensation[2] -Cuff sign (foot spared)

[1]Negative Stemmer's sign occurs when you can grasp thin skin by pinching the upper surface of the second toe (lipedema). A positive test is when you can only grasp a lump of tissue (lymphedema), not the thin skin.
[2]Not to be confused with Dercum's disease with is painful lipomas affecting those with obesity

Reference: Okhovat JP, Alavi A. Lipedema: A Review of the Literature. Int J Low Extrem Wounds. 2015;14(3):262-267. doi:10.1177/153473461455428A

12. (Content: I-B-1) A 33-year-old female recently underwent a sleeve gastrectomy and is losing weight appropriately. She is most impressed by her decreased appetite, irrespective of meals, which has helped maintain a significant calorie deficit. The hormone most likely responsible for her decreased appetite initially acts on what area of the brain?

A. Dorsal vagal complex
B. Amygdala
C. Nucleus of the tractus solitarius
D. **Arcuate nucleus**
E. Lateral hypothalamus

(D) Sleeve gastrectomy, with the removal of up to 80% of the fundus of the stomach, reduces ghrelin levels, thereby significantly decreasing appetite via decreased activation of the NPY/AgRP orexigenic pathway. All peripheral hormones from the intestines and adipose tissue, as well as nutrients, act on first-order central neurons in the **arcuate nucleus of the hypothalamus.** These peripheral hormones either activate the weight-gaining (NPY/AgRP) pathway or the weight-loss (POMC/CART) neuron systems.

The arcuate nucleus is the location of the first-order appetite neurons, which relay signals to second-order neurons deeper within the hypothalamus, ultimately activating or inhibiting certain regions of the brain to manage hunger and satiety.

Many peripheral hormones are affected after bariatric surgery. The predominant hormone impacting weight and appetite for the two most common bariatric surgeries are discussed below:

- **Gastric bypass:** Significant increase in GLP-1 (both basal levels and post-prandial), activating the POMC/CART anorexigenic pathway
- **Sleeve gastrectomy:** Significant decrease in ghrelin and increase in peptide YY (PYY), which decreases the activation of the NPY/AgRP orexigenic pathway

Reference: Ochner CN, Gibson C, Shanik M, Goel V, Geliebter A. Changes in neurohormonal gut peptides following bariatric surgery. Int J Obes (Lond). 2011;35(2):153-166. doi:10.1038/ijo.2010.132

13. (Content: I-D-1) A dietician is reviewing terminology with one of her students. She discusses a term that describes the value of the amount of a nutrient estimated to meet the requirement of half of all healthy individuals in a population. What term is she defining?

A. **Estimated average requirement**
B. Adequate intake
C. Recommended daily allowance
D. Tolerable upper intake level
E. Daily value

(A) The definition of **estimated average requirements (EAR)** refers to the amount of a nutrient estimated to meet the requirement of half of all healthy individuals in the population.

Nutrient requirements and safety thresholds are commonly reported in terminology that must be understood. Some of these are discussed below:

- **Tolerable upper intake level (UL):** This is the highest intake of a nutrient that is likely to pose no risk of toxicity for almost all individuals.
- **Recommended dietary allowance (RDA):** This is the average daily dietary intake of a nutrient sufficient to meet the requirements of nearly all healthy persons within a particular population (age, gender, pregnancy, elderly, etc.).
- **Adequate intake (AI):** This definition is only used if an RDA cannot be determined. It is the recommended intake value based on observed or experimentally determined approximates for a group of healthy persons.
- **Daily value (DV):** A recommended amount an individual should consume for a specific nutrient (i.e., fat, calcium, etc.).

Reference: National Agricultural Library: U.S. Department of Agriculture

14. (Content: I-B-7) A human research study is ongoing and is recruiting patients with a body mass index > 30 kg/m^2 who have not previously been diagnosed with thyroid disease and do not have symptoms of overt hypothyroidism. Inclusion criteria requires a thyroid-stimulating hormone (TSH) level > 5 mcU/mL (reference range 0.4-4.2 mcU/mL). At the end of the study, 130 patients met the above criteria. The patients were then provided resources to assist in losing 5% of their total body weight. Which lab finding would be expected after they achieved their weight-loss goal?

    A. Increased thyroid-releasing hormone
    B. Increased T$_4$ (thyroxine) levels
    C. Decreased T$_3$ (triiodothyronine) levels
    D. Unchanged thyroid level changes

(C) Leptin, produced by adipose tissue, is thought to play a role in thyroid hormone production and levels. It is theorized that leptin stimulates thyroid releasing hormone, thereby stimulating thyroid-stimulating hormone and subsequent T$_4$ and T$_3$, acting similar to mild secondary hyperthyroidism- not subclinical hypothyroidism as previously thought. Therefore, with weight loss (decreased adipose tissue), the decreased leptin would reduce thyroid stimulation and **thus decrease thyroid hormone, including T$_3$ (triiodothyronine) levels.**

A study appears to confirm this theory. Participants lost 10% of their body weight, with a proportional decrease in T$_3$ levels. At their decreased weight, leptin was then exogenously administered, with a subsequent increase in T$_3$ levels, correlating to the notion that leptin (whether endogenous or exogenous) contributes to increased thyroid levels.

Note: Anorexic patients tend to have the lowest TSH and T$_3$ levels.

Reference: Rosenbaum M, Goldsmith R, Bloomfield D, et al. Low-dose leptin reverses skeletal muscle, autonomic, and neuroendocrine adaptations to maintenance of reduced weight. J Clin Invest. 2005;115(12):3579-3586. doi:10.1172/JCI25977
Reference: Blüher S, Mantzoros CS. Leptin in humans: lessons from translational research. Am J Clin Nutr. 2009;89(3):991S-997S. doi:10.3945/ajcn.2008.26788E

15. (Content: I-B-4) A 49-year-old male presents to the office to discuss weight-related complications. He states he was recently promoted to chief operating officer of a Fortune 500 company and the fear of messing up and losing the associated lifestyle, prestige, and salary is "driving me mad." Per chart review, it is noted that since starting this new position, he has gained nearly 45 lbs (20.4 kg). Compared to before the promotion and now, which hormonal change is most likely?

A. Insulin sensitivity increase with glucagon suppression
B. Activation of α-MSH and increased levels of leptin
C. Poor quality of sleeping activating the POMC/CART pathway
D. **NPY activation related to excess cortisol section**
E. Suppressed ghrelin levels due to vagal nerve suppression

(D) Even in the absence of confirmed Cushing's disease, a pathologic hypercortisolism disease, patients with chronic stress have many similar pro-obesity hormonal changes. An elevated baseline stress-level causes increased cortisol release and hyper-responsiveness to the hypothalamic-pituitary axis. This chronic state has been shown to increase the risk of both metabolic syndrome and heart disease.

Increased cortisol levels associated with the stressed state affect neuroendocrine hormones, including increasing insulin and leptin resistance. In addition, cortisol has a direct and indirect effect on the orexigenic pathway in the central nervous system, **leading to activation of the NPY/AgRP pathway.**

Not only does stress increase factors that play a role in promoting obesity, but obesity is a cause of stress for many patients. This cycle can feed into itself, synergistically having an impact on weight.

Treatment in this situation is focused on stress reduction. This could include reducing stressors, increasing wellness activities, therapy, and pursuing stress-relieving hobbies. If these are unlikely to improve symptoms long-term, career changes and more drastic measures may provide the best long-term medical benefits for the patient.

Reference: van der Valk, E.S., Savas, M. & van Rossum, E.F.C. Stress and Obesity: Are There More Susceptible Individuals?. Curr Obes Rep 7, 193–203 (2018). https://doi.org/10.1007/s13679-018-0306-y

16. (Content: I-C-1) A researcher is looking to evaluate different climates' effects on obesity rates. He believes warmer temperatures should allow more outdoor activity, thus lowering obesity rates. He wants to begin his research in the state with the lowest obesity rates. Which state should he start his research?

A. **Colorado**
B. Mississippi
C. Oklahoma
D. Florida
E. West Virginia

(A) Climate does not seem to play as strong of a role in decreasing obesity, although the landscape and outdoor activities may, to some extent. **Colorado** has consistently been one of the states with the lowest rate of obesity, while states in the Southeast tend to have the highest rate.

Obesity is the most common chronic disease in the U.S. with 41.9% of adults having obesity (BMI ≥ 30 kg/m^2) and nearly 73.6% meeting the criteria for overweight or obesity (BMI ≥ 25 kg/m^2).

The image below shows the percent of self-reported obesity data for the United States from the 2021 BRFSS data.

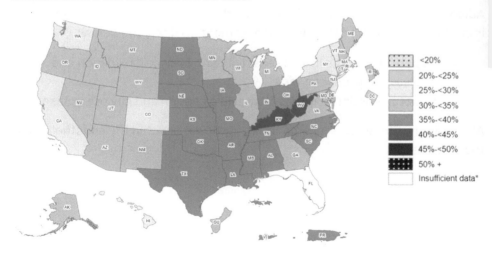

Note: The NHANES survey does in-person weighing (smaller cohort) and is considered more accurate compared to the BRFSS survey, which is self-reported over the phone, and tends to under-report weight.

Reference: https://www.cdc.gov/obesity/data/prevalence-maps.html

17. (Content: I-B-6) An endocrinologist is discussing with a medical student the vast number of hormones that play a role in obesity and satiety. In particular, one hormone is an insulin sensitizer, in which levels are inversely related to body fat mass. In addition, the endogenous levels of this hormone decrease in the setting of type 2 diabetes. The hormone described above most likely originates from which of the following structures?

A. **Adipose tissue**
B. Gastric fundus
C. Duodenum
D. Beta cells of the pancreas
E. Alpha cells of the pancreas

(A) Adiponectin is exclusively produced in the **white adipose tissue; it is the** most abundantly produced and secreted hormone from this tissue. Its levels increase in the setting of lower weight and decrease in the context of high body fat composition. Also, adiponectin levels are strongly inversely related to systemic inflammation and insulin resistance.

Note: Amylin is secreted by the beta islet cells of the pancreas and is co-secreted with insulin. In type 2 diabetes, insulin and amylin levels are increased, although they are less effective (i.e., resistance).

Adiponectin has many different effects on different organs, with the most important being related to insulin management, as discussed below:

- **Hepatic:** Enhances insulin sensitivity and fatty acid oxidation and decreases gluconeogenesis
- **Skeletal muscle:** Increases fatty acid oxidation and glucose uptake

Also, adiponectin reduces inflammation, particularly within the endothelium of the vasculature.

Reference: Erin E. Kershaw, Jeffrey S. Flier, Adipose Tissue as an Endocrine Organ, The Journal of Clinical Endocrinology & Metabolism, Volume 89, Issue 6, 1 June 2004, Pages 2548–2556, https://doi.org/10.1210/jc.2004-0395

18. (Content: I-B-4) A 44-year-old male with a past medical history of insomnia presents for an annual wellness exam. He denies any current complaints, but does admit to right knee pain that is worsened with prolonged walking. He has a moderate score on the Epworth sleepiness scale. His body mass index is 31 kg/m^2, his waist circumference is 81.3 cm (32 inches), and his body fat composition is 24%. Laboratory work, including a hemoglobin A1c, complete metabolic panel, and lipid panel, is unremarkable. An x-ray of his right knee shows moderate osteophytes and joint space narrowing. Which of the following best describes his condition?

A. Sick fat disease
B. Obesity class II
C. Obesity based on % body fat
D. **Fat mass disease**
E. Abdominal obesity

(D) This patient's knee osteoarthritis and moderate probability of obstructive sleep apnea are direct effects of his excess body weight, causing increased mechanical forces. This is consistent with **fat mass disease**.

Both fat mass disease and sick fat disease (adiposopathy) are pathogenic components of obesity. Fat mass refers to the mechanical forces acting on the body, whereas sick fat disease refers to the inflammatory/hormonal effects.

Other components that may be seen in fat mass disease are listed below:

- Heart failure with a preserved ejection fraction
- Obesity hypoventilation syndrome (external restrictive lung disease)
- Thrombotic events due to tissue compression of pelvic and lower extremities which directly impairs venous return
- Hypertension (perivascular adipose tissue restricting vessel wall expansion)

Often, comorbidities of obesity have a component of both sick fat disease and fat mass, which are not mutually exclusive.

Reference: De Lorenzo A, Soldati L, Sarlo F, Calvani M, Di Lorenzo N, Di Renzo L. New obesity classification criteria as a tool for bariatric surgery indication. World J Gastroenterol. 2016;22(2):681-703. doi:10.3748/wjg.v22.i2.681

19. (Content: I-A-3) A 6-year-old male is being seen by a pediatric endocrinologist subspecialist for severe obesity. The mother states that the patient had a normal birth weight and even required nutrient supplementation due to failure to thrive early on. However, since age three, he has had extreme hunger, which has led to progressive weight gain. The child currently weighs 178 lbs (80.7 kg). A genetic mutation is discovered, and subsequent treatment with hormone replacement is initiated with impressive results. Which of the following neuromodulators was most likely activated with the hormone replacement?

   A. Orexin A and B
   B. Alpha melanocyte-stimulating hormone
   C. Agouti-related peptide
   D. Melanin-concentrating hormone

(B) This patient's findings are most consistent with leptin deficiency, an infrequent genetic cause of secondary obesity due to a mutation of the LEP gene. Treatment with exogenous leptin causes drastic weight loss by activating the anorexigenic pathway, which stimulates different **neurotransmitters and neuromodulators, including α-MSH,** thus leading to satiety.

Neurotransmitters associated with Hunger/Satiety	
Orexigenic	Anorexigenic
-Neuropeptide Y (NPY)[1] -Agouti-related peptide (AgRP)[1] -Orexin A and B[2] -Melanin-concentrating hormone[2]	-Proopiomelanocortin (POMC)[3] -Cocaine and amphetamine regulated transcript (CART)[3] -α-Melanocyte-stimulating hormone -Serotonin

[1]Inhibited by insulin, leptin, PYY, and serotonin
[2]Inhibited by leptin, stimulated by NPY/AgRP
[3]Inhibited by NPY and GABA, stimulated by serotonin, leptin, and insulin

Reference: Varela L, Horvath TL. Leptin and insulin pathways in POMC and AgRP neurons that modulate energy balance and glucose homeostasis. EMBO Rep. 2012;13(12):1079-1086. doi:10.1038/embor.2012.174
Reference: Up to Date: "Physiology of leptin"

20. (Content: I-B-1) Researchers are looking at potential intravenous medications to assist in weight loss. One treatment that has shown promise is a synthetic form of a gastrointestinal hormone produced in both the large and small intestines and is found to be elevated within 1 hour after meals. Its contributions to weight loss are due to its potent appetite suppressant and ability to delay gastric emptying and intestinal transit time. The hormone level increases irrespective of macronutrient intake. What is the hormone most likely being studied?

A. Ghrelin
B. Cholecystokinin
C. Glucagon-like peptide 1
D. Oxyntomodulin
E. **Peptide YY**

(E) In clinical research, **peptide YY (PYY)** is being studied as a pharmacologic therapy for obesity. Daily intravenous infusions show decreased appetite and short-term weight loss. This endogenous hormone is usually produced and secreted from the distal small bowel, colon, and rectum, acting as a natural potent appetite suppressant. In addition, it delays gastric and intestinal motility.

Note: Thus far, intranasal and oral formulations of synthetic PYY have been unsuccessful in leading to prolonged weight loss.

Most anorexigenic hormones have been or are currently being studied for pharmaceutical-targeting therapy. Oxyntomodulin is still under investigation, while cholecystokinin has been ineffective long-term due to tachyphylaxis.

Glucagon-like peptide 1 (GLP-1) has been the most successful pharmacologic anorexigenic hormone in causing weight loss thus far. While all formulations are used for diabetes management, two GLP-1 receptor agonist monotherapies are explicitly FDA-approved for weight loss: liraglutide (Saxenda®) and semaglutide (Wegovy®).

Reference: Daily, intermittent intravenous infusion of peptide YY(3-36) reduces daily food intake and adiposity in rats. Prasanth K. Chelikani, Alvin C. Haver, Joseph R. Reeve Jr., David A. Keire, and Roger D. Reidelberger 01 Feb 2006; https://doi.org/10.1152/ajpregu.00674.2005

21. (Content: I-A-4) A previously healthy 9-year-old female presents to her pediatrician for a well-child check. Her growth chart is shown below. Her percentile BMI has steadily increased over the last four visits despite lifestyle changes incorporated within her family. She has breast bud development. Which of the following conditions may be contributing to these findings?

A. Excessive caloric intake
B. Precocious puberty
C. Bulimia
D. Achondroplasia
E. **Hypothyroidism**

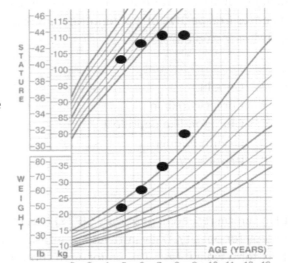

(E) This patient presents with increased weight despite decreased linear bone growth or linear bone growth arrest, which is concerning for an endocrinopathy such as **hypothyroidism.**

In contrast to children with excess weight due to increased caloric intake, those with endocrinopathies such as hypercortisolism (i.e. Cushing syndrome) or thyroid disorders will significantly increase weight compared to height. This mismatch should prompt further evaluation with consideration of the following labs:

- TSH and free T$_4$
- Dexamethasone suppression test and 24-hour urine cortisol

In contrast, excessive caloric intake and precocious puberty tend to cause accelerated linear bone growth proportionate to weight gain. Although syndromic obesity could cause decreased bone growth, excessive weight gain usually occurs earlier and is often accompanied by developmental delay. Also, remember that MC4R deficiency (monogenetic) causes tall stature.

Reference: Obesity medicine association: Pediatric Obesity Algorithm (2020-2022)

22. (Content: I-A-1) A 7-year-old female presents with her mother for a dietician evaluation and education session. The family drinks a lot of sweetened tea in the home and inquires about changing from sugar to nonnutritive sweeteners (NNS). The best response to her inquiry would be that NNS:

    A.   are a preferred alternative to sucrose
    B.   increase the risk of ADHD in children
    C.   may help with weight loss, as they are calorie-neutral
    D.   can cause a dysregulation in appetite
    E.   are regarded as "not safe for children" by the FDA

(D) Although nonnutritive sweeteners (NNS) seem like a good alternative on the surface level as a caloric-neutral option, they should be used cautiously, as some are up to 20,000 times sweeter than natural sugar (i.e., sucrose). This can lead **to a dysregulation in appetite**, especially in children, leading to craving and preferring sweeter tasting foods.

Although deemed safe by the Food and Drug Administration (FDA), NNS tend to promote dietary preferences for sweet foods, often leading to calorie-dense foods that promote weight gain. Therefore, NNS are generally not considered effective for weight loss.

Contrary to initial concerns, NNS are not associated with children developing ADHD, psychiatric conditions, congenital disabilities, malignancies, or autoimmune conditions when exposed as a child or in utero.

Reference: Obesity medicine association: Pediatric Obesity Algorithm (2020-2022)

23. (Content: I-A-3) A 5-year-old male with the disease of obesity is seen in the pediatric clinic for follow-up after meeting with a childhood obesity specialist. This patient has had many difficulties, including significant intellectual disability, retinal dystrophy, and polydactyly. Renal malformations have led to polyuria and polydipsia, requiring a percutaneous endoscopy gastrostomy tube to be placed to keep up with fluid replenishment. Given these findings, the patient most likely carries which of the following diagnoses?

A. Prader-Willi syndrome
B. Cohen syndrome
C. Borjeson-Forssman-Lehmann syndrome
D. Albright hereditary osteodystrophy
E. **Bardet-Biedl syndrome**

(E) All of the above syndromes are associated with genetic mutations that lead to obesity and intellectual disability. However, autosomal recessive **Bardet-Biedl syndrome (BBS)** is also characterized by microorchidism (men), retinal dystrophy, polydactyly, renal malformations, polyuria, and polydipsia.

New: As of 2022, setmelanotide is approved for the treatment of BBS.

The other obesity-related genetic syndromal causes associated with concurrent intellectual disability are as follows:

- **Prader-Willi:** Not inherited; loss of function on chromosome 15. Hyperphagia, short stature, hypotonia, "almond-shaped" eyes. It is the most common <u>syndromal cause</u> of genetic obesity.
- **Albright Hereditary Osteodystrophy:** Short stature, round face, pseudohypoparathyroidism, shortened fourth metacarpals
- **Cohen syndrome:** Autosomal recessive. Small head size, narrow hands and feet, joint hypermobility, "open mouth" expression, low white blood cell count, retinal dystrophy, thick hair and eyebrows
- **Borgeson-Forssman-Lehmann Syndrome:** X-linked (males), seizures, large earlobes, short toes, gynecomastia, and small genitals

Note: Be familiar with the genetic patterns (i.e., autosomal dominant, autosomal recessive, X-linked, etc.) of obesity. These will show up on test day!

Reference: Up To Date: "Genetic contribution and pathophysiology of obesity"

24. (Content: I-B-5) A previously healthy 29-year-old male with a diagnosis of obesity presents to the clinic for a physical examination. He is an accountant and thus is relatively inactive during the day. Vital signs are within normal limits. His BMI is 35 kg/m². He is frustrated that despite exercising and eating similarly to his identical twin brother, he is nearly 40 lbs (18.1 kg) heavier than his brother, who is a mail carrier. Which of the following best explains the weight difference between him and his twin brother?

    A. Basal metabolic rate
    B. Non-exercise activity thermogenesis
    C. Intentional exercise
    D. Resting energy expenditure
    E. Dietary thermogenesis

(B) **Non-exercise activity thermogenesis (NEAT)** is the energy expended for everything that does not include sleeping, eating, or dedicated physical exercise. For this patient, given other similar variables, his sedentary work (accountant) compared to his brother's occupation (mail carrier) most likely explains the difference in energy expenditure and weight differences.

NEAT includes many daily activities, ranging from yard work to fidgeting. These cumulative events increase metabolic rate substantially, impacting an individual's non-resting energy needs (150-500 kcal/day), and may explain the difference in weight amongst individuals.

In order to increase NEAT in individuals, a pedometer can be used to monitor and encourage increased daily steps.

- < 5000 steps daily is considered sedentary (average for a US adult)
- 5000-7500 steps daily is low active
- 7500-1000 steps daily is somewhat active
- > 10,000 steps daily is considered active

In addition to helping with weight, increased NEAT also reduces the risk of cardiovascular disease compared to those with a more sedentary lifestyle.

References: Non-exercise activity thermogenesis (NEAT). Author: Levine, James. MD, PhD. Best Practice and Research Clinical Endocrinology and Metabolism. 2002 Dec; 16 (4):679-702.

25. (Content: I-D-1) On a medical mission trip, a 7-year-old patient is being seen in the clinic. He appears very malnourished, but he seems unphased by his lack of nutrition. His abdomen is distended, and anasarca is present. He is supplemented with low doses of protein in incremental amounts to prevent refeeding syndrome. Which of the following must be consumed in his diet, as his body cannot produce it?

    A. Alanine
    B. Aspartate
    C. Glycine
    D. Leucine
    E. Proline

(D) This patient is presenting with Kwashiorkor, a severe <u>protein</u> malnourishment (not <u>total calorie</u> deficiency). The question essentially asks which of the above is an essential amino acid. Of the options, only **leucine** is considered an essential amino acid.

Severe malnutrition can be differentiated into the following:

- **Marasmus:** Total calorie deficit. Emaciated, irritable, thin sparse hair, low weight, no edema.
- **Kwashiorkor:** Protein deficiency, weight variable, anasarca with ascites, typically apathetic, stripes in the hair (flag sign).

The table summarizes the amino acids.

Amino Acids			
Essential Amino Acids[1]		**Non-essential Amino Acids**	
-Histidine	-Phenylalanine	-Alanine	-Glutamine
-Isoleucine	-Threonine	-Arginine	-Glycine
-Leucine	-Tryptophan	-Asparagine	-Ornithine
-Lysine[2]	-Valine	-Aspartate	-Proline
-Methionine		-Cysteine	-Serine
		-Glutamate	-Tyrosine

[1]Must be consumed (the human body cannot make them)
[2]Lysine deficiency is relatively common in vegans.

Reference: Up to Date: "Malnutrition in children in resource-limited countries: Clinical assessment"

146

26. (Content: I-A-5) A researcher is trying to create a calculator that will take into account epigenetic factors contributing to childhood obesity rates to predict which children are most prone to obesity. He plans to have a smartphone application that contains a checklist of risk factors for childhood obesity, thus providing a percent risk of obesity based on current risk factors. Practitioners would then be able to discuss with the parents how reducing certain risk factors could improve the odds of a healthy-weight in their children. Which of the following should be taken into account for his predictive calculator?

A. Kids have similar obesity rates whether one/both parents have obesity
B. Cesarean-section babies are more likely to be affected by obesity
C. Maternal smoking leads to decreased childhood obesity rates
D. Breastfed infants have fewer infections but increased obesity rates
E. Insufficient gestational weight gain is protective against obesity

(B) Epigenetics is the study of changes caused by gene expression rather than the genetic code (i.e., how the environment affects people). Many correlations have been discovered between childhood obesity and maternal and early infancy environment. Of the above, **newborns delivered via cesarean section are linked with a future increased childhood obesity rate.**

Other significant correlations that increase childhood obesity rates are:

- Maternal insulin resistance and increased preconception BMI
- Both extremes of gestational weight
- Tobacco abuse during pregnancy
- Premature infants
- Bottle-fed (compared to breast-fed) due to lack of self-regulation
- Parents: 1 with obesity (3x risk), both with obesity (10x risk)

In addition, many studies on the neonatal intestinal microbiome are underway, including the association of C-sections, with infants having higher maternal skin microbes in the gut versus vaginal delivery.

Reference: Obesity medicine association: Pediatric Obesity Algorithm (2020-2022)

27. (Content: I-D-2) A 36-year-old female status post sleeve gastrectomy six years prior presents to her primary care physician complaining of numbness to her lower extremities. She has lost 120 lbs (54.4 kg) postoperatively. She is currently taking prenatal vitamins. Physical examination reveals diminished vibratory sense bilaterally in her lower extremities and a positive Romberg test. What is the most likely underlying cause of this patient's clinical presentation?

    A. Decreased intrinsic factor production
    B. Anti-parietal antibodies
    C. Tissue transglutaminase antibodies
    D. Impaired terminal ileum absorption
    E. Decreased dietary intake

(A) This patient is presenting with subacute combined degeneration consistent with the diagnosis of vitamin B_{12} deficiency. The most likely cause is related to her sleeve gastrectomy. Vitamin B_{12} is absorbed in the terminal ileum, with assistance from the co-factor intrinsic factor, which is produced by parietal cells in the stomach. After a sleeve gastrectomy (80% stomach resection), a majority of these parietal cells are also resected, thus **decreasing intrinsic factor production.**

B_{12} deficiency is relatively uncommon in those with normal dietary intake. Some common causes of cyanocobalamin deficiency (B_{12}) are listed below:

- **Pernicious anemia:** Autoimmune condition that leads to antibodies directed at parietal cells, leading to decreased intrinsic factor.
- **Medications:** Metformin (long-term use) interferes with B_{12} absorption in the ileum, and proton pump inhibitors decrease acid secretion.
- **Vegans:** Insufficient supplementation, as B_{12} is usually found in animal protein. This takes years to develop.
- **Malabsorption:** Inflammation that affects the terminal ileum, such as celiac disease (tissue transglutaminase antibodies) or Crohn's disease, can prevent the absorption of B_{12}.

Reference: Up to Date: "Causes and pathophysiology of vitamin B_{12} and folate deficiencies"

28. (Content: I-B-1) A 31-year-old female presents to her dietician's office five months after undergoing a sleeve gastrectomy. During this period, she has lost 43 lbs (19.5 kg) and is encouraged and motivated to continue working toward weight loss. She has followed all dietary recommendations and vitamin replacement. What is the most accurate statement regarding the hormone most affected by this surgery, contributing to her weight loss?

    A. Patients with Prader-Willi syndrome have normal levels
    B. Those with a vagotomy would have similar qualitative levels
    C. Glucose suppresses the hormone for extended periods
    D. Sleep deprivation reduces this hormone, while stress increases it
    E. Leptin levels are directly proportionate to this hormone

(B) Ghrelin is the only gastrointestinal orexigenic hormone made in the gastric fundus and body, as well as the proximal small intestines. A large portion of the cells that secrete this hormone during a sleeve gastrectomy are removed, leading to decreased ghrelin levels. This **decrease is also seen in those who have undergone a vagotomy,** which inhibits ghrelin production.

Ghrelin increases hunger by stimulating the orexigenic pathway through NPY/AgRP receptors in the central nervous system and, to some extent, through the vagal nerve. Important characteristics of Ghrelin are discussed below.

Characteristics of Ghrelin	
Factors that ↑ levels	An empty stomach, fasting, weight loss, stress, sleep deprivation, Prader-Willi syndrome
Factors that ↓ levels	Stretched stomach, post meals, status post vagotomy or sleeve gastrectomy, weight gain, leptin, carbohydrates (fast rebound), protein (prolonged suppression)
Ghrelin level mechanism	Increases gut motility and food intake (through hunger), leading to increased weight gain. Decreases energy expenditure and decreases insulin secretion.

Reference: Miller GD. Appetite Regulation: Hormones, Peptides, and Neurotransmitters and Their Role in Obesity. Am J Lifestyle Med. 2017;13(6):586-601. Published 2017 Jun 23. doi:10.1177/1559827617716376

29. (Content: I-B-7) A pathophysiologist is lecturing medical students on the hormones secreted by adipose tissue. In particular, one of these hormones plays a role in energy balance and is directly proportionate to the amount of adipose tissue in the body. As adipose increases, this hormone increases, signaling satiety and increasing the rate of energy expenditure. Patients with a deficiency of this hormone have obesity at an early age. Which of the following is most similar to the described hormone in both duration of action, and effects on satiety?

    A. Pancreatic polypeptide
    B. Cholecystokinin
    C. Insulin
    D. Glucagon-like peptide 1
    E. Ghrelin

(C) Leptin and **insulin** are the two <u>long-acting</u> adiposity signaling hormones in contrast to the short-acting meal-terminating hormones secreted by the intestines. Although less potent than leptin, insulin causes central satiety, an effect that may be diminished in those with insulin resistance pathology (i.e., diabetes, polycystic ovarian syndrome, etc.).

Note: Pancreatic polypeptide hormone is secreted by the F cells of the endocrine pancreas in response to food intake (calories). This hormone reduces gastric emptying and hunger (centrally) and is associated with low levels in obesity and Prader-Willi syndrome.

Leptin has a role in central signaling regarding energy sufficiency. As adipose tissue increases, leptin increases, thus signaling satiety and increasing energy expenditure. Its levels are proportionate to body fat mass, and thus with weight loss, levels will decrease, leading to increased appetite. It also:

- Stimulates the anorexigenic neuron system (POMC/CART)
- Inhibits the orexigenic neuron system (NPY/AgRP)

Interestingly men have lower levels of leptin compared to women at similar body mass index values, which may indicate more leptin resistance in females.

Reference: Erin E. Kershaw, Jeffrey S. Flier, Adipose Tissue as an Endocrine Organ, The Journal of Clinical Endocrinology & Metabolism, Volume 89, Issue 6, 1 June 2004, Pages 2548–2556, https://doi.org/10.1210/jc.2004-0395

30. (Content: I-B-1 and I-A-1) A 33-year-old female presents to her primary care physician for follow-up regarding her polysomnography results. Her results reveal her apnea-hypopnea index was > 30, indicating severe obstructive sleep apnea; the test was split with continuous positive airway pressure (CPAP) titration. She has a prescription for a CPAP machine but has not picked it up yet. Given these findings, which neurohumoral hormone would be expected to be decreased?

A. Ghrelin
B. Orexin
C. **Leptin**
D. Neuropeptide Y

(C) This patient with severe obstructive sleep apnea has a decreased duration of quality sleep, which has been shown to have adverse health outcomes directly related to obesity. Sleep deprivation and/or reduced sleep quality is associated with decreased leptin levels, leading to increased appetite and reduced energy expenditure.

In a study completed in 2004, those who consistently slept 5 hours, compared to those receiving 8 hours of quality sleep, had the following findings:

- BMI increase of 3.6%
- Leptin decrease of 15.5%
- Ghrelin increase of 14.9%

Note: Ghrelin is produced by the stomach in fasting states and stimulates hunger (i.e., appetite), whereas leptin is one of the many inhibitors of ghrelin.

Sleep apnea is the most common sleep-related breathing disorder, with obesity being the strongest risk factor. Untreated, this condition can lead to increased blood pressure, cardiovascular disease, pulmonary hypertension, and ultimately increased morbidity and mortality. It decreases sleep quality.

Reference: Mignot, Emmanuel, et al. Stanford.edu/med-sleep-1208.html, Dec 2004

31. (Content: I-C-1) A physician is discussing with a medical student the ethnic disparities within obesity. Of the following ethnicity and gender combinations in adults, which would likely have the most significant disparity of increased obesity (based on percentage)?

A. Asian males
B. Hispanic males
C. White females
D. Black females

(D) Race/Ethnic disparities seen in obesity are significant, in which Black and Hispanic populations have higher obesity rates compared to Caucasian and Asians. This is seen in both adults and children. When gender is considered, Black females have significantly higher percentages of obesity than Black males.

Interestingly, gender differences in obesity were seen when household income and education level were taken into consideration:

- Women: Increased obesity was seen in those with more poverty and less education.
- Men: More obesity is seen in those with middle-class incomes and those with moderate education (completed some college).

Note: In adults, the highest rate of obesity tends to occur in middle-age from 40-59 years old. In children, prevalence is highest at 12-19 years.

The table summarizes obesity rates (percentage) in different groups.

Obesity: Race/Ethnic Categorization (Percentages)			
Race/Ethnicity	Men (Boys)	Women (Girls)	Both: Adult (Child)
White	44.7 (17.4)	39.8 (14.8)	42.2 (16.1)
Black	41.1 (19.4)	56.9 (29.1)	49.6 (24.2)
Asian	17.5 (12.4)	17.2 (10.1[1])	17.4 (8.7)
Hispanic	45.7 (28.1)	43.7 (23.0)	44.8 (25.6)

[1]This sub category is based on 2016 data as 2017-2018 did not meet reliability standards.

Reference: Ogden CL, Fakhouri TH, Carroll MD, et al. Prevalence of Obesity Among Adults, by Household Income and Education — United States, 2011–2014. MMWR Morb Mortal Wkly Rep 2017;66:1369–1373. DOI:
Reference: NCHS, National Health and Nutrition Examination Survey, 2017–2018.
https://www.cdc.gov/nchs/data/factsheets/factsheet_nhanes.htm

32. (Content: I-B-3) A patient is presenting to discuss weight loss options. He has tried several dietary plans without success and has trouble maintaining a persistent exercise schedule. Which of the following statements would be most accurate?

A. If you consume less calories than what you use, you will lose weight
B. For every 3500 kcal you decrease in your diet, you will lose 1 lb
C. Losing weight is all about willpower and motivation
D. It is easier to maintain weight loss, rather than lose it
E. **Subcutaneous fat can affect health similarly to visceral fat**

(E) Myths related to obesity are rampant not only among our patients but also among physicians. All of the above are incorrect myths except that **subcutaneous fat can affect health similarly to visceral fat.** The weight from adipose (visceral or subcutaneous) causes numerous health problems, often referred to as fat-mass disease, including osteoarthritis, obstructive sleep apnea, heart failure with preserved ejection fraction, and even hypertension. Subcutaneous fat also can secrete pro-inflammatory hormones, similar to visceral fat, although to a somewhat lesser extent.

Obesity is a complex disease process, incorporating neurohormonal, behavioral, and genetics into both central and peripheral signal processing. Findings seen in calorimeters (3500 kcal = 1 lb) do not correlate well in a living being. Although motivation and willpower are helpful in losing weight, these are by no means the answer to weight loss, nor the reason patients fail to lose weight.

In addition, 'calories in= calories out' has also been debunked as one patient may take in the same caloric intake as a patient with excess weight, but energy expenditure, caloric harvesting, and adipose storage can vary vastly. Other common myths that are inaccurate include:

- If you miss breakfast, your body goes into starvation mode and holds onto calories, leading to weight gain
- Lean individuals have less weight only due to a higher metabolism
- 1 lb of added muscle causes 50 kcal/day of energy expenditure (again, our bodies are not calorimeters)
- Slower weight loss leads to more sustained results

Reference: Obesity medicine association: Obesity Algorithm (2021)

33. (Content: I-D-2) A 46-year-old female presents for an annual follow-up with her obesity medicine specialist. She underwent a successful biliopancreatic diversion and duodenal switch seven years ago. She has been adherent with all nutritional visits and supplemental vitamin intake. She had lost 162 lbs (73.5 kg), but has regained 10 lbs (4.5 kg) in the past year. She denies any new symptoms. Laboratory work reveals a microcytic anemia with a decreased ferritin level. Which gastrointestinal area is most likely responsible for this patient's laboratory abnormalities?

A. Stomach
B. **Duodenum**
C. Jejunum
D. Ileum
E. Colon

(B) A biliopancreatic diversion with duodenal switch bypasses both the duodenum and a portion of the jejunum, leading to decreased mineral absorption. This patient has a microcytic anemia with decreased ferritin, most consistent with iron deficiency anemia. Iron is **primarily absorbed in the duodenum** (and some in the proximal jejunum).

Areas of vitamin and mineral absorption within the gastrointestinal tract are discussed below:

- **Duodenum:** Iron (majority) and calcium
- **Jejunum:** Folate, carbohydrates, amino acids, and potassium. The proximal portion can absorb iron as well.
- **Ileum:** B_{12}, potassium, minerals, salts, fats, and fat-soluble vitamins
- **Colon:** Vitamin K, biotin, B_1, B_3, water, sodium, and chloride

Iron supplementation can be attempted orally. Hemoglobin should improve within two weeks; however, iron stores (i.e., ferritin) can take up to 6 months. If no improvements are seen, consider parenteral replacement.

Reference: Up to Date: "Bariatric surgery: Postoperative nutritional management"

34. (Content: I-B-5) A nutritionist is discussing how energy relates to food intake and nutrition labels. How much energy would it take to raise 1 kilogram of water by 1 °C?

A. **1 Calorie**
B. 10 kilocalories
C. 100 Calories
D. 1,000 Calories
E. 10,000 calories

(A) Calories are a measure of energy. In particular, one calorie is the amount of heat required to raise the temperature of 1 gram of water by 1 °C. Therefore, to raise 1,000 grams (1 kilogram) of water 1 °C, it would take 1000 calories, which is equivalent to **1 Calorie** (notice the capitalization).

Note: 1,000 calories = 1 Calorie = 1 kilocalorie

When referencing food (i.e., food labels) or exercise, often the term Calorie is used, which refers to 1 kilocalorie (kcal). As this is a unit of energy, it should be noted that one kcal = 4.184 kilojoules of energy.

Reference: Obesity medicine association: Obesity Algorithm (2021)

35. (Content: I-D-3) A 23-year-old male presents to his family practice physician after he read an article on high-dose calcium intake related to weight loss. He is currently taking twice the recommended daily allowance, but hasn't noticed a significant weight loss at this point. He asks if this is an effective obesity treatment. His current BMI is 27 kg/m². His only complaint is constipation. Given his current status, which of the following is most likely increased in this patient?

    A. Parathyroid hormone activity
    B. Vitamin D levels
    C. Lipogenesis
    D. Lipolysis
    E. Fat storage levels

(D) Patients with high calcium intake tend to have **increased lipolysis** (fat breakdown) and decreased lipogenesis (fat production) and fat storage. In fact, epidemiologic data suggest a lower prevalence of overweight, obesity, and insulin resistance in people with high calcium intake.

Note: This study does not recommend taking above the recommended daily allowance for calcium, but instead taking adequate calcium intake. Also, this plays a small role when compared to exercise and diet.

The two mechanisms proposed to explain calcium intake on body weight is that increased dietary calcium suppresses PTH and vitamin D, thereby decreasing intracellular calcium in adipocytes, which inhibits lipogenesis and stimulates lipolysis (the opposite is true with low calcium intake).

The other mechanism is that dietary calcium intake binds and inhibits fatty acid absorption in the gastrointestinal tract.

Note: The prevalence of vitamin D (a fat-soluble vitamin) deficiency in obesity is > 30% due to body dilution, as skin surface area is not proportionate to patient volume. This deficiency does not increase weight.

Reference: Dietary Calcium Intake and Obesity; Sarina Schrager. The Journal of the American Board of Family Practice May 2005, 18 (3) 205-210; DOI: https://doi.org/10.3122/jabfm.18.3.205

36. (Content: I-B-3) A group of physicians are developing a program to address patients with coronary artery disease who are at the highest risk of mortality within the next five years. To simplify the program, they only evaluate the body mass index and waist circumference. Those with the highest mortality risk will be entered into an intensive physical, dietary, and behavioral modification program. Which of the following parameters of patients should receive priority entrance into this class?

A. BMI 22 kg/m²; Waist circumference 85 cm
B. **BMI 22 kg/m²; Waist circumference 101 cm**
C. BMI 26 kg/m²; Waist circumference 85 cm
D. BMI 30 kg/m²; Waist circumference 85 cm
E. BMI 30 kg/m²; Waist circumference 101 cm

(B) A large study (> 15,000 participants) of patients with coronary artery disease were evaluated to see which group had the highest mortality rate. Interestingly, they discovered that patients with increased waist circumference had higher associated 5-year mortality throughout all BMI ranges. Even more interestingly, **patients with a normal BMI but increased waist circumference had the highest 5-year mortality risk.** This displayed the importance of visceral fat as it relates to adiposopathy.

The hazard ratio (HR) of those with normal weight but increased waist circumference, compared to the other mentioned patients, are as follows (all statistically significant with P < 0.0001):

- BMI 22 kg/m²; Waist circumference 85 cm: **HR 1.10**
- BMI 26 kg/m²; Waist circumference 85 cm: **HR 1.20**
- BMI 30 kg/m²; Waist circumference 85 cm: **HR 1.61**
- BMI 30 kg/m²; Waist circumference 101 cm: **HR 1.27**

Reference: Combining Body Mass Index With Measures of Central Obesity in the Assessment of Mortality in Subjects With Coronary Disease; Thais Coutinho, Kashish Goel, Daniel Corrêa de Sá, Rickey E. Carter, David O. Hodge, Charlotte Kragelund, Alka M. Kanaya, Marianne Zeller, Jong Seon Park, Lars Kober, Christian Torp-Pedersen, Yves Cottin, Luc Lorgis, Sang-Hee Lee, Young-Jo Kim, Randal Thomas, Véronique L. Roger, Virend K. Somers, Francisco Lopez-Jimenez; J Am Coll Cardiol. 2013 Feb, 61 (5) 553-560.

37. (Content: I-B-8) A 49-year-old female is discussing a recent incident with her health coach. She states that she recently dropped off her only child at college. A week later, she walked by a bakery and the smell brought back memories of her and her child baking bread on the weekends. Despite recently finishing up lunch and not being hungry, she indulged in two large pieces of bread. Which area of activation played the largest role in this incident?

A. Amygdala
B. **Hippocampus**
C. Pre-frontal cortex
D. Hypothalamus
E. Occipital lobe

(B) This patient's desire to eat bread was triggered by memories, not internal hunger stimuli. The **hippocampus** is activated with memories and in the setting of food, can override physiologic satiety. Obesity is very complex, with several areas affecting energy expenditure and food intake. Two primary paths are discussed below:

- **Homeostatic:** This consists of the complex POMC/CART and NPY/AgRP pathways located in the hypothalamus, which responds to peripheral neurohormonal inputs. This is the body's primary regulatory center.
- **Hedonic:** These pathways can override the homeostatic pathway. In other words, activation of the centers below can activate hunger, promoting food intake even if not initially hungry.
  - *Limbic system:* This is primarily driven by dopamine and mediates cravings, rewards, compulsions, and food addiction.
  - *Emotion/Memories:*
    - Amygdala: This area activates in response to food cues (advertisements, visuals, etc.).
    - Hippocampus: Memories or prior experiences activate this area (i.e., the smell of a dessert reminds you of a family celebration).
  - *Pre-frontal cortex:* This area is involved in impulse control, spontaneity, planning, and decision-making.

Reference: Farr OM, Li CR, Mantzoros CS. Central nervous system regulation of eating: Insights from human brain imaging. Metabolism. 2016 May;65(5):699-713. doi: 10.1016/j.metabol.2016.02.002. Epub 2016 Feb 6. PMID: 27085777; PMCID: PMC4834455.

38. (Content: I-A-3) A 4-year-old male with weight and height consistently in the 95th percentile presents to his pediatrician for follow-up regarding tumor surveillance. He recently underwent an abdominal ultrasound showing hepatosplenomegaly without concerning findings for malignancy. What genetic characteristic is most likely associated with this condition?

    A. Autosomal recessive inheritance
    B. Chromosome 15q deletion
    C. Chromosome 8q22 mutation
    D. Chromosome 11p15.5 dysregulation
    E. ALMS 1 mutation

(D) This patient presents with excess weight at a young age, hepatosplenomegaly, and requires tumor surveillance. These findings are associated with Beckwith-Wiedemann syndrome, which is due to **genetic dysregulation of chromosome 11p15.5.**

Beckwith-Wiedemann syndrome is a fetal overgrowth syndrome that commonly presents with enlarged organs (hepatomegaly, splenomegaly, nephromegaly, and macroglossia) and predisposes the patient to tumor growth. Therefore, frequent surveillance with abdominal ultrasounds and tumor markers are necessary, as Wilms tumors and hepatoblastoma are possible.

Note: Expect to see genetic inheritance patterns on obesity medicine boards.

Genetic Patterns of Early-Onset Childhood Obesity	
Autosomal recessive	-Bardet-Biedl syndrome -POMC deficiency -Congenital leptin deficiency -Cohen syndrome (8q22 mutation)
X-linked	-Fragile X syndrome -Wilson-Turner syndrome
Paternal chromosome 15q deletion	Prader-Willi syndrome
ALMS 1 mutation	Alstrom syndrome
Chromosome 11p15.5 dysregulation	Beckwith-Wiedemann syndrome
MC4R mutation	MC4R deficiency

Reference: Up to Date: "Beckwith-Wiedemann Syndrome"
Reference: Obesity medicine association: Pediatric Obesity Algorithm (2020-2022)

39. (Content: I-A-5) A 32-year-old pregnant female presents for education regarding her recent diagnosis of gestational diabetes mellitus (GDM). In particular, she wants to know the risk factors for her infant developing the disease of childhood obesity in order to make appropriate changes. Which would be the most accurate information to provide to this patient?

A. **High protein intake early in life increases BMI at age 2**
B. Breastfeeding only for the first week of life reduces toddler weight
C. Gestational diabetes does not influence childhood obesity rates
D. Early complementary feedings result in reduced caloric intake at 12 months
E. A cesarean section reduces unfavorable microbiota leading to reduced childhood weight

(A) Epigenetics plays a role in childhood obesity rates due to gene expression. Several perinatal risk factors influence weight gain in infants. Feeding habits such as **high protein intake**, early complementary feedings, and added sugars raise the risk of increased toddler weight.

In females who have excess weight before pregnancy and develop gestational diabetes (i.e., insulin resistance), childhood obesity rates are the highest. Thus parental education, strict insulin control, demonstrating healthy habits, and reducing high-density and carbohydrate-rich foods should be emphasized.

Interestingly, although breastfeeding overall reduces the risk of childhood obesity, mothers with GDM produce milk rich in glucose initially, which has been shown to increase weight at two years compared to infants provided with donor milk during the first week of life. This effect seems less pronounced if infants are breastfed over a more extended period, compared to only breastfeeding the first few weeks.

Reference: Obesity medicine association: Pediatric Obesity Algorithm (2020-2022)

40. (Content: I-B-6) A 37-year-old female presents to her surgeon for a 12-month follow-up after a successful sleeve gastrectomy. She has followed all diet and exercise regimens as prescribed by her dietician and electrophysiologist. However, she has noticed that even though she has increased her exercise time to 220 minutes weekly, she has not seen a significant decrease in weight as expected. She has lost 95 lbs (43 kg) postoperatively but has plateaued. Which of the following most likely explains this plateau effect?

    A. Increased total energy expenditure
    B. Increased muscle efficiency
    C. Adaptive thermogenesis
    D. Modified set-point
    E. Increased leptin levels

(B) This patient who fails to lose additional weight, despite increased exercise, is experiencing **increased muscle efficiency,** in which her muscles burn fewer cumulative calories, although exercising for longer durations of time. This occurs because of muscle hypertrophy (efficiency) and less body weight to move. Another way to think of this is a 300 lb patient will burn more calories than a 200 lb patient (more mass, thereby increasing the required energy to move). Although she is likely experiencing adaptive thermogenesis, this does not explain her lack of weight loss with additional exercise.

There are many reasons why patients plateau or experience weight gain, as discussed below:

- **Neurohormonal:** Leptin, cholecystokinin, peptide YY all decrease, thus removing inhibitory actions on ghrelin, increasing appetite
- **Energy:** Decrease in resting energy expenditure due to weight loss
- **Adaptive thermogenesis:** Reduction in resting metabolic rate
- **Set-point fallacy:** Incorrect belief that once you achieve a lower weight, your body will maintain this decreased weight naturally
- **Commitment amnesia:** Lack of maintaining behavior, dietary, and physical activity levels that were required to lose the initial weight

Reference: Obesity medicine association: Obesity Algorithm (2021)

41. (Content: I-E-1) A 29-year-old male plans to run a marathon in the next four months. He has been training daily and can run nearly 18 miles without stopping. What is true of the muscle fibers he predominantly utilizes to prepare for this marathon?

A. Energy is from glycolysis
B. Creates forceful contractions
C. Fatigue susceptible
D. **Increased mitochondria are present**

(D) A person training for longevity is working on strengthening their slow-twitch or type 1 muscle fibers. These fibers produce their energy by utilizing adenosine triphosphate (ATP) made within the **mitochondria, which are abundant** in these slow-twitch muscle fibers.

Skeletal muscles are made up of bundles of individual muscle fibers called myocytes. These myocytes each contain many myofibrils, which are strands of actin and myosin proteins (making up the contractile component of the muscle, the sarcomere). These grab onto each other and pull together, cumulatively shortening the muscle and causing muscle contractions.

Muscle fibers respond to training, developing more type I or type II fibers based on the forces imposed on them. For example, a weightlifter will likely generate more slow-twitch muscles (heavy weights, repetitions) whereas a boxer will develop more fast-twitch (acceleration, speed). These fibers are further compared in the table below.

Muscle Fiber Types		
Muscle type	Slow Twitch (Type I)	Fast Twitch (Type II)
Energy	Oxidative metabolism	Anaerobic glycolysis
Fatigue	Resistant	Susceptible
Physical activity	Prolonged (marathon)	Forceful (sprinting)

Reference: Ørtenblad N, Nielsen J, Boushel R, Söderlund K, Saltin B, Holmberg HC. The Muscle Fiber Profiles, Mitochondrial Content, and Enzyme Activities of the Exceptionally Well-Trained Arm and Leg Muscles of Elite Cross-Country Skiers. Front Physiol. 2018;9:1031. Published 2018 Aug 2. doi:10.3389/fphys.2018.01031

42. (Content: I-A-4) A 66-year-old female presents to the clinic for worsening vision. She states that this has been progressing for the past six months, but recently nearly caused a car accident. She has also had daily headaches, which she attributes to the vision changes, and reports she always feels hungry. Her vital signs are normal except for her BMI, which has increased from 31 to 33 kg/m^2 since last year. Physical exam reveals bilateral loss of the lower peripheral visual fields. Laboratory work reveals a TSH is 0.1 µU/mL (reference range: 0.5–5.0 µU/mL) and a T$_4$ is 2 µg/dL (reference range: 5–12 µg/dL). Prolactin levels are normal. Which of the following is the most appropriate next step?

A. **Brain imaging**
B. Levothyroxine replacement
C. Ophthalmology referral
D. Radioactive iodine scan of the thyroid
E. Growth hormone and ACTH levels

(A) This patient is presenting with bilateral hemianopsia, central hypothyroidism, and hyperphagia concerning for hypothalamic obesity. One likely cause is a craniopharyngioma, a rare, slow-growing cystic lesion that develops from the remnants of Rathke's pouch. Compression and damage of the pituitary, hypothalamus, and optic chiasm lead to symptoms. An **MRI of the pituitary** is the most important next step if this condition is suspected.

Hypothalamic obesity occurs due to damage of the ventromedial hypothalamus (VMH), leading to loss of homeostatic inputs, and thus causing decreased energy expenditure, hyperphagia, and subsequent obesity.

Craniopharyngioma is the most common tumor to cause hypothalamic obesity, with other etiologies including brain radiation, trauma, intracranial surgeries, increased intracranial pressure, or other brain tumors. Most patients will have concurrent vision changes, headaches, nausea, and endocrine pathology, including diabetes insipidus, central hypothyroidism, and deficiencies of growth hormone and adrenocorticotropic hormone. Amenorrhea and erectile dysfunction are common.

Memory aid: Masses in the ventromedial hypothalamus lead to more weight, whereas lesions in the lateral hypothalamus lead to less weight.

Reference: Up To Date: "Craniopharyngioma" and "Obesity in adults: Etiologies and risk factors"

43. (Content: I-B-3) A double-blinded study is performed with patients who have a body mass index between 25-30 kg/m^2. They receive either a placebo or an intravenous medication theorized to increase brown adipose tissue (BAT) activation. At the end of the infusion, patients undergo a positron emission tomography (PET) scan to evaluate the presence of BAT. After the trial, there was an 11% increased tracer uptake, as evidenced by the PET scan, in those receiving the medication compared to the placebo group. Which of the following most accurately describes the studied adipose tissue?

A. Its brown color is due to increased lysosomes
B. It couples oxidative phosphorylation, increasing ATP production
C. It is stimulated by acetylcholine of the parasympathetic system
D. Resting metabolic rate is inversely proportional to BAT levels
E. It utilizes glucose and free fatty acids to increase lipolysis

(E) BAT is different from white adipose tissue, as it contains numerous large mitochondria (giving it its brown color) and serves as a warming mechanism for vital organs by uncoupling oxidative phosphorylation, thereby generating heat, instead of energy (ATP) via non-shivering thermogenesis. This process increases the resting metabolic rate proportionately to levels of BAT by **utilizing glucose and free fatty acids to increase lipolysis**.

Although thought to be present in infants only and decreasing until no longer present in adulthood, a study published in the New England Journal of Medicine in 2009 revealed that BAT (biopsy-confirmed) could be activated by cold exposure, as displayed on a PET scan.

Studies are underway to evaluate pharmacotherapy that could activate brown fat. Most recently, mirabegron was shown in a small study (n=14) to increase BAT with increased resting metabolism by 6% and improved insulin sensitivity. However, it did not change their weight or body composition.

Beiging is another theory in which white adipose tissue can act like brown adipose tissue (upregulating an uncoupling protein seen in brown fat), leading to increased energy expenditure. Beige is indistinguishable from BAT on scans.

Reference: Chronic mirabegron treatment increases human brown fat, HDL cholesterol, and insulin sensitivity. O'Mara et al. J Clin Invest. 2020 Jan 21. pii: 131126. doi: 10.1172/JCI131126. [Epub ahead of print]. PMID: 31961826.
Reference: Virtanen et al. NEJM 4/9/2009; 360:1518-1525; DOI: 10.1056/NEJMoa0808949

44. (Content: I-D-4) A 29-year-old health-conscious female is discussing her diet with a nutritionist. Although not focused on weight loss, she is interested to see if her diet matches the recommendations based on the acceptable macronutrient distribution range, as set forth by the United States Department of Agriculture (USDA). Which of the following would meet that criteria if the macronutrient was listed as a percentage of her total calories?

   A. Protein 45%
   B. Carbohydrate 60%
   C. Fat 40%
   D. Linoleic acid (Ω -6 fatty acid) 15%
   E. α-Linolenic acid (Ω-3 fatty acid) 5%

(B) Acceptable macronutrient distribution ranges (AMDR) is the percent of energy intake associated with a reduced risk of chronic disease yet provides adequate amounts of essential nutrients. Of the options, only **carbohydrates are within AMRD for adults, which is 45-65%.**

Note: The AMRD references are not often followed by those attempting weight loss, which may differ drastically from these recommendations.

Obviously, there is no AMRD for alcohol, but it contains 7 kcal/gm, whereas water contains 0 kcal/gm.

Acceptable Macronutrient Distribution Ranges			
Macronutrient	% of Total Calories for Adults	Kcal/gm	Recommended Daily Allowance (Grams/day)
Protein	10-35%	4	56 (men) 46 (women)
Carbohydrate	45-65%	4	130
Fat[1]	25-35%	9	NA

[1] AMDR of polyunsaturated fatty acids: linoleic acid (Ω -6 fatty acid) is 5-10%, and α-linolenic acid (Ω-3 fatty acid) is 0.6-1.2%. AMDR of saturated fat, cholesterol, and trans-fat are not determined.

Reference: Dietary Reference Intakes for Energy, Carbohydrate, Fiber, Fat, Fatty Acids, Cholesterol, Protein, and Amino Acids (2005)

45. (Content: I-B-8) A 29-year-old female presents for a follow-up appointment with her primary care physician. Over the past year, she has lost 40 lbs (18.1 kg), which she attributes to meal replacements and an effective exercise regimen. A recent body composition scan revealed a 3% reduction in adipose tissue. However, over the past two months, she has regained 5 lbs (2.3 kg). She denies a change in her diet or exercise regimen but does admit to "sneaking a few extra snacks here and there," as she states her hunger has increased. Which of the following neurohormonal changes is most likely contributing to her increased weight gain?

    A. Increased leptin levels
    B. Loss of inhibition of the NPY/AgRP pathway
    C. Melanocortin 4 receptor activation
    D. Orexin A and B hormone suppression
    E. Inhibition of neurotrophic factor

(B) Adipose tissue is hormonally active, with one of its primary secreted hormones being leptin. Therefore, a decrease in adipose through weight loss would lead to decreased leptin levels. Because leptin is an inhibitor of the orexigenic (i.e., weight-gaining) pathway, this reduces **the inhibition of the NPY/AgRP (orexigenic) pathway,** leading to increased hunger, decreased energy expenditure, and ultimately weight gain.

Leptin hormone is an anorexigenic hormone secreted by white adipose tissue. Its two main functions include:

- Stimulating anorexigenic neuron system (POMC/CART)
- Inhibiting orexigenic neuron system (NPY/AgRP)

Note: Decreased leptin is a strong contributor to the weight plateau and regains often seen in patients who lose significant weight.

Reference: Erin E. Kershaw, Jeffrey S. Flier, Adipose Tissue as an Endocrine Organ, The Journal of Clinical Endocrinology & Metabolism, Volume 89, Issue 6, 1 June 2004, Pages 2548–2556, https://doi.org/10.1210/jc.2004-0395

46. (Content: II-B-4) A 34-year-old female with a BMI of 29 kg/m² presents to her primary care physician with overeating concerns. She states that she often eats a large amount of food, lacking control while eating during these episodes. She hides this behavior from her roommate as she feels intense embarrassment and guilt. Given the most likely diagnosis, what other finding would most likely be expected?

    A. Eating more rapidly than normal
    B. Compensatory purging
    C. Consuming > 25% of calories after dinner
    D. Repetitive behaviors
    E. Eating small, unplanned amounts of food

(A) This patient's diagnosis is most consistent with binge eating disorder (BED), the most common eating disorder, affecting up to 3.5% of the general population and up to 50% of individuals with severe obesity. It is associated with **eating more rapidly than usual.**

BED is a compulsive eating disorder that should be treated before targeting treatment for obesity alone (i.e., pharmacotherapy or surgery).

Diagnosis Criteria for Binge Eating Disorder

Recurrent episodes of binge eating marked by:
  • Eating large amounts of food in a discrete amount of time
  • A sense of lack of control with eating during these episodes

Associated with 3 or more of the following:
  • Eating more rapidly than normal
  • Eating until uncomfortably full
  • Eating large amounts of food when not physically hungry
  • Hiding eating behaviors due to embarrassment
  • Feeling disgusted, depressed, or guilty after episodes

Marked distress about binge eating
Occurs on average at least 1 time per week for 3 months
Not associated with compensatory purging behaviors

Reference: DSM-5: Diagnostic and Statistical Manual of Mental Disorders, Fifth Edition

47. (Content: II-D-3a) A 43-year-old female is presenting with increased thirst and urination. She states that over the past 2-3 months, she has woken up multiple times in the night to urinate and feels like she cannot "drink enough water". She has a past medical history of autoimmune hemolytic anemia and obesity class II. In addition to other age-appropriate screenings, which laboratory test is most sensitive to diagnose her with the most likely condition?

A. Hemoglobin A1c
B. Fasting glucose levels
C. HOMA-IR levels
D. **Oral glucose tolerance test**
E. Fructosamine levels

(D) The **oral glucose tolerance test** is the most sensitive test to diagnose diabetes mellitus. This consists of consuming a glucose load followed by subsequent serum glucose levels 2 hours after the glucose ingestion. It is more likely to diagnose diabetes and pre-diabetes but is less commonly done due to the inconvenience compared to hemoglobin A1c (HbA1c) levels. Importantly, HbA1c levels are most accurate in patients with a red blood cell life span of 3 months. If shorter, such as this patient with hemolytic anemia, the test will underestimate the true hemoglobin A1c values.

The American Diabetes Association defines the criteria for diabetes as follows:

- Hemoglobin A1c ≥ 6.5%
- Fasting glucose levels of ≥ 126 mg/dL
- Classic symptoms of diabetes with a random glucose of ≥ 200 mg/dL
- Oral glucose tolerance test (OGTT) displaying a glucose level of ≥ 200 mg/dL two hours after ingestion of 75 grams of glucose

Note: The HOMA-IR can be calculated by obtaining a fasting glucose insulin and glucose level to determine insulin resistance. Its clinical utility is controversial.

Reference: Up to Date: "Clinical presentation, diagnosis, and initial evaluation of diabetes mellitus in adults"

48. (Content: II-C-5) A 3-year-old male is brought into the pediatric office, as the mother has recently noticed increased weight gain and an insatiable appetite that was not previously present. After reviewing the growth chart, it is noted that his height has maintained the 60th percentile. However, his weight has increased from the 50th percentile to the 90th percentile in the past 1.5 years. A speech therapist has seen him for delayed speech, and he is scheduled to see a therapist for late motor development. Which of the following would most likely be seen on physical examination?

A. Short 4th and 5th metacarpals
B. Hepatosplenomegaly
C. Polydactyly
D. Macroglossia
E. **Almond-shaped eyes**

(E) This patient with neurodevelopmental delays and apparent intellectual disability with excessive weight gain, most likely has Prader-Willi syndrome, a paternal chromosome 15q partial deletion (i.e., under-expressed gene). Physical examination findings include thin upper lips and **almond-shaped eyes.** At birth, they are often smaller, with bitemporal narrowing of the head, hypotonia, and characteristic "floppiness."

Other characteristics of Prader-Willi syndrome are discussed below:

- **Diagnosis:** DNA methylation studies
- **Age of obesity:** Onset between 2-5 years of age
- **Treatment:** Calorie restriction and behavioral therapy are the mainstays for obesity, with growth and sex hormone replacement at puberty.

Note: Other conditions causing some of the above findings include Beckwith-Wiedemann syndrome (macroglossia and hepatosplenomegaly), Albright Hereditary Osteodystrophy (shortened 4th and 5th metacarpal bones), and Bardet-Biedl syndrome (polydactyly).

Reference: Cassidy SB, Driscoll DJ. Prader-Willi syndrome. Eur J Hum Genet. 2009;17(1):3-13. doi:10.1038/ejhg.2008.165
Reference: Up to Date: "Clinical features, diagnosis, and treatment of Prader-Willi syndrome"

49. (Content: II-C-2) A 33-year-old Caucasian female is presenting to her primary care physician for an annual exam. She is up to date on her preventative screenings and immunizations. Although she exercises and avoids eating at fast-food restaurants, she is concerned about her cardiovascular risk, as her father had a heart attack at age 42. In this patient, at which body mass index would a waist circumference provide the most useful information regarding cardiovascular risk?

    A. 18 kg/m^2
    B. 24 kg/m^2
    C. 33 kg/m^2
    D. 40 kg/m^2

(C) In patients with a **body mass index between 25-34.9 kg/m^2**, the abdominal circumference is recommended to provide additional information on cardiovascular risk. In those with a BMI ≥ 35 kg/m^2, waist circumference is unlikely to add further risk stratification.

Abdominal obesity indicates excess adiposity and infers an increased risk of cardiometabolic risks such as diabetes, metabolic syndrome, hypertension, etc. Cut-off values for abdominal obesity in the U.S. and Canada are as follows:

- Males: > 102 cm (> 40 in)
- Females: > 88 cm (> 35 in)

Note: A BMI cut-off value of ≥ 23 kg/m^2 should be used for screening and confirmation of excess adiposity in South Asian, Southeast Asian, and East Asian adults. Waist circumference cut-offs of ≥ 85 cm for men and ≥ 74-80 cm for women are consistent with abdominal obesity in these populations. These ethnic populations have similar cardiovascular and diabetes risks at these lower BMIs compared to Caucasians at higher thresholds.

For the most accurate results, abdominal waist circumference should be obtained at the level of the iliac crest. The measuring tape should be snug but not compress the skin and be kept parallel to the floor. The measurement taken at the end of normal expiration is most precise.

Reference: AACE/ACE Guidelines: AMERICAN ASSOCIATION OF CLINICAL ENDOCRINOLOGISTS AND AMERICAN COLLEGE OF ENDOCRINOLOGY COMPREHENSIVE CLINICAL PRACTICE GUIDELINES FOR MEDICAL CARE OF PATIENTS WITH OBESITY (2016). Recommendation 6-7, and Figure 2.

50. (Content: II-D-2) Researchers are performing a study on obesity and the effects on the associated comorbidities as weight fluctuates over two years. They desire the most accurate fat composition measurements at a molecular level, regardless of cost. Which of the following measurement modalities would meet these criteria?

    A. Skinfold calipers
    B. Deuterium dilution hydrometry
    C. Bioelectric impedance analyses
    D. Dual-energy x-ray absorptiometry
    E. Body mass index

(B) For research purposes, **isotope dilution hydrometry** is considered the most accurate test to determine body fat composition at the molecular level, although this method is not utilized in clinical practice. The principle behind this test is that all cells in the body will take up an administered water isotope tracer, except body fat. Therefore, measurement of the isotope dilution allows for the calculation of non-fat mass, which can be subtracted from total body weight, resulting in fat mass.

Note: Percent body fat can assist in diagnosing patients with obesity, defined as ≥ 25% percent body fat in males and ≥ 32% in females. Caucasian males and Hispanic females generally have higher % body fat.

Body Fat Measurements		
Method	**Pros**	**Cons**
Calipers	Inexpensive	-User-dependent/variable -Not accurate at ↑ BMI
DXA	-Accurate -Relatively inexpensive -Considered the gold standard	-May not accommodate those with extreme BMI
BIA	-Relatively accurate -Inexpensive -Commonly used	-Hydration dependent -Avoid if the patient has electrical cardiac devices
Underwater densitometry	Very accurate	-Time-consuming -Cumbersome
CT/MRI	Very accurate	-Expensive -Radiation exposure (CT)

DXA: Dual-energy x-ray absorptiometry; **BIA:** Bioelectrical impedance analysis.

Reference: Obesity Medicine Association: Obesity Algorithm (2021)

51. (Content: II-B-3) A 23-year-old healthy female presents for an annual examination at her family practice physician's clinic. She has decided to pursue a vegan diet in place of the pescatarian diet she had previously consumed. She wants to ensure she does not become malnourished and asks about vitamin supplementation. What deficiency will most likely be present if supplementation is not initiated within the next year?

A. Vitamin C
B. Cyanocobalamin
C. Vitamin D
D. Folate
E. Vitamin K

(C) Patients consuming a vegan diet (no animal products) are most likely to become deficient and require supplementation of vitamin B_{12}, vitamin D, and omega-3. Of those, **vitamin D** will most likely be deficient within a year, as vitamin B_{12} takes years to deplete stores in the absence of pernicious anemia.

Note: Other vitamin deficiencies vegans are at risk for include iron, zinc, and calcium.

There are many benefits of vegetarian and vegan diets, which are considered low fat by definition, as < 20% of total calories come from fat. Some benefits include weight loss, lower risk of certain cancers, cardioprotection, improved lipid profile, and decreased diabetes risk.

Variants of this diet include the following:

- Lacto-ova: Consume dairy and eggs
- Pescatarian: Eat fish (no red meat or poultry)
- Vegans: Consume absolutely no animal products
- Vegetarians: May eat animal products (milk, eggs), but not meat

Reference: Up to date: "Vitamin supplementation in disease prevention"

52. (Content: II-D-3a) A 61-year-old male diagnosed with hypertension and obesity class II presents to his sleep specialist to discuss his overnight polysomnography results. His primary care physician referred him after he was experiencing unrefreshing sleep and waking up holding his breath. His spouse also had concerns about loud snoring with pauses in his breathing. Given this patient's history, what is the minimal apnea-hypopnea index (AHI) needed to diagnose obstructive sleep apnea?

A. **5 per hour**
B. 15 per hour
C. 30 per hour
D. 60 per hour

(A) This patient is presenting with severe symptoms of obstructive sleep apnea, **requiring an AHI ≥ 5 episodes of apnea or hypopnea per hour** to meet diagnostic criteria for obstructive sleep apnea.

OSA severity and diagnosis are based on the apnea-hypopnea index (AHI), which is the summation of the following events per one-hour period (total events/total hours of sleep):

- **Apnea:** Respiratory pauses that last ≥ 10 seconds
- **Hypopnea:** Shallow breathing leading to oxygen desaturation of ≥ 4%

An additional diagnostic criterion is the respiratory disturbance index (RDI), which adds respiratory effort-related arousals (RERA) to hypopnea and apnea. RDI, therefore, is more sensitive.

Diagnostic Criteria for Obstructive Sleep Apnea	
AHI or RDI > 15/hr **or** > 5/hr with severe symptoms (one or more):	
• Daytime sleepiness • Unrefreshing sleep • Waking up breath-holding, gasping, or chocking	• Fatigue • Insomnia • Witnessed apneic episodes • Loud snoring
Severity (AHI): Mild (5-15); Moderate (15-30); Severe > 30	

AHI: Apnea-hypopnea index; **RDI:** Respiratory disturbance index

Reference: Up To Date: "Clinical manifestations and diagnosis of OSA in adults"

53. (Content: II-A-1) A physician is working in a weight loss clinic and seeing a patient with inadequate insurance coverage. The patient meets criteria for pharmacologic therapy and is interested, but cannot afford name-brand combination medications. Therefore, the physician discusses the off-label use of medications, including emulating the newer combination medications by prescribing the two medications separately. The patient comes back one month later with no weight loss. He explains that he lost one of the two prescriptions. Which medications did he most likely take for the past month?

A. Topiramate
B. Phentermine
C. Bupropion
D. Liraglutide
E. **Naltrexone**

(E) Of the options above, the only medication that is used in a combination anti-obesity medication for its synergistic effect, but is ineffective alone in causing weight loss, is **naltrexone.**

Bupropion and naltrexone are used for their synergistic effects in weight loss. Bupropion works by stimulating the cleavage of POMC, while increasing the agonism of melanocortin-4 receptors, by releasing α-MSH, assisting the anorexigenic pathway. However, another cleavage product from POMC, β-endorphin, causes a negative feedback loop within the POMC neuron when it binds the μ-opioid receptor, thereby decreasing the neuronal activity. This opioid receptor and subsequent downstream effects of β-endorphin are blocked by naltrexone, thus amplifying the α-MSH effects and reducing further food intake.

Without the effects of bupropion, the counter effects are not present, and therefore naltrexone, by itself, is ineffective.

Reference: The burden of obesity in the current world and the new treatments available: focus on liraglutide 3.0 mg Marcio C. Mancini1,2,3 and Maria Edna de Mel. Mancini and de Melo Diabetol Metab Syndr (2017) 9:44 DOI 10.1186/s13098-017-0242-0

174

54. (Content: II-C-7) A 9-year-old female is brought to her pediatrician for a well-child check. A few years ago, she was diagnosed with depression. Although the medications prescribed have helped with her mood symptoms, her appetite has significantly increased. She eats approximately 3500 kcal/day and admits to playing on the computer and watching more television than previously. Lab work including thyroid hormone levels are normal. Her weight is displayed on the growth chart below. Which stature curve would best correlate with her height?

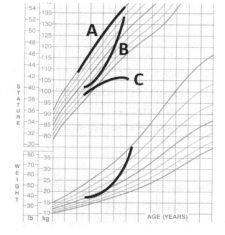

A. Line A
B. **Line B**
C. Line C

(B) Children consuming excess calories leading to weight gain would have an upward trajectory on both the height and weight curves in a proportional manner, consistent with **line B**. In contrast, those with endocrinopathies such as hypothyroidism or Cushing's disease would develop increased weight with decreased growth velocity, leading to flattening of the growth curve (line C).

Exceptions to the generalized statements above occur in various genetic etiologies of obesity:

- **Tall stature:** Melanocortin 4 receptor deficiency leads to persistently tall stature with increased weight. This would likely cause a growth curve similar to line A.
- **Short stature:** Turner syndrome, Down syndrome, Prader-Willi, and Albright Hereditary Osteodystrophy would cause a patient to be persistently on a lower percentile growth curve.

Reference: Styne DM, Arslanian SA, Connor EL, Farooqi IS, Murad MH, Silverstein JH, Yanovski JA. Pediatric Obesity-Assessment, Treatment, and Prevention: An Endocrine Society Clinical Practice Guideline. J Clin Endocrinol Metab. 2017 Mar 1;102(3):709-757. doi: 10.1210/jc.2016-2573. PMID: 28359099; PMCID: PMC6283429.

55. (Content: II-C-3) A 27-year-old female with a history of hypertension and recently diagnosed obstructive sleep apnea (OSA) presents for evaluation after having failed many name-brand diets. She states she has always been "on the heavier side," but needing a CPAP machine for OSA motivated her to lose weight. Physical examination reveals a rounded face and truncal obesity with widened abdominal striae. Laboratory work reveals a hemoglobin A1c in the pre-diabetes range. What other findings would most likely be present on physical exam?

A. Scalloped tongue
B. Hirsutism
C. Decreased deep tendon reflexes
D. Periumbilical hernia
E. Superficial ecchymosis

(E) This patient presenting with hypertension, OSA, wide (> 1 cm) abdominal striae, and moon facies has physical exam findings consistent with the diagnosis of Cushing's syndrome. Facial acne and **easy bruising** are also commonly seen. Clinical and physical findings are related to hypercortisolism.

Cushing's syndrome is a rare cause of secondary obesity, but essential to consider in the right clinical scenario. Clinical pearls are listed below:

- **Clinical manifestations:** Facial plethora, moon/round face, dorsal fat pad (buffalo hump), hypertension, truncal obesity (thin extremities), proximal muscle weakness, osteoporosis, glucose intolerance, acne, and ecchymosis.
- **Etiology:** The most common cause of hypercortisolism is iatrogenic, although central (excess ACTH secretion), peripheral (adrenal adenoma), and paraneoplastic etiologies are possibilities.
- **Initial screening:** 24-hour urinary-free cortisol excretion (x2), overnight 1 mg dexamethasone test, or late-night buccal salivary swab (x2).

Reference: Up to Date: "Establishing the diagnosis of Cushing's syndrome"

56. (Content: II-D-1) A female sprinter undergoes indirect calorimetry to determine her respiratory quotient (RQ), which is obtained by measuring carbon dioxide eliminated divided by oxygen consumed. It is determined that when the athlete is slowly jogging, she mostly consumes lipids. However, during sustained sprinting, her RQ would be expected to be near which of the following values?

A. 0.5
B. 0.7
C. 1.0
D. 1.3

(C) The respiratory quotient (RQ) equals eliminated carbon dioxide divided by oxygen consumed, measured on indirect calorimetry. The RQ can determine which macronutrients are being metabolized (energy utilized by the body). If energy consumption is only from lipids, the RQ will be 0.7, whereas if solely from carbohydrates, it will be closer to 1.0.

The respiratory quotient allows you to determine which macronutrients are being consumed for energy in a steady state.

- If low-energy but sustainable exercise is being performed (jogging in a marathon), then the RQ will be closer to 0.7, as stored fats are primarily being used for energy. In addition, inactivity tends to be closer to 0.7.
- If high-intensity, high-energy exercise is being performed (sprinting), carbohydrates are mainly used for energy, and the **RQ is near 1.**

Note: This topic will likely be tested in a simple form; thus, memorizing the respiratory quotients in the table below and having a basic understanding will be sufficient.

Respiratory Quotient	
Carbohydrates	1
Proteins	0.8
Fats	0.7
Mixed	0.8

Reference: Patel H, Kerndt CC, Bhardwaj A. Physiology, Respiratory Quotient. 2020 Sep 16. In: StatPearls. Treasure Island (FL): StatPearls Publishing; 2021 Jan–. PMID: 30285389.

57. (Content: II-C-6) A 44-year-old female presents for a follow-up three years after undergoing a Roux-en-Y gastric bypass. She is pleased with her results, having lost nearly 55% of her total body weight loss and she states she continues to lose weight despite no longer following the dietician's recommendations or exercising. She denies depression and says she feels well but admits to diarrhea. Preoperative BMI was 47.3 kg/m^2, and today it is 22.7 kg/m^2. Physical exam is normal except for some excess skin in the abdomen and arms. She has not followed up with her surgeon after the first year. Which of the following may explain her weight loss?

A. Vitamin deficiency
B. Anastomotic stricture
C. Small intestinal bowel overgrowth
D. **A shorter common intestinal channel**
E. Expected post-surgical weight loss

(D) The common channel is the portion of the intestine after the digestive and alimentary tracts connect. A shorter channel (as seen in biliopancreatic diversion with a duodenal switch) leads to decreased absorption of nutrients. This otherwise asymptomatic patient has lost an excessive amount of weight (35% expected after Roux-en-Y gastric bypass) in the setting of not adhering to dietary or physical activity recommendations. This is concerning for an anatomical cause, most likely **a shorter common channel** leading to malabsorption, which also explains this patient's persistent diarrhea. Other causes of excess weight loss are discussed below:

- Eating disorders such as bulimia or anorexia nervosa
- Underlying malignancy, which is usually associated with increased fatigue, night sweats, and potentially localizing symptoms etc.
- Small intestinal bowel overgrowth of which symptoms would include bloating, nausea, early satiety, abdominal discomfort, and diarrhea
- Anastomotic stricture with symptoms including localized abdominal pain, food aversion, and possible dysphagia
- Depression or other psychiatric conditions

Reference: Akusoba I, Birriel TJ, El Chaar M. Management of Excessive Weight Loss Following Laparoscopic Roux-en-Y Gastric Bypass: Clinical Algorithm and Surgical Techniques. Obes Surg. 2016 Jan;26(1):5-11. doi: 10.1007/s11695-015-1775-7. PMID: 26105983.

58. (Content: II-D-3a) A 14-year-old female with a BMI of 39 kg/m² presents to her family practitioner for recurrent headaches. She states the headaches are pulsatile and occasionally cause loss of appetite. In addition, she now has difficulty seeing the board during school and must sit toward the front of her class. She has intermittent loss of vision and diplopia when standing up. Which of the following would be the best test to determine her cause of headaches?

    A. Orthostatic vital signs
    B. Overnight sleep study
    C. Ophthalmologic evaluation
    D. Brain imaging
    E. Cerebral spinal fluid studies

(E) This adolescent female with obesity class II has intermittent headaches, vision changes, and positional diplopia. She likely has a diagnosis of idiopathic intracranial hypertension (IIH), also known as pseudotumor cerebri. Although many options are valid, only a **lumbar puncture displaying elevated opening pressure** will definitively diagnose this patient with IIH.

Note: Imaging may be necessary to exclude secondary causes for headaches, while an ophthalmology examination is necessary to document the degree of papilledema. Although sleep apnea can cause headaches, it should not cause vision changes.

IIH is most commonly seen in women with excess weight and is characterized by vision loss, papilledema, and headaches caused by elevated intracranial pressures with otherwise normal cerebral fluid studies.

Treatment options should include weight loss of >5-10% (lifestyle modifications and/or medical or surgical options) with a low-sodium diet. In addition, carbonic anhydrase inhibitors such as acetazolamide and topiramate (which also help with weight loss) lower cerebral fluid pressure.

Surgical interventions such as optic nerve sheath fenestration and shunting procedures should be pursued for deteriorating vision or intractable headaches.

Reference: Up to Date: "Idiopathic intracranial hypertension (pseudotumor cerebri): Clinical features and diagnosis & prognosis and treatment"

59. (Content: II-C-7) A mother brings her 9-year-old son to his pediatrician for evaluation, as she is concerned that his height and weight are increased in comparison to his peers. The mother states that her son does tend to watch 4-5 hours of television daily and is "constantly snacking." The son has no known health concerns, and overall appears happy. Physical examination reveals a BMI of 19.75 kg/m^2, which is the 86th percentile for his age and gender. Which of the following most accurately describes his weight categorization?

A. Underweight
B. Healthy weight
C. Overweight
D. Class 1 obesity
E. Class 2 obesity

(C) Unlike adults, in which absolute BMI is used to categorize weight, in children aged 2-20, weight status is based on a percentile range of BMI, taking into consideration gender and age. For this patient, who is in the 86th percentile range for BMI, this places him in the **overweight category.**

Importantly, BMI is not used until children reach 2 years of age. Instead, weight for length is used in those ages 0-2 years of age.

Childhood Obesity Classification (Age 2-19 years)	
Classification	Percentile Range[1] (% BMI)
Underweight	Less than 5%
Healthy weight	5 to < 85%
Overweight	85 to < 95%
Obesity	95 to < 99%
Severe Obesity	≥99th percentile
Expanded Definition (Splits Obesity into Class I, II, and III)	
Class 1 Obesity	≥ 95th percentile to < 120% of the 95th percentile
Class 2 Obesity	≥ 120% to < 140% of the 95th percentile or BMI ≥ 35 to ≤ 39 kg/m^2
Class 3 Obesity	≥ 140% of the 95th percentile or BMI ≥ 40 kg/m^2

[1]Percentile range based on age and gender.

Reference: Obesity medicine association: Pediatric Obesity Algorithm (2020-2022)

60. (Content: II-A-3) A 19-year-old male presents to his primary care physician for an annual physical evaluation. He admits to eating significantly more since he started college. He relates this to stress and a change in sleep habits since moving to the dormitories. He states he has gained approximately 20 lbs (9.1 kg) over the past five months. His BMI is 29 kg/m². Laboratory findings include a hemoglobin A1c of 5.9% (reference range: < 5.7%), and his fasting cholesterol panel is consistent with dyslipidemia. To diagnose him with metabolic syndrome, what additional finding is necessary?

A. Abdominal circumference of 100 cm (39 inches)
B. Diagnosis of obstructive sleep apnea
C. Diastolic blood pressure of 82 mmHg
D. **Being treated with amlodipine**

(D) This patient with pre-diabetes (HbA1c 5.7-6.5%) and dyslipidemia nearly meets the criteria for metabolic syndrome. Of the answer options, the additional **presence of hypertension, with or without treatment**, would meet the National Cholesterol Education Program (NCEP) Adult Treatment Panel III (ATP III) criteria for metabolic syndrome. Diagnostic criteria for metabolic syndrome requires 3 of the following 5 to be present:

- Abdominal obesity, defined as a waist circumference ≥ 102 cm (40 in) in men and ≥ 88 cm (35 in) in women
- Serum triglycerides ≥ 150 mg/dL or drug treatment for elevated triglycerides
- Serum high-density lipoprotein (HDL) cholesterol < 40 mg/dL in men and < 50 mg/dL in women, or drug treatment for low HDL cholesterol
- Blood pressure ≥ 130/85 mmHg, or drug treatment for elevated blood pressure
- Fasting plasma glucose (FPG) ≥ 100 mg/dL, or drug treatment for elevated blood glucose

Reference: Up to Date: "Metabolic syndrome (insulin resistance syndrome or syndrome X)"

61. (Content: II-B-5) A 14-year-old female presents to her pediatrician's office for an annual examination. She denies any concerns but appears withdrawn. She states school is "going okay." When asked about diet, she says she hardly eats because she is "fat and ugly." Physical examination reveals a BMI of 17 kg/m^2, with a global cachectic appearance. Which of the following is most associated with her underlying condition?

A. Tachycardia
B. Urinary phosphate wasting
C. Increased osteoblast activity
D. **Decreased luteinizing hormone**
E. Respiratory alkalosis

(D) This patient is presenting with restricted calorie intake due to a distorted body image, consistent with the diagnosis of anorexia nervosa. This condition is associated with many findings, including:

- Central hypogonadism (functional amenorrhea) with **low luteinizing hormone (LH)** and follicular stimulating hormone (FSH)
- Bradycardia
- Electrolyte disturbances, especially hypomagnesemia, hypokalemia, and metabolic alkalosis
- Osteoporosis (decreased osteoblast and osteoclast activity)

Diagnostic Criteria for Anorexia Nervosa[1]	
Restriction of energy intake relative to requirements leading to ↓ weight	
Intense fear of gaining weight or becoming overweight or persistent behavior that interferes with weight gain	
Body image distortion/lack of recognition of the seriousness of ↓ weight	
Specifiers • Restricting type (i.e., diet) • Binge eating/purging type	**Severity** • Mild: BMI ≥ 17-18.5 kg/m^2 • Moderate: BMI 16-17 kg/m^2 • Severe: BMI 15-16 kg/m^2 • Extreme: BMI < 15 kg/m^2

[1]Amenorrhea is no longer a diagnostic criterion

Reference: DSM-5: Diagnostic and Statistical Manual of Mental Disorders, Fifth Edition

62. (Content: II-D-1) A sports medicine physician is working with athletes to optimize their performance. He has them undergo testing to determine the VO_2 maximum, in order to calculate their cardiorespiratory fitness level. Which of the following statements is most accurate regarding VO_2 max?

A. VO_2 max increases with age
B. Professional athletes have low levels of VO_2 max
C. **Decreasing body fat percentage improves VO_2 max**
D. VO_2 max is similar among genders

(C) The volume of oxygen consumed (VO_2) is a marker of oxygen utilization, with higher levels indicating increased efficiency. Efficiency includes oxygen absorption (lungs), oxygen distribution (heart), and oxygen utilization (muscles). Pathology or inefficiency of any of these systems would decrease VO_2 max.

VO_2 max is measured by cardiopulmonary exercise testing. Patients breathe through a closed loop system containing a mask and tubing, with the tubes connected to an oxygen and carbon dioxide analyzer. Measurements of oxygen consumption are in mL/kg/min.

Generalizations about VO_2 max include:

- Levels decrease with age (approximately a 30% decrease at age 65 compared to age 20).
- Athletes have higher levels
- **Decreasing body fat percentage increases levels**
- Males generally have higher VO_2 levels when compared to females

VO_2 max is often looked at as a marker of cardiorespiratory health and endurance, with some of the fittest athletes having levels in the 90 mL/kg/min range. In contrast, the average female and male are in the 35 and 45 mL/kg/min range, respectively.

Reference: Lundby C, Montero D, Joyner M. Biology of VO2 max: looking under the physiology lamp. Acta Physiol (Oxf). 2017 Jun;220(2):218-228. doi: 10.1111/apha.12827. Epub 2016 Nov 25. PMID: 27888580.

63. (Content: II-D-3a) A 34-year-old male presents to the clinic after attending a bariatric seminar. He is interested in weight loss surgery. He takes amlodipine for hypertension and is adherent with continuous positive airway pressure (CPAP) for his obstructive sleep apnea. He denies any tobacco or alcohol history. Which of the following would be the most appropriate initial screening test for metabolic-associated fatty liver disease at this time?

A. History
B. Physical exam findings
C. **Laboratory work**
D. Right upper quadrant ultrasound
E. Liver biopsy

(C) All patients diagnosed with overweight or obesity, type 2 diabetes mellitus, or metabolic syndrome should be screened for metabolic-associated (nonalcoholic) fatty liver disease (MAFLD). Screening should be completed with a **liver enzyme (AST/ALT) evaluation.** ALT is the most specific enzyme for NAFLD in adults and children.

Although the physical examination is essential, it is not sensitive nor specific for diagnosing MAFLD. Therefore, initial laboratory testing with a complete metabolic panel is indicated, followed by imaging modalities such as a right upper quadrant ultrasound if liver transaminases are elevated.

MAFLD includes a spectrum of fatty liver diseases as follows:

- Hepatosteatosis is fatty liver
- Hepatosteatitis is fatty liver with inflammation
- Metabolic-associated steatohepatitis (MASH) is the presence of > 5% hepatic fat, with inflammation and hepatocyte injury, +/- cirrhosis

No FDA drugs are explicitly approved to treat MAFLD, although GLP-1 receptor agonists and PPAR (i.e., thiazolidinediones) have shown some potential.

Update: Recent changes to nomenclature have changed nonalcoholic fatty liver disease (NAFLD) to metabolic-associated liver disease (MAFLD) to better describe the underlying physiology of this condition.

Reference: AACE/ACE Guidelines: AMERICAN ASSOCIATION OF CLINICAL ENDOCRINOLOGISTS AND AMERICAN COLLEGE OF ENDOCRINOLOGY COMPREHENSIVE CLINICAL PRACTICE GUIDELINES FOR MEDICAL CARE OF PATIENTS WITH OBESITY (2016). Recommendation 16.
Reference: Obesity medicine association: Obesity Algorithm (2021)

64. (Content II-C-1) A 22-year-old male is frustrated by his recent diagnosis of "overweight," which was made at an insurance screening exam. He weight-lifts for 3-4 hours daily and competes at the state and national level for body-building. Prior testing reveals an 18% body fat composition. What other condition would act similarly to this patient in terms of an increased BMI with a discordant obesity-related risk association?

A. **Congestive heart failure**
B. Increased age
C. Southeast Asian ethnicity
D. Sarcopenia
E. Osteoporosis

(A) **Congestive heart failure** or any condition that increases excess water through third spacing (i.e., cirrhosis, nephrotic syndrome) tends to overestimate body mass index (BMI) but not increase adiposity-related risk factors that are usually associated with an increased BMI. The other listed choices tend to underestimate the adiposity risk associated with a particular BMI.

Note: Body mass index does not consider body composition, which is a better measurement for obesity in those with fluid overload or extremes of muscle mass (i.e., bodybuilders or those with sarcopenia).

BMI is generally the first step in determining the degree of excess weight to estimate adiposity. However, this does not always accurately determine cardiovascular risks, as this may be better predicted by waist circumference, waist-to-hip ratio, or body-mass composition in certain populations.

Regardless, BMI is overall easy to obtain, reproducible, cheap, and for the general population correlates with adiposity. Therefore many insurance companies (and the FDA) rely on this almost exclusively for determining inclusivity for bariatric surgery and anti-obesity medications.

Reference: Obesity medicine association: Obesity Algorithm (2021)
Reference: Up to Date: "Obesity in adults: Prevalence, screening, and evaluation"

65. (Content: II-C-6) A 63-year-old female presents to her primary care physician's office for follow-up after starting methotrexate with complaints of a sore tongue and irritability. She was diagnosed with polymyalgia rheumatic two years ago and was placed on 15 mg of prednisone daily. However, she had gained nearly 60 lbs (27.2 kg) while on prednisone. Eight months ago, she was transitioned to methotrexate for glucocorticoid-sparing therapy. Her BMI is 35 kg/m^2. Which of the following is most responsible for her current condition?

- A. Vitamin B_1
- B. Vitamin B_2
- C. Vitamin B_3
- **D. Vitamin B_9**
- E. Vitamin B_{12}

(D) This patient, who is on methotrexate without mention of folate supplementation, presenting with glossitis and irritability, most likely has developed **functional folic acid deficiency (B_9)**. Although the intention to treat secondary obesity was appropriate, the lack of proper vitamin supplementation was not. B_9 deficiency can also be seen in patients with alcohol use disorder and other medications such as phenytoin, sulfasalazine, and TMP-SMX.

Water Soluble B Vitamin Deficiencies		
$B_\#$	Name	Deficiency
B_1	Thiamine	Wernicke's encephalopathy, Korsakoff syndrome, Beriberi: wet (cardiovascular) and dry (neurologic)
B_2	Riboflavin	Sore throat, cheilitis, stomatitis, glossitis, itchy eyes
B_3	Niacin	Pellagra (dermatitis, diarrhea, dementia, death)
B_5	Pantothenic acid	Rare! Paresthesia, restlessness, apathy, hypoglycemia
B_6	Pyridoxine	Peripheral neuropathy, microcytic anemia
B_7	Biotin[1]	Facial dermatitis, neurologic findings (depression, neuropathy, hallucinations)
B_9	Folate	Macrocytic anemia without significant neurologic findings, mouth ulcers, irritability. Fetal neuro tube defects in pregnancy.
B_{12}	Cyanocobalamin	Subacute combined degeneration, macrocytic anemia, glossitis, neurologic manifestations

[1]Consumption of large quantities of raw egg whites can bind to biotin, preventing its absorption, leading to a deficiency.

Reference: Up to Date: "Overview of water-soluble vitamins"

66. (Content: II-C-4) A 14-year-old male presents to his family practice physician for his annual physical examination. He is in the 105th percentile for weight and the 65th percentile for height. His upper arm circumference is 37 cm. Which of the following would likely cause an inaccurately elevated systolic blood pressure?

    A. Using a large adult-sized cuff (16x36 cm)
    B. Sitting in a chair with back support
    C. Having the patient rest his arm by his side
    D. Telling the patient not to talk during inflation
    E. Deflating the cuff at 5-10 mmHg per second

(C) Understanding blood pressure monitoring is vital to ensure accurate results and avoid overtreatment and overdiagnosing hypertension. Systolic blood pressure may appear artificially elevated if the patient is supine, the patient's legs are crossed, **the arms are allowed to rest unsupported by the patient's side**, or when using an undersized blood pressure cuff.

Note: ABOM will ask questions on the appropriate evaluation of comorbidities of obesity, including proper techniques. Expect these questions on test day!

Accurate blood pressure monitoring is essential in determining a disease that often requires medications. Proper techniques are described below:

- Patients should be seated comfortably. The back should be supported, and the legs should be uncrossed.
- The blood pressure cuff should be on bare skin.
- The patient's arm should be supported at the level of the heart.
- The cuff bladder should encircle 80% of the arm circumference.
- There should be no talking while obtaining the measurement.

An appropriately sized blood pressure cuff for the patient's arm size is required. The term "large adult" for a blood pressure cuff is a misnomer, as it should be based on the arm circumference, not a subjective adult size.

References: New AHA Recommendations for Blood Pressure Measurement; Am Fam Physician. 2005 Oct 1;72(7):1391-1398.
Reference: 2017 ACC/AHA/AAPA/ABC/ACPM/AGS/APhA/ASH/ASPC/NMA/PCNA Guideline for the Prevention, Detection, Evaluation, and Management of High Blood Pressure in Adults

67. (Content: II-B-4) A 44-year-old female presents to the office with concerns about weight-gain. She rarely eats breakfast but instead eats from the time she gets home from work until bedtime. She occasionally awakens and consumes calories at night. The only medication she takes is zolpidem for insomnia. Which of the following questions would be most helpful to determine if the nocturnal caloric intake is caused by zolpidem versus night eating syndrome?

A. Are you aware during your nocturnal eating episodes?
B. What is the dose of your zolpidem?
C. Do you have a prior history of sleep walking?
D. Do you take any other over-the-counter medications?
E. Are you drowsy in the mornings after taking zolpidem?

(A) Night eating syndrome (NES) is often associated with depression and insomnia. One of the characteristic features of NES is waking up in the night to eat. Importantly, **patients are awake and aware they are eating,** which differentiates this from sleep-related eating disorders (SRED) caused by sleep-medications (e.g., zolpidem). SRED is a parasomnia where patients unknowingly "sleep-eat" with no memory of this in the morning.

Diagnostic Criteria for Night Eating Syndrome
Increased intake after evening meal: • At least 25% of caloric intake occurs after the evening meal   • Two episodes of nocturnal eating per week
Three of the following: • Lack of desire to eat breakfast (≥4 times per week)   • Increased appetite after supper and/or throughout the night   • Sleep onset and/or sleep maintenance insomnia present   • Feeling that one must eat in order to fall back to sleep   • Mood is often depressed or worsens in the evening
Awareness of nocturnal episodes present (excludes SRED)
Marked distress or impairment in functioning
Pattern of eating is present for at least 3 months
Findings not attributed to substance use, medication, or other disorders

SRED: sleep-related eating disorder

Reference: Allison KC, Lundgren JD, O'Reardon JP, Geliebter A, Gluck ME, Vinai P, Mitchell JE, Schenck CH, Howell MJ, Crow SJ, Engel S, Latzer Y, Tzischinsky O, Mahowald MW, Stunkard AJ. Proposed diagnostic criteria for night eating syndrome. Int J Eat Disord. 2010 Apr;43(3):241-7. doi: 10.1002/eat.20693. PMID: 19378289; PMCID: PMC4531092.

68. (Content: II-F) A university hospital is working with the Centers for Medicare and Medicaid Services (CMS) regarding billing and repayments. The current system allows for an increased hospital length of stay based on body mass index alone. The new proposal is to establish repayments and recommended appropriate length of stay on comorbidities and functional limitations. Which of the following would be the best categorization method to initiate?

    A. New York Heart Association Classification
    B. Edmonton Obesity Staging System
    C. Epworth Sleepiness Score
    D. World Health Organization Obesity Classification
    E. King's Obesity Staging Criteria

(B) **The Edmonton Obesity Staging System (EOSS)** is used to categorize patients based on the severity of obesity-related comorbidities, psychologic symptoms, and functional limitations rather than focusing strictly on anthropometric measurements such as waist circumference and body mass index.

Therefore, this staging system provides better insight into the patient's long-term impact of obesity and may help determine the level of appropriate treatment (along with established metrics).

For example, if there are two patients, both with a BMI of 32 kg/m², and one is EOSS stage 0 (asymptomatic and no risk factors), and the other is EOSS stage 2 (moderate, established comorbidities), prioritizing more frequent visits, anti-obesity medication management, dieticians, etc. for the latter patient may have a more substantial health impact, especially if resources are limited.

Note: The King's Obesity Staging Criteria staging system was designed to compare baseline pre-operative and post-operative variables in bariatric surgery patients. Some variables are more subjective (i.e., perceived health status and body image) and thus would be less helpful in this vignette.

Reference: Using the Edmonton obesity staging system to predict mortality in a population-representative cohort of people with overweight and obesity. Raj S. Padwal, Nicholas M. Pajewski, David B. Allison and Arya M. Sharma. CMAJ October 04, 2011 183 (14) E1059-E1066; DOI: https://doi.org/10.1503/cmaj.110387
Reference: "Assessment of obesity beyond body mass index to determine benefit of treatment." E. T. Aasheim, S. J. B. Aylwin, S. T. Radhakrishnan, A. S. Sood, A. Jovanovic, T. Olbers, C. W. le Roux, First published: 05 July 2011 https://doi.org/10.1111/j.1758-8111.2011.00017.x

69. (Content: II-D-2) A physician is discussing the different terminology used in body composition to a rotating internal medicine resident. She describes a term that encompasses muscles, organs, water, bones, ligaments, tendons, and essential fat, but does not include nonessential or storage adipose tissue. Which of the following terms is she most likely describing?

    A. Fat mass
    B. Fat-free mass
    C. Lean body mass
    D. Total body mass
    E. Percent body fat

(C) **Lean body mass** is the total body mass (including muscles, internal organs, water, bones, ligaments, and tendons) minus nonessential or storage adipose tissue. It slightly differs from fat-free mass because lean body mass includes the essential fat in the bone marrow, central nervous system, and internal organs. Lean body mass makes up approximately 75% of total body mass (40% muscle, 25% organs, and 10% bone).

Note: Fat-free mass does not include **<u>ANY</u>** body fat in its calculation.

Importantly, lean body mass is less in females, less in those who are sedentary, and decreases as age increases. Higher lean body mass is associated with increased health, whereas increased fat mass is associated with increased health risks.

Although most dual-energy x-ray absorptiometry (DXA) scans measure fat, soft tissue, and bone, more advanced ones will decipher the type of fat, thus allowing for lean body mass calculations. In those that do not, fat-free mass (FFM) is calculated by taking total mass minus fat mass. FFM is often within 5% of LBM, given that lean body mass includes only a limited subset of adipose tissue (i.e., essential fat).

Different formula calculations are discussed below:

- Total body mass = fat mass + lean mass + bone mass
- Fat-free mass = total body mass – fat mass
- % body fat = fat mass/(total body mass – bone mass)

Reference: Obesity medicine association: Obesity Algorithm (2021)

70. (Content: II-B-4) A 37-year-old mother of two presents to her primary care physician's office for follow-up after recently being diagnosed with binge-eating disorder (BED). She has started cognitive behavioral therapy and has noticed improvements. She states that upon researching BED, she has seen a lot of the same tendencies and characteristics of her condition in her 11-year-old daughter. Her daughter is scheduled to meet with her pediatrician and will likely be diagnosed with which of the following?

    A. Grazing
    B. Anorexia nervosa
    C. Loss of control eating disorder
    D. Night eating syndrome
    E. Bulimia nervosa

(C) This patient's daughter, who has many of the same symptoms of BED, will likely be diagnosed with **loss of control eating disorder (LOC-ED).** This condition is nearly identical to BED, but is only diagnosed in children < 12 years old. First-line treatment for LOC-ED is interpersonal psychotherapy.

Diagnosis Criteria for Loss of Control Eating Disorder (age < 12 years old)
Recurrent episodes of binge eating marked by: • Eating large amounts of food in a discrete amount of time   • A sense of lack of control with eating during these episodes
Associated with 3 or more of the following: • Eating more rapidly than normal   • Eating until uncomfortably full   • Eating large amounts of food when not physically hungry   • Hiding eating behaviors because embarrassed by behavior   • Feeling disgusted, depressed, or guilty after episodes
Marked distress about binge eating
Occurs on average at least 1 time per week for 3 months
Not associated with compensatory purging behaviors

Reference: Tanofsky-Kraff M, Marcus MD, Yanovski SZ, Yanovski JA. Loss of control eating disorder in children age 12 years and younger: proposed research criteria. Eat Behav. 2008;9(3):360–365. doi:10.1016/j.eatbeh.2008.03.002

71. (Content: II-C-1) A patient is discussing with a physician a news story that was heard earlier in the day. The report stated patients who have a BMI ≥ 25 kg/m² have a longer life expectancy than those with a BMI < 25 kg/m². The patient now questions the utility of obtaining a BMI at each visit. Which is a true statement regarding the correlation between BMI and obesity-related comorbidities?

A. A BMI of 35 kg/m² decreases life expectancy the same as smoking
B. BMI is the best indicator of cardiovascular disease
C. 50% of type 2 diabetes is directly related to obesity-range BMI
D. **A 5-unit increase in BMI increases ischemic stroke risk by 20%**

(D) The obesity paradox states that increased BMI has a favorable effect on mortality, as shown in some limited studies. However, these studies do not consider fat distribution (visceral fat) or the concept of "sick fat disease," which significantly affects mortality/comorbidities.

Both extremes of BMI have increased mortality, but BMI alone does not account for cardiovascular risk in individuals with a BMI 25-30 kg/m² (overweight). Visceral (or truncal) obesity incurs a higher cardiovascular risk than BMI alone in these moderate BMI ranges; cardiovascular risk is better predicted by waist circumference or waist-to-hip ratio than BMI alone.

Regardless, BMI does have many direct correlations, discussed below:

- **Mortality:** A BMI between 25-35 kg/m² reduces life expectancy by 2-4 years, and a BMI of 40-45 kg/m² by 8-10 years (similar to smoking).
- **Heart failure:** Risk increases 2-fold with a BMI ≥ 30 kg/m².
- **Atrial fibrillation:** For every ↑ of 1 unit BMI, risk increases by 4%.
- **Diabetes type 2:** 80% of cases are directly related to obesity.
- **Cerebral vascular accident:** For **every ↑ 1 unit BMI, there is an increase in ischemic stroke by 4%** and hemorrhagic stroke by 6%.
- **Sleep apnea:** BMI > 30 kg/m² incurs a 30% risk of sleep apnea.

Note: There are 230 comorbidities associated with obesity, including malignancy.

Reference: Up to Date: "Overweight and obesity in adults: Health consequences"

72. (Content: II-C-5) A 3-year-old female is referred to a geneticist for evaluation after persistent milestone delays and a recent seizure. The child appears very happy, smiling, and frequently laughing during the examination. Her movements are spastic and she is only able to pull herself up to a seated position and stand with assistance. She does not talk and only babbles intermittently. What would the genetic workup most likely reveal?

A. **Angelman syndrome**
B. Turner syndrome
C. Borjeson-Forssman-Lehmann syndrome
D. Albright hereditary osteodystrophy
E. Fragile-X syndrome

(A) This patient presents with seizures, speech and balance issues, and an overly happy affect, consistent with **Angelman syndrome.** This syndrome often occurs de novo due to errors in maternal imprinting. In addition, these patients may have increased appetites leading to obesity (one-third of patients).

Patients with Angelman syndrome have some unique characteristics:

- A very happy personality, with frequent smiling and laughing
- Development delays, including walking
- Minimal talking (often babbling)
- Seizures between 2-3 years of age
- Spastic and jerky movements with microcephaly
- Sleep disorders, including insomnia

This condition is caused by a genetic abnormality of chromosome 15 called the ubiquitin protein ligase E3A (UBE3A), which is normally inherited from the mother (maternal imprinting). However, if the mother's gene is missing or defective, this causes Angelman syndrome. A similar paternal deletion of a gene on the same chromosome causes Prader-Willi syndrome.

Reference: Up To Date "Microdeletion syndromes (chromosomes 12 to 22)"
Reference: https://www.mayoclinic.org/diseases-conditions/angelman-syndrome/symptoms-causes/syc-20355621

73. (Content: II-A-3) A 68-year-old female with a history of type 2 diabetes presents to the clinic following a bariatric seminar. Although she understands there is no definitive age limit to surgery, she elects to undergo medical management. Her current diabetic medication regimen includes a maximum dose of metformin. Her hemoglobin A1c is 9.6%. The risks and benefits of a daily FDA-approved injectable, anti-obesity medication for long-term use is discussed. What medical history would be necessary for the physician to inquire about before starting this medication?

    A. Papillary thyroid carcinoma
    B. Suicidal ideation
    C. History of cholelithiasis
    D. Diabetic gastroparesis

(D) This patient with a history of obesity and diabetes would be a great candidate for liraglutide, a daily FDA-approved long-term-use anti-obesity drug. However, given the mechanism (GLP-1 receptor agonist), it can slow gastrointestinal motility and gastric emptying. Therefore it should be avoided in those with a **history of severe gastroparesis.**

Liraglutide (Saxenda®)	
Dose	Inject 0.6 mg subcutaneously daily. Increase by 0.6 mg daily at weekly intervals to a target dose of 3.0 mg/day
Mechanism	Glucagon-like peptide 1 receptor agonists activate the hypothalamus, reducing food intake, increasing satiety, decreasing caloric intake and improving glucose metabolism (incretin).
Contraindications	Prior hypersensitivity to liraglutide, history of or family history of medullary thyroid carcinoma (black box warning), patients with multiple endocrine neoplasia type 2, and pregnancy. *Relative contraindication: Severe gastroparesis and increased risk of pancreatitis[1]
Side Effects	Gastrointestinal distress (abdominal pain, nausea, vomiting), dizziness, hypoglycemia, increased lipase (increased risk of pancreatitis[1])

[1]Meta-analysis has shown no increased risk of pancreatitis or pancreatic cancer with GLP-1 use.

Reference: Liraglutide package insert

74. (Content: II-C-3 and I-B-4) An 11-year-old male presents to his pediatrician for complaints of right lower extremity pain. He states the pain has worsened over the past month, describing it as a dull ache. There was no preceding trauma. His mother brought him in after she noticed him walking with a limp. His BMI is in the 120th percentile for his age and gender. Physical examination reveals limited internal rotation of his right hip and an antalgic gait. Which of the following is most likely the culprit of his presenting condition?

    A. Blount disease
    B. Slipped capital femoral epiphysis
    C. Osgood-Schlatter disease
    D. Legg-Calve-Perthes disease
    E. Aseptic necrosis

(B) This adolescent patient with excess adipose tissue presents with a new-onset unilateral limp and external rotation (i.e., resistance to internal rotation) of the hip. These findings are most consistent with **slipped capital femoral epiphysis (SCFE).**

SCFE results from the instability of the growth plate of the proximal femur, resulting in a Salter-Harris fracture. This is most commonly from fat mass disease (i.e., mechanical overload), although it can also be from a growth spurt. It requires urgent surgical evaluation.

Other differentials and their characteristics are discussed below:

- Blount disease is the bowing of the tibia (varus) and can be seen in children with obesity.
- Legg-Calve-Perthes disease is idiopathic avascular necrosis of the femoral head and can present similarly to SCFE, including impaired internal rotation; however, it usually affects younger patients (ages 5-6 years old). It may be painless and present only as a limp.
- Osgood-Schlatter disease is seen in young, active patients and presents with a pronounced tibial tuberosity.

Reference: Up to Date: "Evaluation and Management of Slipped Capital Femoral Epiphysis (SCFE)"

75. (Content: II-B-1) A mother of three children presents to her family practitioner for well-child examinations. Two of the children have been diagnosed with obesity. The mother has not followed up with the dietician as recommended, and the children are still consuming high-caloric density packaged food. Which of the following would be the most appropriate question to ask now?

A. **Do you run out of food towards the end of the month?**
B. Is your transportation adequate for making appointments?
C. Do you feel like you are suited to take care of your children?
D. What sweets could be eliminated from your children's diets?
E. How can we incorporate physical activity?

(A) Food insecurity can lead to excessive weight due to poor quality of food intake (calorie-rich food, but poor nutritional value) and food deserts (inadequate grocery stores within a reasonable parameter of home). Screening questions for food insecurity include:

- In the past 12 months, have you been worried about whether food would run out before you got money to purchase more?
- In the past 12 months, **has the food you purchased run out,** and you didn't have the money to buy more?

These two questions can clue you into the potential financial constraints the patient is experiencing and the underlying etiology of childhood obesity. Poorer quality food tends to be less expensive, is packaged (better preservation), and may be preferential to higher-quality foods (increased spoilage and cost).

Nearly 1 out of 5 children meet the definition of food insecurity (75 million families), often related to household poverty, parents' educations (highest correlation), single-parent homes, and larger families.

Having a working knowledge of local and federal resources may bridge the gap and provide improved nutrition leading to long-term benefits.

Reference: Obesity medicine association: Pediatric Obesity Algorithm (2020-2022)

76. (Content: II-A-4) A 25-year-old male presents to his primary care physician's office with the complaint of weight gain. Over the past two years, he has gained nearly 35 lbs (15.9 kg). He states that he first noticed the weight gain once he began to work the night shift. He says he still exercises 30 minutes daily before work but does admit to increased hunger and snacking throughout his shift. Compared to 4 years ago, which of the following would most likely be observed in the patient at this visit?

    A. Decreased orexin
    B. Increased cortisol
    C. Suppressed ghrelin
    D. Increased melatonin
    E. Increased adiponectin

(B) Patients who work rotating or night shifts have circadian misalignment, which increases their risk of obesity, diabetes, depression, hypertension, and hyperlipidemia. Of the list above, these patients have **increased cortisol levels**, as well as the following:

- Decreased energy expenditure
- Increased inflammatory cytokines (IL-6, TNF-α, IL-1β)
- Decreased adiponectin
- Decreased leptin, melatonin, and metabolic rate
- Blunted post-meal suppression of ghrelin
- Increased insulin resistance and risk of diabetes

There appears to be a cumulative effect on circadian misalignment, with those working > 10 years on the night shift having the highest risk of obesity and obesity-related comorbidities.

Options to help with circadian rhythm dysfunction that arise with rotating shifts include incorporating sleep hygiene, using melatonin before sleep and stimulants such as caffeine during work shifts. This allows for a quicker adjustment of sleep/work cycles, mitigating the negative effects above.

Reference: Kim, Tae Won & Jeong, Jong-Hyun & Hong, Seung-Chul. (2015). The Impact of Sleep and Circadian Disturbance on Hormones and Metabolism. International Journal of Endocrinology. 2015. 1-9. 10.1155/2015/591729.
Reference: Peplonska B, Bukowska A, Sobala W. Association of Rotating Night Shift Work with BMI and Abdominal Obesity among Nurses and Midwives. PLoS One. 2015;10(7):e0133761. Published 2015 Jul 21. doi:10.1371/journal.pone.0133761

77. (Content: II-B-2) A 31-year-old male presents as a 2-week follow-up to his weight-loss clinic. Since being seen previously, he has decreased his soda consumption and has reduced the number of times he eats fast food from three times weekly to once. Also, he has started to briskly walk around his neighborhood for approximately 30 minutes three times weekly. He has lost 4 lbs (1.8 kg) since his last appointment. According to current minimum recommendations, what goal should be set regarding his 30-minute exercise sessions?

A. Increase to daily sessions
B. **Increase to 5 sessions weekly**
C. Change from walking to jogging
D. Set a goal in terms of miles, not minutes
E. No changes necessary

(B) This patient is making significant initial progress in his lifestyle changes. Per recommendations by many entities, aerobic physical activity should be prescribed to patients who carry a diagnosis of overweight or obesity. **The minimum goal should be ≥ 150 min/week of moderate-intensity exercise, performed during 3-5 sessions per week.**

Other essential recommendations regarding exercise are as follows:

- Resistance training should be prescribed to those undergoing weight-loss therapy to promote fat loss while preserving fat-free mass (goal 2-3x weekly).
- To reduce a sedentary lifestyle, encourage increasing non-exercise and active leisure activities.
- Exercise should be individualized based on patient capabilities and preferences, considering physical limitations.

Note: Higher levels of physical activity (200-300 minutes/week) are recommended to prevent weight regain in the long term (> 1 year).

Reference: AACE/ACE Guidelines: AMERICAN ASSOCIATION OF CLINICAL ENDOCRINOLOGISTS AND AMERICAN COLLEGE OF ENDOCRINOLOGY COMPREHENSIVE CLINICAL PRACTICE GUIDELINES FOR MEDICAL CARE OF PATIENTS WITH OBESITY (2016): Recommendation 67- 70

78. (Content: II-B-5) A 16-year-old female presents to her family practitioner at the request of her mother after being found to be self-inducing vomiting. The patient states this is something she has done for the past few months, most often after she eats more than she intends to, saying it helps with the guilt. She is active in sports, has several close friends, and is getting good grades. Given the underlying diagnosis, which of the following abnormalities is most likely to develop in this patient if left untreated?

A. Anion gap metabolic acidosis
B. Shortened corrected QT interval
C. **Mallory-Weiss tear**
D. Melanosis coli
E. Keratoconjunctivitis sicca

(C) This patient is presenting with concerning findings for bulimia nervosa, a predominantly female eating disorder that can lead to esophageal tears **(i.e., Mallory-Weiss tears),** melanosis coli (if laxative-induced), fluid and electrolyte disturbances (metabolic alkalosis in the setting of emesis), arrhythmias, dental erosions, swollen salivary/parotid glands, and loss of the gag reflex.

The diagnosis criteria for bulimia nervosa is summarized below.

Diagnostic Criteria for Bulimia Nervosa
Recurrent episodes of binge eating characterized by BOTH: • Eating in a discrete amount of time an amount of food that is larger than most would eat during a similar time/circumstance   • Sense of lack of control over eating during an episode
Recurrent inappropriate compensatory behaviors, such as: • Self-induced vomiting   • Misuse of laxatives, diuretics, enemas, or other medications   • Fasting or excessive exercise
Binge eating/compensatory behavior occurs once weekly x 3 months
Self-evaluation is unduly influenced by body shape and weight
The disturbance does not occur exclusively during episodes of anorexia nervosa.

Reference: DSM-5: Diagnostic and Statistical Manual of Mental Disorders, Fifth Edition

79. (Content: II-D-3b) A 26-year-old female is presenting to her family practitioner for an infertility evaluation. She states that although she has unprotected sex approximately three times weekly, she has not become pregnant for the past two years. She says she averages one heavy menstrual cycle every three months. Her BMI is 34 kg/m². Physical examination reveals facial hair stubble. Pelvic examination is unremarkable; however, clitoromegaly is noted. An ovarian ultrasound is unrevealing. Given these findings, which lab test would most likely be present?

A. **Increased luteinizing hormone**
B. Decreased free thyroxine levels
C. Decreased androgen levels
D. Elevated cortisol levels
E. Elevated vitamin D (25-OH) levels

(A) This patient who has findings of hirsutism and virilization (clitoromegaly) with amenorrhea meets the criteria for the diagnosis of polycystic ovarian syndrome (PCOS), the most common endocrine disorder in women (affecting 10%). This condition is an imbalance of hormones characterized by **an increased luteinizing hormone (LH): follicular stimulating hormone (FSH) ratio** and increased androgens.

Notably, nearly 50% of women with PCOS have insulin resistance and are affected by excess weight/obesity. Metformin and anti-obesity medications are effective treatment options for weight and insulin resistance.

Rotterdam Consensus states patients must meet 2 of the 3 for diagnosis:

- Hyperandrogenism (biochemical or clinical)
- Menstrual irregularities (anovulation)
- Polycystic ovaries by ultrasound

Note: A 5-10% decrease in weight increases the chance of ovulation and fertility. It is essential to discuss this with patients.

Reference: Up to Date: "Diagnosis of polycystic ovary syndrome in adults"

80. (Content: II-B-3) A 45-year-old female presents to her internist with concerns of bleeding within her mouth. She states that she has been utterly frustrated with her weight and has decided to go on an "extreme diet" for the past three months. She has been consuming water and only small amounts of protein and carbohydrates. She lost nearly 45 lbs (20.4 kg) during this time. A physical exam shows dried blood on her gums and spiral hair on her arms. Given her most likely deficiency, which of the following is a potential complication?

A. Peripheral neuropathy
B. Hallucinations
C. High-output cardiac failure
D. Dermatitis
E. **Poor wound healing**

(E) Vitamin deficiencies are common after malabsorptive procedures but can also be seen in extreme dieting. Given this patient's lack of fruits or vegetables in her diet, gum disease, and spiral hairs (corkscrew hairs), she has most likely developed scurvy due to severe vitamin C deficiency. Symptoms include anemia, perifollicular microhemorrhages, and weakness. Also, **poor wound healing** can occur as vitamin C is involved in the hydroxylation of collagen.

In addition to poor dietary intake of fruits and vegetables, overcooking these sources of vitamin C can also result in a deficiency. Vitamin C deficiency may also lead to the following:

- Petechia[1]
- Ecchymosis[1]
- Bleeding gums
- Dry skin

[1]Also consider vitamin K deficiency with these findings

Another life-threatening concern in those who are malnourished is refeeding syndrome. This occurs in the setting of prolonged malnutrition leading to depleted phosphate storage. If provided nutrition, especially high carbohydrate loads, insulin release causes phosphate to shift intracellularly. Because phosphate is used for energy in the form of ATP, muscle weakness (including cardiac and diaphragm) and fatal arrythmias can occur.

Reference: Léger D. Scurvy: reemergence of nutritional deficiencies. Can Fam Physician. 2008;54(10):1403–1406.

81. (Content: II-D-3a) A 63-year-old female presents to her primary care office for a routine evaluation. Her lab results reveal a TSH level of 11.1 mU/L (reference range: 0.4-4.5 mU/L) with a normal T4 level. She had similar lab values two months prior, completed for insurance screening purposes. She feels well overall and denies fatigue, constipation, or cold intolerance. Which of the following would be the next best step?

A. Start levothyroxine if the patient begins having symptoms
B. Order thyroid peroxidase antibodies levels
C. **Initiate weight-based synthetic thyroxine replacement**
D. Repeat TSH, T3, and T4 levels in 3 months
E. Discuss desiccated thyroid replacement therapy

(C) This patient is presenting with subclinical hypothyroidism, defined as an elevated thyroid stimulating hormone (TSH) with normal thyroid hormone levels (T4). TSH levels ≥ 10 mU/L are an indication to **initiate weight-based levothyroxine** regardless of symptoms. Importantly, desiccated thyroid should not be used for the treatment of hypothyroidism as dosages vary and contain active (T3) hormone in significant amounts.

Note: T3 is generally not tested in patients with hypothyroidism. Even in profound hypothyroidism, T3 levels can be normal.

Subclinical hypothyroidism is common, affecting approximately 5-10% of the general population and 1 out of 5 women older than age 60. Treating with thyroid replacement is indicated in the following situations:

- Primary hypothyroidism (elevated TSH with decreased T4)
- Central hypothyroidism (decreased or inappropriately normal TSH in the setting of decreased T4)
- Asymptomatic subclinical hypothyroidism with a TSH ≥ 10 mU/L
- Subclinical hypothyroidism with a TSH 4.5-10 mU/L with symptoms (cold intolerance, etc.). Treating in this TSH range if asymptomatic is controversial and, therefore, not testable.

Reference: Hossein Gharib, R. Michael Tuttle, H. Jack Baskin, Lisa H. Fish, Peter A. Singer, Michael T. McDermott, Subclinical Thyroid Dysfunction: A Joint Statement on Management from the American Association of Clinical Endocrinologists, the American Thyroid Association, and The Endocrine Society, The Journal of Clinical Endocrinology & Metabolism, Volume 90, Issue 1, 1 January 2005, Pages 581–585, https://doi.org/10.1210/jc.2004-1231

82. (Content: II-C-3) A 27-year-old male presents to a new primary care physician's office for evaluation of fatigue. He has not been seen by a physician "since high school," as he has felt well and has not been seriously ill. He denies alcohol or tobacco use and states that he tries to avoid fast-food. Vital signs are within normal limits, besides a BMI of 28 kg/m². Physical examination reveals hyperpigmented skin in his axillary folds and the nape of his neck. Other physical exam findings are unremarkable. A cholesterol panel reveals total cholesterol to be 220 mg/dL (reference range < 200 mg/dL), and an HbA1c of 6.0% (reference range: < 5.7%). What other physical examination finding is most likely present?

    A. Xanthoma
    B. Easy bruising
    C. Acrochordons
    D. Dry skin
    E. Corkscrew hairs

(C) This patient presenting with an elevated hemoglobin A1c within the prediabetic range and acanthosis nigricans (hyperpigmentation of the neck, axilla, or groin), has findings consistent with insulin resistance. Other findings associated with insulin resistance include **acrochordons (skin tags)**.

Skin findings associated with obesity are discussed below:

Skin Findings Associated with Obesity-Related Conditions	
Exam Findings	**Associated Condition**
Acanthosis nigricans and skin tags	Insulin resistance/diabetes
Acne	Polycystic ovarian syndrome and Cushing's syndrome/disease
Xanthelasmas or xanthomas	Hyperlipidemia (very elevated)
Moon facies, buffalo-hump, wide-based striae, easy bruising, facial plethora	Cushing's syndrome/disease
Dry and cracked skin, thinning of eyebrows, periorbital edema	Hypothyroidism

Reference: Up to Date: "Overweight and obesity in adults: Health consequences"

83. (Content: II-C-7) A mother brings her child to the pediatrician for his 18-month well-child exam. He has met all of his age-appropriate milestones, including starting to walk at 12 months old. She states that he has gained more "rolls" in the arms and legs and seems to be gaining weight faster than she recalls of her other children. Which would be the most accurate way to track this patient's weight parameters?

A. Weight-for-height
B. Body mass index
C. Age-adjusted growth
D. Weight-for-length
E. CDC growth charts

(D) Weight assessment in those under 2 years old is done by evaluating **weight-for-length** using the World Health Organization charts, taking into account gender and age. The body mass index percentile is not used until two years of age.

Growth charts are available from 2 different organizations:

- **Centers for Disease Control and Prevention (CDC):** These charts are based on a cohort of primarily non-breastfed, Caucasian American children. The CDC chart cohort data was unavailable for the first three months of age, and the sample sizes were limited for sex and age for the first six months, limiting its utility in those under 2 years of age.
- **World Health Organization (WHO):** This is based on cohorts from more diverse ethnic backgrounds, predominantly breastfed children. These children were breastfed for at least four months, with most still breastfeeding at 12 months.

The recommendations from the CDC are to use the WHO growth standards for infants 0-2 years of age and the CDC growth charts thereafter. The WHO charts more accurately reflect the recommended standards for infant feeding in the early population.

Reference: https://www.cdc.gov/growthcharts/who_charts.htm

84. (Content: II-E and II-A-3) A 46-year-old male with a BMI of 38 kg/m² presents for follow-up regarding his diabetes. He is being treated with metformin and empagliflozin; his last HbA1c was 6.8%. He has mild knee pain with prolonged exercise but otherwise feels well. According to the Edmonton Obesity Staging System, he would be classified as which of the following?

A. Stage 0
B. Stage 1
C. **Stage 2**
D. Stage 3
E. Stage 4

(C) The Edmonton Obesity Staging System (EOSS) is a tool that considers comorbidity and functional limitations to better determine obesity cardiometabolic risks and treatment aggressiveness compared to anthropometric-based categorization alone. A patient with a BMI of 38 kg/m² (class 2 obesity) with diabetes would be classified as **EOSS stage 2.**

A patient that meets the criteria for obesity but has no risk factors, symptoms, or functional limitations would be EOSS stage 0. The other stages are below:

EOSS Staging System	
Stage 1	**Stage 2**
Subclinical risk factors with **mild** symptoms such as borderline hypertension, pre-diabetes, or mild osteoarthritis	Established comorbidities requiring medical treatment with **moderate** symptoms such as depression, HTN, T2DM, GERD, OSA, and HLD
Stage 3	**Stage 4**
Significant obesity-related comorbidities with **significant** limitations, end-organ damage, or impairment, such as myocardial infarction, suicidal ideation, reduced mobility, stroke, and diabetic complications	**Severe** (i.e., end-stage) disabling symptoms and limitations such as wheelchair or bed-bound, pulmonary hypertension from OHS, end-stage renal disease from DM nephropathy, and decompensated cirrhosis from MAFLD

Reference: Using the Edmonton obesity staging system to predict mortality in a population-representative cohort of people with overweight and obesity. Raj S. Padwal, Nicholas M. Pajewski, David B. Allison and Arya M. Sharma. CMAJ October 04, 2011 183 (14) E1059-E1066; DOI: https://doi.org/10.1503/cmaj.110387

85. (Content: II-B-4) A 21-year-old male with a past medical history of depression and obesity presents to a dietician for a nutrition evaluation. He states that he has overeaten at night for as long as he can remember. He admits to craving sweets and even sometimes wakes up throughout the night to get a snack. Given his most likely underlying diagnosis, which of the following findings is likely to be seen in this patient?

    A. Daytime fatigue
    B. Excessive daily protein intake
    C. Pica
    D. Frequent daytime grazing
    E. Morning anorexia

(E) This patient's history is most consistent with the diagnosis of night eating syndrome (NES), a condition seen in 1.5% of the general population and approximately 30% of those seeking bariatric surgery. NES is classically characterized by the triad of **morning anorexia**, evening hyperphagia, and insomnia. It is also associated with the following:

- Nocturnal awakening and food consumption
- Increased carbohydrate-to-protein ratio (7:1)
- Consumption of 25-50% of daily calories after the evening meal

NES is commonly associated with those with low self-esteem or self-image, depression, and those with increased perceived stress.

Treatment for NES is focused on encouraging regular meal consumption earlier in the daytime, with increased protein intake being very effective. Cognitive-behavioral therapy can help with many eating disorders, including NES. Pharmacotherapy may be considered, including selective serotonin reuptake inhibitors, with a very high response rate to sertraline.

Reference: Allison KC, Tarves EP. Treatment of night eating syndrome. Psychiatr Clin North Am. 2011;34(4):785–796. doi:10.1016/j.psc.2011.08.002

86. (Content: II-D-1) An electrophysiology study is being performed, which evaluates the resting metabolic rate of individual organs in an average person without excess body weight. A radiotracer is injected into a patient who is lying still, and a subsequent body scan is performed. The tissue with the highest metabolic rate displays the brightest on body scan imaging, with quantitative data extrapolated. Based on this scan, which of the following tissue would most likely display the brightest on imaging?

    A. Kidneys
    B. Heart
    C. Digestive system
    D. Liver
    E. Fat

(D) Resting metabolic rate (RMR) refers to energy expended at rest and accounts for 70% of total daily expenditure. Of the components that make up RMR, **skeletal muscle and the liver** comprise the most substantial portion, accounting for 20% of RMR each.

Note: Basal metabolic rate (BMR) is similar to RMR, but requires the individual to be fasting, resting, and supine in a thermoneutral environment. Thus, RMR is more frequently used due to its ease of obtainability with indirect calorimetry. Both BMR and RMR are increased in the setting of excess weight.

Total energy expenditure is made up of resting metabolic rate (RMR), physical activity (PA), and dietary thermogenesis, with contributions of 70%, 20%, and 10%, respectively, for each component.

Note: RMR = 1 metabolic equivalent of task (MET).

Resting Metabolic Rate by Organ System			
Organ	Component	Organ	Component
Skeletal muscle	20%	Digestive system	10%
Liver	20%	Kidneys	5%
Brain	15%	Fat	5%
Heart	10%	Remaining	15%

Reference: Reference: Obesity medicine association: Obesity Algorithm (2021)

87. (Content: II-A-4) A 33-year-old male presents to his family practice physician at his wife's request for "sleep-eating." He states that his wife has caught him multiple times in the middle of the night eating large amounts of food before returning to bed. He has no recollection of this in the morning but has noticed that he has consistently been gaining weight, despite a relatively healthy diet and exercise. He does admit to working rotating shifts. Given this history, which medication is this patient most likely taking?

A. Diphenhydramine
B. Eszopiclone
C. Ramelteon
D. Trazodone
E. Ginkgo biloba

(B) This patient is experiencing a sleep-related eating disorder, a misnomer as it is not an actual eating disorder but rather a parasomnia. Patients taking sedatives such as **eszopiclone (Lunesta®)** are most likely to experience this.

Sleep-related eating disorder (SRED) is a variant of sleepwalking, affecting approximately 3% of the general population. It most commonly occurs in the first one-third of the sleep period.

Its associations are listed below:

- Occurs with increased frequency in those with high stress
- The majority (80%) have associated restless leg syndrome (RLS), periodic limb movement disorder (PLMD), obstructive sleep apnea (OSA), or somnambulism.
- Medications correlating with incidence are sedative-hypnotics, such as antipsychotics and psychotropic medications.

Treatment is targeted at removing the offending agent and treating any underlying associated disorders (RLS, OSA, PLMD). Topiramate, SSRIs, and trazodone also have some efficacy in treatment.

Reference: Up To Date: "Disorders of arousal from non-rapid eye movement sleep in adults"

88. (Content: II-D-3a) A 51-year-old female is undergoing a preoperative evaluation for a planned Roux-en-Y gastric bypass. She admits to often feeling tired during the day, occasionally falling asleep during conversations. Her spouse has told her that she snores very loudly, sometimes requiring him to sleep in another bedroom. Vital signs are within normal limits. BMI is 39 kg/m^2, and her neck circumference is 17 inches (43.2 cm). What is the next best step in evaluating for obstructive sleep apnea?

    A. Inquire if she has stopped breathing during sleep
    B. Place a referral for an overnight pulse-oximetry test
    C. Place a referral for polysomnography
    D. Perform a physical exam, focusing on the oral exam
    E. Order a daytime arterial blood gas

(C) This patient meets the criteria for a positive screening for obstructive sleep apnea (OSA) via the "STOP-BANG" questionnaire. She scored 5 points (snores, fatigued, increased body mass index, neck circumference, and age), placing her at high risk and warranting further evaluation with **polysomnography**.

The STOP-BANG screening tool was validated in preoperative evaluation, with a score ≤ 2 adequately excluding a diagnosis of OSA, whereas a score of ≥ 5 makes OSA highly likely (specificity 80%).

STOP-BANG Score (1 point for each positive)			
S	Snore loudly	B	BMI ≥ 35 kg/m^2
T	Tiredness (daytime fatigue)	A	Age > 50 years old
O	Observed apnea	N	Neck circumference > 40 cm
P	Pressure (elevated BP)	G	Gender: Male
Risk: Low (0-2), Intermediate (3-4), High[1] (5-8)			

[1]Some recommendations state that ≥ 3 is considered high risk and warrants further evaluation

Note: Another clinical pretest probability scoring system that may be used for OSA is the Epworth Sleepiness Scale, which includes a series of questions about the likelihood of them falling asleep during certain activities throughout the day.

Reference: AACE/ACE Guidelines: AMERICAN ASSOCIATION OF CLINICAL ENDOCRINOLOGISTS AND AMERICAN COLLEGE OF ENDOCRINOLOGY COMPREHENSIVE CLINICAL PRACTICE GUIDELINES FOR MEDICAL CARE OF PATIENTS WITH OBESITY (2016). Recommendation 21.

89. (Content: II-A-1) A 17-year-old female presents to her family medicine doctor for a sports physical. She has no prior medical history, although she feels more fatigued than average. Vital signs reveal a heart rate of 60 BPM and a BMI of 22 kg/m². A physical exam reveals parotid gland enlargement and scrapes over the dorsum of her second metacarpal phalangeal joint. She is elusive when asked questions about her eating habits. Which medications is contraindicated given her most likely underlying diagnosis?

    A. Trazodone
    B. Bupropion
    C. Topiramate
    D. Sertraline
    E. Buspirone

(B) This patient presents with findings of Russell's sign (callouses or cuts on the knuckles due to repetitive self-induced vomiting) and parotid gland enlargement. In the setting of a normal BMI, this is concerning for the diagnosis of bulimia nervosa. **Bupropion is contraindicated in eating disorders**, epilepsy, or other conditions that lower the seizure threshold.

Bulimia affects up to 10% of women over their lifetime, with 16-22 years old being the most common age group affected. The vast majority are females (90%), often with a concurrent mood disorder or history of abuse, especially sexual abuse (25%).

Treatment options for bulimia nervosa should include nutritional rehabilitation and cognitive behavioral therapy. Often these are combined with medications for a synergistic effect. Fluoxetine is FDA-approved for bulimia nervosa, whereas other SSRIs, such as sertraline, are effective but used off-label.

90. (Content: II-B-5) A 29-year-old male presents to an internist to establish care. His chief concern is related to his lack of upper body strength, in particular the muscle size. He states despite working out his arms for nearly 3 hours daily, his arms still appear smaller than he would like. He has difficulty focusing on his work as a car salesman, as he feels people notice his arms and admits to being very self-conscious. A physical exam reveals a healthy, muscular-appearing male in no distress. If inquired, the patient most likely would admit to experiencing which of the following?

A. **Compulsive behaviors**
B. Anxiety attacks
C. Severe calorie restriction
D. Nocturnal eating
E. Delayed sleep onset

(A) This patient's preoccupation with his appearance (i.e., arm size) is consistent with the diagnosis of body dysmorphic disorder with muscle dysmorphia. This condition is closely related (and treated similarly) to **obsessive-compulsive disorders**.

Body dissatisfaction responds well to cognitive behavioral therapy, whereas medications (SSRIs, topiramate, lamotrigine) are used off-label.

Diagnostic Criteria for Body Dysmorphic Disorder
Preoccupation with ≥ 1 flaw in physical appearance that is not observable or appears slight to others.
Performed repetitive behaviors: • Mirror checking • Excessive grooming • Skin picking • Reassurance seeking • Compares his/her appearance with others
Preoccupation causes distress/impairment in areas of functioning
Preoccupation is not better explained by another eating disorder

Reference: DSM-5: Diagnostic and Statistical Manual of Mental Disorders, Fifth Edition

91. (Content: II-D-3b) A university is conducting a research study. The primary objective is to correlate quantitative sex hormone binding globulin (SHBG)) levels with different patient characteristics. In particular, age, weight, and comorbid conditions such as polycystic ovarian syndrome (PCOS) are analyzed. Which of the following patients would have an increased SHBG level compared to their comparative matched cohort?

A. A patient with a BMI of 45 kg/m^2
B. A female with a diagnosis of PCOS
C. A younger individual
D. A male with decreased total testosterone
E. **A patient six months status post gastric bypass**

(E) Sex hormone binding globulin directly correlates with several conditions, including comorbidities of excess weight. Older patients and those who have lost weight (**through bariatric surgery** or other means) have higher levels of SHBG compared to younger patients or those with a similar BMI who have not lost weight.

Correlations between patient characteristics/comorbidities and corresponding SHBG levels should be understood, as discussed below:

- SHBG is decreased in patients with obesity. However, with weight loss, these levels will increase.
- Patients with PCOS have decreased SHBG levels due to the increased levels of insulin inhibiting hepatic SHBG production.
- Males with obesity have decreased total testosterone levels due to decreased SHBG, although free testosterone is similar amongst variations in BMI in the absence of other conditions.
- SHBG increases proportionally with age.

Reference: Zhu JL, Chen Z, Feng WJ, Long SL, Mo ZC. Sex hormone-binding globulin and polycystic ovary syndrome. Clin Chim Acta. 2019 Dec;499:142-148. doi: 10.1016/j.cca.2019.09.010. Epub 2019 Sep 13. PMID: 31525346.
Reference: Cooper LA, Page ST, Amory JK, Anawalt BD, Matsumoto AM. The association of obesity with sex hormone-binding globulin is stronger than the association with ageing--implications for the interpretation of total testosterone measurements. Clin Endocrinol (Oxf). 2015 Dec;83(6):828-33. doi: 10.1111/cen.12768. Epub 2015 May 11. PMID: 25777143; PMCID: PMC4782930.

92. (Content: II-C-1 and 5) A pediatrician is evaluating a young patient in the office and determines that the body mass index charts utilized for most children in her practice is inadequate for this patient, and a specialized BMI chart is utilized. The patient most likely has which of the following findings on physical examination?

    A. Bicuspid aorta
    B. Macrocephaly
    C. Macroglossia
    D. Ovarian agenesis
    E. Upslanting palpebral fissures

(B) Certain populations have unique pediatric BMI curves, including patients with achondroplasia, which presents with short stature, brachydactyly, **macrocephaly,** and frontal bossing.

Notably, although patients with Down syndrome (presenting with macroglossia and upslanting palpebral fissures) have an increased risk of obesity and use different charts for weight and height, the BMI guidelines from the CDC recommend using charts for normally developing children. This is recommended to provide early detection of excess weight in order to incorporate earlier intervention.

In addition, those with Turner's syndrome (with physical examination findings displaying ovarian agenesis and having a correlation with a bicuspid aorta) commonly have abnormal glucose metabolism and a higher prevalence of diabetes mellitus. Although there are unique BMI charts for this population, they are very specific to locality (i.e., Turkey and Japan) and are not universally accepted by the CDC.

Note: All of the above conditions have associations with shorter stature and increased weight, as well as complications including obstructive sleep apnea, cardiovascular disease, and potentially early-onset impaired motility.

Reference: Up to Date: "Achondroplasia"
Reference: Obesity medicine association: Pediatric Obesity Algorithm (2020-2022)

93. (Content II-C-1) A 41-year-old Caucasian male presents to his primary care physician for an annual health screen. His immunizations are up to date. A recent diabetes and hypertension screening completed through work were within normal limits. His height is 70 inches (178 cm), and his weight is 260 lbs (117 kg). By utilizing the chart below, his weight would best be described as being in which of the following categories?

BMI	28	29	30	31	32	33	34	35	36	37	38	39	40	41	42	43	44	45	46
5'4"	163	169	174	180	186	192	197	204	209	215	221	227	232	238	244	250	256	262	267
5'5"	168	174	180	186	192	198	204	210	216	222	228	234	240	246	252	258	264	270	276
5'6"	173	179	186	192	198	204	210	216	223	229	235	241	247	253	260	266	272	278	284
5'7"	178	185	191	198	204	211	217	223	230	236	242	249	255	261	268	274	280	287	293
5'8"	184	190	197	203	210	216	223	230	236	243	249	256	262	269	276	282	289	295	302
5'9"	189	196	203	209	216	223	230	236	243	250	257	263	270	277	284	291	297	304	311
5'10"	195	202	209	216	222	229	236	243	250	257	264	271	278	285	292	299	306	313	320
5'11"	200	208	215	222	229	236	243	250	257	265	272	279	286	293	301	308	315	322	329

(Note: Weight is in pounds)

A. Normal weight
B. Overweight
C. Class I obesity
D. **Class II obesity**
E. Class III obesity

(D) This patient has a body mass index of 37.3 kg/m^2, placing him in the range of **class II obesity.** The classification of weight based on BMI includes:

Classification of BMI			
Classification	BMI (kg/m^2)	Classification	BMI (kg/m^2)
Underweight	< 18.5	Class I obesity	30-34.9
Normal weight	18.5- 24.9	Class II obesity	35-39.9
Overweight	25-29.9	Class III obesity	≥ 40

Reference: AACE/ACE Guidelines: AMERICAN ASSOCIATION OF CLINICAL ENDOCRINOLOGISTS AND AMERICAN COLLEGE OF ENDOCRINOLOGY COMPREHENSIVE CLINICAL PRACTICE GUIDELINES FOR MEDICAL CARE OF PATIENTS WITH OBESITY (2016)

94. (Content: II-D-3a) A 49-year-old female with a history of severe obesity is following-up with her pulmonologist regarding her pulmonary hypertension, confirmed with a right-heart catheterization. She has no prior tobacco or occupational exposures, and her polysomnography test was negative. Given this information, which of the following would most likely be seen in this patient?

A. Class 4 Mallampati score
B. Increased Epworth sleepiness scale
C. FVC/FEV$_1$ < 0.70
D. Increased respiratory disturbance index
E. **Arterial blood gas PaCO$_2$ > 45 mmHg**

(E) This patient is presenting with pulmonary hypertension in the setting of severe obesity, with obstructive sleep apnea (OSA) ruled out through polysomnography (the gold standard). Given this, the next most likely diagnosis is obesity hypoventilation syndrome, which requires **an increased carbon dioxide level** on a daytime arterial blood gas for diagnosis.

Obesity hypoventilation syndrome (OHS), also referred to as Pickwickian syndrome, is a restrictive lung disease that carries high mortality rates. Although 90% have concurrent OSA, it can occur independently. It is associated with pulmonary hypertension and right-sided heart failure.

Diagnostic criteria include:

- Obesity (body mass index > 30 kg/m^2)
- PaCO$_2$ > 45 mmHg
- Exclusion of other causes

First-line treatment is non-invasive positive airway pressure, whereas definitive treatment focuses on weight loss.

Reference: Up to Date: "Treatment and prognosis of the obesity hypoventilation syndrome"

95. (Content: II-D-3) A mother brings her previously healthy 10-year-old daughter to her family medicine physician for an annual examination. The patient has been spending more time on the computer and watching television, with decreased physical activity. Her weight has steadily increased. Her body mass index is in the 86th percentile for age and gender. The patient denies any symptoms or concerns, including fatigue, polyuria, or hirsutism. Given this, which test should be ordered for screening purposes?

A. **Fasting lipid profile**
B. Aspartate aminotransferase
C. Fasting glucose
D. Creatinine
E. Thyroid-stimulating hormone

(A) The Expert Committee provides laboratory screening tests that should be considered in children with overweight or obesity. In this patient in the overweight category without risk factors[1], only **a fasting lipid panel** is recommended. Laboratory work to obtain based on recommendations is listed below.

- **BMI 85th- 94th percentile (no risk factors[1]):** Fasting lipid panel
- **BMI 85th- 94th percentile (risk factors[1]):** Add AST, ALT, and fasting glucose
- **BMI ≥ 95th percentile:** All of the above, in addition to BUN and creatinine

In children with obesity, nearly 1/3 will have fatty liver disease, with ALT being the best initial screening test. Although a liver biopsy is considered the gold standard for confirmation, more commonly, imaging is utilized (ultrasound, MRI, transient elastography, etc.). Initial treatment includes intense lifestyle modifications, including diet, exercise, and elimination of sugary drinks, in addition to further evaluation by a subspecialist.

[1]Risk factors include prediabetes/diabetes, hyperlipidemia, sleep apnea, central adiposity, or family history of metabolic accociated fatty liver disease.

Reference: Expert Committee Recommendations Regarding the Prevention, Assessment, and Treatment of Child and Adolescent Overweight and Obesity: Summary Report and APPENDIX. Sarah E. Barlow and the Expert Committee; Pediatrics December 2007, 120 (Supplement 4) S164-S192; DOI: https://doi.org/10.1542/peds.2007-2329C.

96. (Content: II-C-3 and 5) After injuring his finger, a 6-year-old male with class III obesity presents to the emergency department. The mother states that the child was trying to swing at a local park when his finger became stuck in the chain. The patient has full range of motion but increased swelling of his third digit. An x-ray is shown below. Which other finding is most likely?

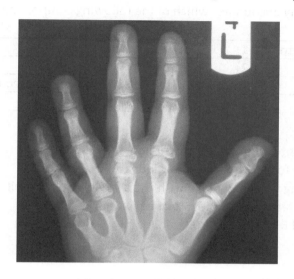

A. **Pseudohypoparathyroidism**
B. History of seizures
C. Almond-shaped eyes
D. Microorchidism

(A) This patient presents with early-onset obesity and shortened 4th and 5th digits (as seen on the hand x-ray) and likely carries the diagnosis of Albright Hereditary Osteodystrophy. This condition is characterized by a shorter stature, round facies, shortened fourth and fifth metacarpals, intellectual disability, impaired olfaction, and **pseudohypoparathyroidism.**

Pseudohypoparathyroidism is characterized by renal resistance to parathyroid hormone (PTH), leading to hypocalcemia, hyperphosphatemia, and elevated PTH levels.

Image Reference: Hasani-Ranjbar S, Jouyandeh Z, Amoli MM, Soltani A, Arzaghi SM. A patient with features of albright hereditory osteodystrophy and unusual neuropsychiatric findings without coding Gsalpha mutations. *J Diabetes Metab Disord*. 2014;13:56. Published 2014 May 22. doi:10.1186/2251-6581-13-56
Reference: Obesity medicine association: Obesity Algorithm (2021)

97. (Content: III-B-1) A 44-year-old female presents to her primary care physician with dysuria and malodorous urine. She denies abdominal pain. She has type 2 diabetes and was recently started on a medication to help with weight loss and diabetes control. In addition, she initiated a new diet this week. Her urinalysis dipstick results are below. Given these findings, the diet she has started most likely encourages which of the following components?

Leukocyte	1+	Specific gravity	1.011
Nitrite	2+	Ketone	2+
Protein	Trace	Bilirubin	Not detected
Blood	1+	Glucose	3+

A. **Significant carbohydrate restriction**
B. Avoiding foods with a glycemic index > 70
C. Increasing omega-3 intake with extra virgin vegetable oil
D. Limiting fat intake to 20-25% of daily calories
E. Intake of 5 servings of fruit minimum

(A) A ketogenic diet **significantly restricts carbohydrate** intake, promoting fat for energy and thus placing the patient in a ketotic state. Therefore, her diet is the most likely cause of ketones in her urine. The patient's recent introduction of an SGLT-2 inhibitor may increase her risk of urinary tract infections, cause glucosuria, and may even cause euvolemic diabetic ketoacidosis. However, she has no other symptoms (nausea, abdominal pain, etc.) to indicate ketoacidosis as her cause of ketosis.

The key points of the ketogenic diet are listed below:

- Carbohydrates are generally reduced to 60-90 grams daily in a ketogenic diet. Some may do an initial induction phase (20 g daily).
- A ketogenic and the Atkin's diet are examples of carbohydrate-restrictive diets (< 45% calories from carbs).
- Fruits, dairy, carbohydrates, and starchy vegetables are restricted.

Note: Extreme caution should be used if a patient is starting a ketogenic diet and is currently taking an SGLT-2 inhibitor due to the risk of ketoacidosis. Insulin should also be decreased, with hypoglycemic education provided.

Reference: Obesity medicine association: Obesity Algorithm (2021)

98. (Content: III-G-4) A 14-year-old male presents for his annual checkup at his pediatrician's clinic. He has no prior medical history. His BMI is 31 kg/m². The pediatrician discusses healthy eating choices, exercise, and lifestyle changes to prevent weight-related complications. This discussion is an example of which of the following phases of prevention in chronic obesity?

    A. Primary prevention
    B. Secondary prevention
    C. Tertiary prevention

(B) This pediatrician is trying to prevent future weight gain, as well as weight-related complications of obesity, in a patient that _already_ meets obesity criteria, meeting the definition of **secondary prevention.**

The three phases of chronic disease prevention apply to obesity, which guides the intensity and modality of disease intervention.

- **Primary prevention:** Prevent the development of overweight and obesity through education, environment, and promoting healthy eating and regular physical exercise.

- **Secondary prevention:** Prevent future weight gain and the development of weight-related complications in patients with excess weight or obesity by initiating lifestyle and behavioral intervention (+/- pharmacologic therapy).

- **Tertiary prevention:** Target weight loss to eliminate or mitigate weight-related complications and prevent disease progression by initiating lifestyle/behavioral interventions, weight-loss medication, and/or potentially considering metabolic surgery.

Reference: AACE/ACE Guidelines: AMERICAN ASSOCIATION OF CLINICAL ENDOCRINOLOGISTS AND AMERICAN COLLEGE OF ENDOCRINOLOGY COMPREHENSIVE CLINICAL PRACTICE GUIDELINES FOR MEDICAL CARE OF PATIENTS WITH OBESITY (2016): Recommendation 2

99. (Content: III-F-2) A patient had a previous bariatric procedure performed ten years ago in which a band was placed around the top of the stomach, creating a small pouch. Although adjustable, the patient has had difficulty following up and thus is interested in a surgical revision. The patient has had three adjustments during the past decade, initially losing 32 lbs (14.5 kg), but has since regained this weight. Which is true of this bariatric procedure?

A. It is considered a malabsorptive procedure
B. **The minimum BMI required for placement is 30 kg/m²**
C. Mortality rate is similar to other bariatric procedures
D. Adjustment requires conscious sedation
E. It is the most common weight loss procedure worldwide

(B) Laparoscopic adjustable gastric banding (LAGB) is a restrictive procedure in which a stomach pouch is created by placing an adjustable band around the upper portion of the stomach ❶, allowing for decreased food intake. Also, the increased pressure on the stomach prolongs the sensation of fullness, thus helping suppress appetite. A subcutaneous port ❷ is available and allows for fluid to be added, allowing for increased restriction. It has the lowest mortality rate and is considered the least invasive surgical option. It is approved in those with a **BMI of 30 kg/m² with an obesity comorbidity.**

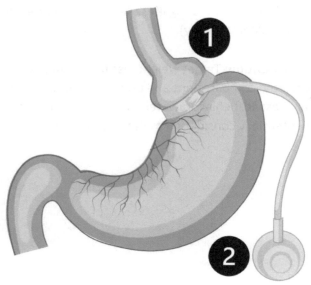

Image citation: Image created by Charu G. Copyright owned by Kevin Smith, DO
Reference: Suter M, Giusti V, Worreth M, Héraief E, Calmes JM. Laparoscopic gastric banding: a prospective, randomized study comparing the Lapband and the SAGB: early results. Ann Surg. 2005;241(1):55-62.
doi:10.1097/01.sla.0000150071.86934.36

100. (Content: III-H-4) A healthy 6-year-old female presents with her father to her primary care physician for an annual exam. She has no prior medical conditions and is up to date on immunizations. Her father has no concerns about her current health but is concerned about preventing weight gain, as her sibling has excess weight. The patient's BMI is in the 50th percentile, with consistent height and weight in the 55th and 60th percentile, respectively. Which of the following is the most appropriate recommendation for this child?

    A. Consume 3 or more fruits and vegetables daily
    B. Minimize screen time to < 3 hours daily
    C. Allow the child to self-regulate meals
    D. Encourage at least 8 hours of sleep nightly
    E. Eat as a family at least 3 times weekly

(C) This patient with a healthy weight is encouraged to maintain healthy eating and lifestyle choices to continue her current projectile (i.e., prevention). There is consistent evidence that allowing children under 12 years old **to self-regulate their meal quantities**, in contrast to promoting restrictive feeding behaviors, is preferred and leads to better weight outcomes. Importantly, this self-regulating applies to meals, not snacking.

In addition to the above recommendation, healthy lifestyle habits for children include healthy eating and decreasing sedentary time, as discussed below:

- Limit screen time to 2 hours daily
- Encourage sleeping ≥ 9 hours nightly
- Intake ≥ 5 servings of fruits and vegetables daily
- Minimize or eliminate (preferred) sugar-sweetened beverages
- Prepare meals at home when possible
- Eat at the table with family ≥ 5 times weekly
- Consume a healthy breakfast every morning
- Perform at least 60 minutes of physical activity daily

Reference: Expert Committee Recommendations Regarding the Prevention, Assessment, and Treatment of Child and Adolescent Overweight and Obesity: Summary Report.. Sarah E. Barlow and the Expert Committee; Pediatrics December 2007, 120 (Supplement 4) S164-S192; DOI: https://doi.org/10.1542/peds.2007-2329C.

101. (Content: III-F-4) A 53-year-old male is presenting for evaluation for weight loss. He has started the bridge-to-transplant program, which requires a BMI of 35 kg/m² or less in order to be listed on the kidney transplant list. His current BMI is 44 kg/m². Both medication and surgical options are discussed. He prefers to undergo bariatric and metabolic surgery. Which of the following surgical options is most preferred?

A. Single anastomosis duodeno-ileal bypass
B. Roux-en-Y gastric bypass
C. **Vertical sleeve gastrectomy**
D. Gastric balloon
E. Aspiration device

(C) In this patient wishing to undergo a renal transplant, the best choice is a **vertical sleeve gastrectomy (VSG).** Temporary measures such as a gastric balloon may not provide enough time for weight loss and being accepted for a transplant, as they have a maximum duration of 6 months. Other malabsorptive procedures should be avoided in those who will require immunosuppressants, due to absorption issues, and those likely to need frequent steroids, due to the increased risk of anastomotic or marginal ulcers.

Selecting an appropriate surgery will ultimately be up to the surgeon to discuss. However, understanding why specific procedures should be avoided or encouraged is helpful. Other patients who may benefit from VSG include:

- Ill-patients: Patients who are more chronically ill, including those with obesity-related comorbidities such as pulmonary hypertension and heart failure with preserved ejection fraction may benefit from a sleeve gastrectomy due to shorter anesthesia times.
- Recurrent renal stones: Malabsorptive procedures increase oxalate absorption.
- Risk of severe nutritional deficiencies
- Organ transplant patients, including those on chronic immunosuppressants or those requiring critical medications that require adequate absorption.

Reference: Veroux M, Mattone E, Cavallo M, Gioco R, Corona D, Volpicelli A, Veroux P. Obesity and bariatric surgery in kidney transplantation: A clinical review. World J Diabetes. 2021 Sep 15;12(9):1563-1575. doi: 10.4239/wjd.v12.i9.1563. PMID: 34630908; PMCID: PMC8472502.

102. (Content: III-F-2) A 34-year-old male with a past medical history of hypothyroidism presents for an initial evaluation regarding weight-loss surgical options. In particular, he is interested in an aspiration device. He affirms this would work well with his lifestyle, as he works remotely at home. He has good family support and performs daily aerobic physical activity for 30 minutes. He has already begun behavioral therapy, including chewing his food slowly and thoroughly. Which of the following would be a contraindication to this device?

A. **Night eating syndrome**
B. Prior hemicolectomy
C. Gastroesophageal reflux disease
D. Diastolic heart failure
E. Zenker diverticulum

(A) The AspireAssist® aspiration device is FDA approved for long-term weight management in adults aged ≥22 years old with a BMI of 35-55 kg/m². Although this device has similar contraindications as other percutaneous endoscopic gastrostomy tubes, it is also contraindicated in those with eating disorders, including **night eating syndrome,** bulimia, or binge eating disorder.

Note: Ensuring the patient is logistically able to perform the aspiration (schedules, mental capacity, time commitment, etc.) is vital for success.

Aspiration devices are a relatively safe and unique option for weight loss. In the PATHWAY study, excess weight loss of 31.5% was observed at 52 weeks, with ongoing studies following out to 5 years.

Important Contraindications to the AspireAssist® Device	
- Prior abdominal surgeries that ↑ risk of gastrostomy tube placement - Esophageal stricture, obstruction, severe gastroparesis, IBD, GOO - History of refractory gastric ulcers, active ulcers, bleeding, or tumors	- Coagulation disorder or anemia - Pregnant or lactating females - Physical/mental disability or psychological illness that may interfere with adherence - Eating disorders (see above)

IBD: Inflammatory bowel disease; **GOO:** Gastric outlet obstruction

Reference: AspireAssist® Clinician guide
Reference: Aspiration Therapy as a Tool to Treat Obesity: 1- to 4-Year Results in a 201-Patient Multi-Center Post-Market European Registry Study. Nystrom et al. Obesity Surgery. Published online Feb 1 2018.

103. (Content: III-H-1 and III-D-6) A mother brings her 6-year-old daughter, who is in the 95th percentile for weight based on her BMI, to her pediatrician's office due to persistent constipation despite increased water intake. They have been using over-the-counter stool softeners without relief. The mother states that the child is not picky regarding food and eats "whatever is available." The physician recommends increasing whole grains. What effect will this indirectly have on the child?

A. Reduce HDL and triglyceride levels
B. Increase risk of irritable bowel syndrome
C. Increase nutrient-rich food intake
D. Increase saturated fat consumption
E. Diarrhea and potential fecal incontinence

(C) Increased fiber intake (including whole grains) has been shown to have several positive effects in both children and adults, including decreased energy-dense food intake and **increased desire for nutrient-rich foods.**

Fiber is preferred to come from the diet, such as fruits, legumes, whole grains, and vegetables, rather than supplementation when feasible. Fiber has many benefits, including:

- Improving blood glucose levels
- Reducing total cholesterol
- Reducing LDL cholesterol
- Improving satiety
- Decreasing constipation (via stool-bulking)

In addition, psyllium (a water-soluble fiber) has been shown to improve the above parameters and abdominal pain in those with irritable bowel syndrome. It is recommended at 6g/day in those aged 6-12 and 12g/day in those ≥12 years old in combination with low saturated fat to improve lipids and possibly help with weight.

Reference: Expert Panel on Integrated Guidelines for Cardiovascular Health and Risk Reduction in Children and Adolescents Full Report. Published Oct 2012.

104. (Content: III-F-5c) A 57-year-old male presents to the emergency department two weeks after a Roux-en-Y gastric bypass for dehydration, nausea, and vomiting. His spouse has also noted some confusion recently. Vital signs reveal a heart rate of 110/min and a blood pressure of 89/58 mmHg. Physical exam reveals dry mucus membranes, nystagmus, and difficulty walking. He is alert and oriented x 1. Given his most likely nutritional deficiency, what other clinical sequelae may be seen if left untreated?

    A. Macrocytic anemia
    B. Dermatitis (pellagra)
    C. Seizure disorder
    D. Glossitis and cheilitis
    E. Peripheral neuropathy

(E) This patient is presenting in the acute post-bariatric surgery period with significant vomiting, confusion, and nystagmus, consistent with thiamine (B_1) deficiency (Wernicke's encephalopathy), a water-soluble vitamin. B_1 deficiency can cause many symptoms, including **symmetric peripheral polyneuropathy.**

Thiamine deficiency presentations vary by chronicity. Some of the more common presentations are discussed below:

- **Wet beriberi:** High-output congestive heart failure, including cardiomegaly, cardiomyopathy, peripheral edema, and tachycardia
- **Dry beriberi:** Symmetric peripheral polyneuropathy (sensory and motor), primarily affecting the distal extremities
- **Wernicke's encephalopathy:** Ataxia, nystagmus, ophthalmoplegia, and confusion; considered reversible
- **Korsakoff syndrome:** Irreversible, a chronic neurological condition characterized by impaired short-term memory and confabulation

Note: It is imperative to give thiamine before glucose to prevent the risk of precipitating Wernicke's encephalopathy.

Reference: Up to Date: "Overview of water-soluble vitamins"

105. (Content: III-D-2) A 59-year-old male presents to his internist with the desire to start pharmacotherapy for weight loss. The physician is interested in starting a particular combination medication but first inquires about a history of calcium oxalate stones, as this medication should be avoided in those with a history of renal nephrolithiasis. Given the most likely medication eluded to, what is a contraindication of this medicine?

A. Chronic malabsorption syndrome
B. Family history of medullary thyroid cancer
C. **Concurrent history of glaucoma**
D. History of epilepsy or risk of seizures
E. Uncontrolled hypertension

(C) The medication being described is phentermine/topiramate, which should be avoided in those with a history of renal calculus. One of the contraindications is a diagnosis of **glaucoma.**

As of 2022, phentermine/topiramate ER is now approved for pediatric patients ≥ 12 years old with a BMI of ≥ 95th percentile for age and sex.

Phentermine/Topiramate ER (Qsymia®)	
Dose	-AM dose 3.75/23 mg x 14 days, then 7.5/46 mg daily. -If weight loss < 3% after 12 weeks, increase to 11.25/69 mg x 14 days, then 15/92 mg (full strength). -D/C if < 5% weight loss after 12 weeks at max dose
Mechanism	-**Phentermine:** This sympathomimetic amine stimulates the hypothalamus to release norepinephrine, resulting in decreased appetite and food intake. -**Topiramate ER:** Potential mechanism: Enhances GABA activity and Na$^+$ channels, leading to appetite suppression and satiety enhancement
Contraindications	Hypersensitivity to phentermine or other formulary components, concurrent MAOI use, hyperthyroidism, glaucoma, and pregnancy. *Avoid in those with renal calculus history, coronary artery disease, and severe anxiety
Side Effects	Paresthesia, insomnia, constipation, dysgeusia, xerostomia, lightheadedness, increased heart rate

Reference: Phentermine/topiramate ER package insert

106. (Content: III-F-7) A 36-year-old female with diabetes mellitus type 2 presents to her primary care physician's clinic for a bariatric surgery evaluation. Her diabetes has been poorly controlled despite being on metformin, liraglutide, empagliflozin, and now high-dose insulin. She exercises 250 minutes weekly and has been on a low glycemic index dietary plan for the past nine months. Despite this, her hemoglobin A1c is 8.9% (reference range: 4.2-5.7%). Her body mass index is 32 kg/m². Regarding her bariatric surgery eligibility question, would she be a good candidate?

    A. No: Her body mass index is not in an appropriate range
    B. No: She only has one obesity-related comorbidity
    C. No: She should pursue an insulin pump instead
    D. Yes: Her diabetes is difficult to control
    E. Yes: She meets the criteria for Roux-en-Y gastric bypass only

(D) Even as early as 2016, a joint statement from 45 professional societies, including the American Diabetes Association, recommended bariatric surgery in those with a **body mass index (BMI) between 30-34.9 kg/m² and type 2 diabetes with inadequate glycemic control,** despite optimal medical therapy and lifestyle changes.

In 2022, the American Society for Metabolic and Bariatric Surgery (ASMBS) and the International Federation for the Surgery of Obesity and Metabolic Disorders (IFSO) updated bariatric surgery criteria, which includes the following key changes regarding metabolic and bariatric surgery (MBS):

- MBS is recommended for patients with a BMI ≥ 35 kg/m² regardless of comorbidities
- MBS should be considered for individuals with metabolic disease with a BMI 30-34.9 kg/m². A trial of nonsurgical management is recommended prior to pursuing surgical options in this population.
- BMI thresholds should be adjusted in the Asian population, allowing those with a BMI ≥27.5 kg/m² to be offered MBS
- Appropriate children and adolescents should be considered for MBS

These changes are based on numerous studies showing the long-term improvement of mortality and obesity-related morbidities.

Reference: 2022 American Society for Metabolic and Bariatric Surgery (ASMBS) and International Federation for the Surgery of Obesity and Metabolic Disorders (IFSO): Indications for Metabolic and Bariatric Surgery. Published:October 20, 2022 DOI:https://doi.org/10.1016/j.soard.2022.08.013

107. (Content: III-G-7) A 52-year-old male presents to his primary care physician with concerns of decreased libido. He states he has no current sexual desire and does not wake up with a morning erection. A physical exam reveals small testicles, gynecomastia, and a BMI of 52 kg/m². Morning testosterone levels are low on two occasions, while a prostate-specific antigen is within normal limits. Starting testosterone in this patient would likely have what effect?

    A. Increase HbA1c
    B. Decrease fertility
    C. Increase weight
    D. Worsening lipid panel
    E. Increasing blood pressure

(B) In patients with confirmed hypogonadism, testosterone replacement and lifestyle modifications should be considered in those not seeking fertility. Appropriate testosterone replacement is associated with weight loss, **reduced fertility,** decreased waist circumference, and improved glucose, HbA1c, and cholesterol panel. If patients who are taking testosterone lose a significant amount of weight, the dosing may need to be reduced.

The etiology of reduced fertility is shown below.

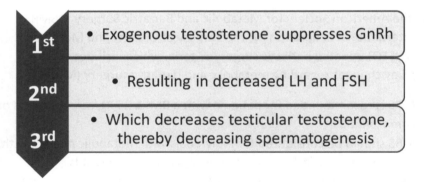

1st	• Exogenous testosterone suppresses GnRh
2nd	• Resulting in decreased LH and FSH
3rd	• Which decreases testicular testosterone, thereby decreasing spermatogenesis

GnRH: Gonadotropin-releasing hormone; LH: Luteinizing hormone; FSH: Follicular stimulating hormone

Reference: AACE/ACE Guidelines: AMERICAN ASSOCIATION OF CLINICAL ENDOCRINOLOGISTS AND AMERICAN COLLEGE OF ENDOCRINOLOGY COMPREHENSIVE CLINICAL PRACTICE GUIDELINES FOR MEDICAL CARE OF PATIENTS WITH OBESITY (2016): Recommendation 54

108. (Content: III-D-2) A 47-year-old male with end-stage renal disease is presenting to his primary care physician's office with the desire to lose weight. To be considered for a renal transplant, he must lose an additional 22 lbs (10 kg). Although he has incorporated lifestyle modifications, he has failed to meet his weight loss goals. He is interested in bariatric medications. Which of the following would be the most appropriate medication to prescribe?

- A. Phentermine/topiramate ER
- B. Naltrexone/bupropion ER
- **C. Liraglutide**
- D. Phentermine monotherapy
- E. Metformin

(C) All FDA-approved anti-obesity medications used for long-term weight loss should be avoided in the setting of end-stage renal disease, except for GLP-1 receptor agonists **(liraglutide or semaglutide),** orlistat, or cellulose and citric acid hydrogel (considered a medical device, not a medication). In addition, metformin is contraindicated if GFR is <30 mL/min.

The use of pharmacologic weight loss treatments in chronic kidney disease is limited and should be used with caution. Significant limitations are summarized below:

- **End-Stage renal failure:** Orlistat, semaglutide, and liraglutide can be used in selected patients with caution. Cellulose and citric acid hydrogel is not systemically absorbed and thus approved at any GFR.
- **GFR < 30 mL/min:** Naltrexone/bupropion ER, and phentermine/topiramate ER are not recommended.
- **GFR 30-49 mL/min:** Naltrexone/bupropion ER should not exceed 8/90 mg BID, and phentermine/topiramate ER is limited to 7.5/46 mg daily.
- **GFR > 50 mL/min:** All weight-loss medications are permissible.

Reference: AACE/ACE Guidelines: AMERICAN ASSOCIATION OF CLINICAL ENDOCRINOLOGISTS AND AMERICAN COLLEGE OF ENDOCRINOLOGY COMPREHENSIVE CLINICAL PRACTICE GUIDELINES FOR MEDICAL CARE OF PATIENTS WITH OBESITY (2016): Recommendation 83-85

109. (Content: III-D-6) A patient presents to her internist with concerns about supplements she has been taking. She was started on L-carnitine and green tea extract at the recommendation of an herbalist. However, since starting, she has noticed increased anxiety, palpitations, and a slight tremor. Both of these supplements theoretically work by which mechanism?

    A. Energy expenditure
    B. Satiety
    C. Carbohydrate metabolism
    D. Blocking fat absorption
    E. Increase in fat oxidation

(E) Both supplements mentioned above have mechanisms of action that include decreasing fat synthesis and **increasing fat oxidation.** Green tea extract in high amounts causes anxiety, tremors, and palpitations.

Note: No legal dietary supplement ingredient has been demonstrated to be effective for weight loss, and these should not be recommended in place of other proven, effective therapies. Also, supplements are often not in a pure form (not regulated) and may contain substances such as stimulants, diuretics, or laxatives that may cause adverse medical effects. Finally, drug-herb interactions are possible.

The table summarizes the mechanism for many different supplements:

Supplement Mechanisms	
↑ Energy expenditure	Yerba mate, ephedra, guarana, Yohimbe, country mallow, bitter orange
↑ Satiety	Guar gum, psyllium, prebiotic fiber
↑ Fat oxidation	L-carnitine, green tea, DHEA, pyruvate, raspberry ketone, hydroxycitric acid, conjugated linoleic acid
↓ Dietary fat absorption	Chitosan
↑ Carbohydrate metabolism	Chromium, ginseng, white kidney bean extract

Reference: Up to Date: "Overview of herbal medicine and dietary supplements"

110. (Content: III-A-1) A 52-year-old female has presented for a follow-up visit to the bariatric clinic. A rotating resident is interviewing the patient and is asking questions such as "What weight-loss techniques have worked for you in the past?" and "So, swimming was an exercise you could do long-term?" After further discussions, the resident expresses hope stating, "It sounds like you are ready to pursue and maintain weight loss." He summarizes the visit, and the patient leaves the office. Which skill did this resident utilize?

    A. OARS
    B. FRAMES
    C. SMART goals
    D. RULE

(A) OARS is an acronym commonly used as a motivational interviewing skill that leads to higher levels of patient engagement and ownership, while decreasing resistance/barriers leading to improved overall outcomes. **OARS** stands for the following:

- **Open-ended questions:** Avoid yes/no answers. This helps explore the patient's reasoning for the change.
- **Affirmations:** Recognize strengths and how these can be applied to future goals to implement change.
- **Reflection:** Careful listening followed by facilitating evocation, developing discrepancy, resolving ambivalence, offering collaboration, and supporting self-efficacy.
- **Summarize:** Recap of discussion, setting realistic future goals, and plans to follow up.

Other acronyms used in motivational interviewing include:

RULE is an acronym focused on the motivation interview principles, and stands for **R**esist the righting reflex, **U**nderstand your patient's motivation, **L**isten to your patient, **E**mpower your patient.

FRAMES is a structural framework for conducting motivational interviewing and stands for **F**eedback about personal risk, **R**esponsibility of patient, **A**dvice to change, **M**enu of strategies, **E**mpathetic style, and **S**elf-efficacy.

Reference: Obesity Medicine Association: Obesity Algorithm (2021)

111. (Content: III-F-4) An obesity medicine specialist is working with an internal medicine resident and discusses ways to improve surgical outcomes, including decreased hospitalization and recovery times. Which of the following should routinely be performed to improve outcomes?

A. **Preoperative carbohydrate loading**
B. Intraoperative low-molecular-weight heparin
C. Nasogastric nutritional supplementation
D. Intraoperative high ventilator tidal volumes
E. Postoperative intravenous opioid administration

(A) Preoperative enhanced recovery after bariatric surgery (ERABS) clinical pathways should be implemented in all patients undergoing bariatric surgery to improve postoperative outcomes. This includes allowing the patient to have **oral nutrition with carbohydrates up to 2 hours preoperatively** to decrease insulin resistance, decrease protein catabolism, decrease hospital length of stay, and experience a faster return of bowel function.

A summary of additional recommendations are below:

ERABS Summary for Improved Surgical Outcomes	
Preoperative	Prehabilitation: Deep breathing exercises, CPAP, incentive spirometry, leg exercises, H_2 blocker/PPI, carbohydrate loading, pre-anesthesia medication
Intraoperative	Opioid-sparing multi-modal analgesia, pulmonary recruitment maneuvers, protective ventilation strategies, silent bleeding detection, avoiding excess fluid administration (goal-directed fluid management), anti-emetic prophylaxis, regional blocks
Postoperative	Thromboprophylaxis (early ambulation, etc.), early return of oral intake, multimodal analgesia regimen

CPAP: continuous positive airway pressure; **PPI:** Proton pump inhibitors

Reference: AACE/TOS/ASMBS/OMA/ASA 2019 Guidelines: CLINICAL PRACTICE GUIDELINES FOR THE PERIOPERATIVE NUTRITION, METABOLIC, AND NONSURGICAL SUPPORT OF PATIENTS UNDERGOING BARIATRIC PROCEDURES – 2019 UPDATE. Recommendation 34, 35, 36, 40. Table 8.

112. (Content: III-F-5a) A surgeon consults an obesity medicine specialist after a 39-year-old female develops a provoked lower extremity deep venous thrombosis (DVT) extending to the femoral artery on post-operative day three from a Roux-en-Y gastric bypass. Post-op complications included persistent nausea and vomiting, which have now subsided. The surgeon requests assistance with anticoagulation therapy. What is the most appropriate recommendation to provide?

    A. Initiate rivaroxaban and check anti-Xa levels in 3 days
    B. Bridge anticoagulation with fondaparinux and warfarin
    C. Start an unfractionated heparin drip and place an IVC filter
    D. Consult vascular surgery for mechanical thrombectomy
    E. Discharge patient with weight-based enoxaparin

(E) This patient, who is otherwise ready for discharge, develops a DVT in the post-operative setting after a malabsorptive procedure. **Weight-based enoxaparin or parenteral options** are preferred due to studies suggesting increased bleeding risk with warfarin, a vitamin K antagonist (VKA), and decreased absorption of direct oral anticoagulants (DOACS).

Bariatric surgery either reduces the stomach volume or bypasses the absorbable intestinal area, leading to unreliable anticoagulation bioavailability.

Recommendations for perioperative VTE treatment is as follows:

- Use parenteral anticoagulation in the early/subacute phase after bariatric surgery (<4 weeks).
- Transitioning to a DOAC or VKA can be considered after at least four weeks of parenteral therapy. It is recommended to closely monitor INR (VKA) to verify absorption and bioavailability.

The bioavailability of DOACS are least likely to be affected in a sleeve gastrectomy, but the guidance above should still be followed. A recent study suggested that DOACs are non-inferior to VTE <u>prevention</u> compared to parenteral options, but this has not been studied in VTE <u>treatment</u>.

Reference: Martin KA, Beyer-Westendorf J, Davidson BL, Huisman MV, Sandset PM, Moll S. Use of direct oral anticoagulants in patients with obesity for treatment and prevention of venous thromboembolism: Updated communication from the ISTH SSC Subcommittee on Control of Anticoagulation. J Thromb Haemost. 2021 Aug;19(8):1874-1882. doi: 10.1111/jth.15358. Epub 2021 Jul 14. PMID: 34259389.

113. (Content: III-E) A recently published study has shown weight-loss success and diabetes improvement with a subcutaneous injectable medication undergoing continued clinical testing. The medication contains GLP-1 and another hormone that is endogenously secreted by the K cells in the proximal small intestines. This dual medication has been shown to have more significant effects on diabetes and weight than with a GLP-1 alone due to its dual incretin effect. The described medication combined with a GLP-1 is

A. Amylin
B. Oxyntomodulin
C. Glucagon
D. Gastric inhibitory peptide
E. Peptide YY

(D) Tirzepatide[1] is a dual GLP-1 receptor agonist and **gastric inhibitory peptide** (which is endogenously secreted by the K cells in the small intestines) medication recently approved for diabetes (Mounjaro®) and expected to be soon FDA-approved for obesity. Compared to GLP-1 monotherapy, patients had improved weight loss and improvements in HbA1c.

Combination medications with different mechanisms of action are being explored, as synergistic properties and sometimes improved tolerability are often seen. Many of these combinations utilize GLP-1 with other anorexigenic hormones. A few other trials that are advancing and showing significant weight loss include:

- Cagrilintide[2] (amylin analogue) + semaglutide
- Bimagrumab[3]: An activin type II receptor blockade monoclonal antibody used to treat inclusion body myositis has shown benefits in reducing fat mass and increasing lean mass.
- Retatrutide: Triad of GLP-1, glucagon, and gastric inhibitory peptide

[1] **Reference:** Tirzepatide versus Semaglutide Once Weekly in Patients with Type 2 Diabetes. Juan P. Frías, M.D., Melanie J. Davies, M.D.; N Engl J Med 2021; 385:503-515 DOI: 10.1056/NEJMoa2107519
[2] **Reference:** Cagrilintide plus semaglutide for obesity management. Sara Becerril, Gema Frühbeck. Published: April 22, 2021 DOI:https://doi.org/10.1016/S0140-6736(21)00944-2
[3] **Reference:** Effect of Bimagrumab vs Placebo on Body Fat Mass Among Adults With Type 2 Diabetes and Obesity: A Phase 2 Randomized Clinical Trial. JAMA Netw Open. 2021 Jan Heymsfield SB, Coleman LA, Miller R, Rooks DSdoi: 10.1001/jamanetworkopen.2020.33457.

114. (Content: III-D-9) A 44-year-old female with a history of ovarian cancer recently completed chemotherapy. During cancer treatment, she lost substantial weight and currently has a BMI of 20 kg/m². She states she does not have a significant appetite and must force herself to remember to drink protein shakes, although she has no nausea. Her diabetes mellitus type 2 initially had improved with the unintended weight loss and she quit all of her medications during treatment. Her most recent hemoglobin A1c is 7.4% (reference range: ≤5.7%). Which is the most appropriate medication to initiate at this time?

A. Semaglutide
B. Sitagliptin
C. Tirzepatide
D. Insulin
E. Dapagliflozin

(B) This patient, who has lost a significant amount of weight in the setting of chemotherapy and has a persistently decreased appetite, would benefit from weight-neutral diabetes medication. Of the options, only **sitagliptin** is weight neutral. Besides insulin, which is obesogenic, the other options are weight-negative.

Sitagliptin (Januvia®)	
Dose	Take 100 mg daily orally. *Renal impairment:* Reduce to 50 mg daily if GFR ≥30 to <45 mL/minute, and 25 mg daily if GFR <30 mL/minute (including if on dialysis).
Mechanism	Dipeptidyl Peptidase 4 (DPP-4) inhibitors prevent the breakdown of incretins glucagon-like peptide 1 and gastric inhibitory peptide, increasing pancreatic insulin synthesis and decreasing glucagon.
Contraindications	Prior serious hypersensitivity reaction to sitagliptin
Side Effects	Gastrointestinal distress (diarrhea or nausea) and nasopharyngitis (5%), pancreatitis[1]

[1]A meta-analysis (TECOSS Study) revealed the incidence of pancreatitis with sitagliptin was similar to placebo

Reference: Sitagliptin package insert

115. (Content: III-G-7) A 26-year-old male is presenting for psychiatric evaluation as part of a multi-disciplinary team approach before bariatric surgery. He admits that he eats until he feels uncomfortably full, even eating large amounts when he doesn't feel hungry. This is something that has caused significant guilt and depression. He eats much more over a short period compared to his friends. He states it feels "like I lose control when food is around." Which of the following classes of medications is FDA approved to treat his underlying condition?

A. **Central nervous system stimulant**
B. Anticonvulsant
C. Atypical antipsychotic
D. Selective serotonin neuromodulator
E. Glucagon-like peptide analog

(A) This patient presents with findings consistent with the diagnosis of binge eating disorder (BED), the most common eating disorder. **Lisdexamfetamine dimesylate, a central nervous system stimulant,** is the only FDA-approved medication to treat this condition.

Cognitive behavior therapy is recommended as first-line therapy to treat BED. While the only FDA-approved pharmacotherapy for BED is lisdexamfetamine dimesylate (brand name Vyvanse®), there are many medications commonly used off-label and have good efficacy, as listed below:

- Topiramate
- Phentermine/topiramate ER
- Selective serotonin reuptake inhibitors
- Bupropion
- GLP-1 receptor agonists

Importantly, BED should be treated before you address obesity with bariatric surgery.

Note: Lisdexamfetamine dimesylate is only FDA-approved for BED and attention deficit/hyperactivity disorder.

Reference: Up To Date "Binge eating disorder in adults: Overview of treatment"

116. (Content: III-A-1) A 14-year-old male presents for a sports physical for the upcoming football season. He has always been at the 95th-100th percentile of his weight compared to his peers. His weight today is 204 lbs (92.5 kg). He has unhealthy eating habits and consumes multiple sodas daily. The concern about his weight is discussed, including the health risks. He seems perplexed by this, as he feels he is at a good weight for football. After further discussion, he agrees to a focused follow-up visit regarding dietary modifications. Which of the following stages of change is this patient experiencing?

A. Pre-contemplation
B. Contemplation
C. Preparation
D. Action
E. Maintenance

(B) Although this patient presented in pre-contemplation related to obesity (unaware of the issue), after further discussion with the practitioner, he is not only aware that the problem exists, but he is interested in hearing about potential solutions, moving him into the **contemplation stage.**

Stages of change are a vital component of the transtheoretical model, a framework for understanding the dynamic process of behavior change.

Stages of Change		
Stage	**Definition**	**Intervention**
Pre-contemplation	Unaware of issue or unwilling to change	MI: Build awareness, discuss risks/benefits
Contemplation	Interested in changing within the next 6 months	MI: Assess/provide info, encourage/support
Preparation	Willing to change in the next 30 days (planning)	CBT: Set SMART[1] goals, and develop an action plan
Action	Initiation of change (approx. 6 months)	CBT: Reward and encourage small changes
Maintenance	Continued change for > 6 months	CBT: Positive reinforcement, lapse/relapse coaching
Relapse	Returning to undesirable behaviors	Normalization and assessing which stage they are in.

MI: Motivational interviewing; **CBT**: Cognitive behavioral therapy
[1]**SMART**: Specific, Measurable, Achievable, Relevant, and Timing

Reference: Obesity Medicine Association: Obesity Algorithm (2021)

117. (Content: III-C-1) A 57-year-old business executive returns to his primary care physician for follow-up regarding his exercise prescription. Although the prescription clearly states 300 minutes of exercise weekly in the form of brisk walking, he does not have that amount of time to devote to exercise and did not fulfill his prescription. His current BMI is 31 kg/m². What would be the most appropriate modification to his exercise prescription?

A. Change to water walking
B. Increase exercise intensity
C. Change to resistance training
D. Focus on dietary components instead
E. Confront him on his priorities

(B) Although this patient was prescribed an appropriate exercise prescription, it did not consider his time constraints. One alternative that would still meet the physical activity guidelines would be to **increase the intensity of exercise from moderate (3-6 METS) to vigorous (> 6 METS),** thereby decreasing exercise time from 150-300 minutes/week to only 75-150.

For substantial health benefits, adults should perform 150-300 minutes per week of moderate-intensity aerobic physical activity or 75-150 minutes per week of vigorous-intensity aerobic exercise.

- **Moderate-intensity:** Conversation takes effort. You can talk but not sing. It is starting to get challenging. Example: Brisk walking.
    - Target heart rate between 64-76% of maximum heart rate, where maximum heart rate is estimated by 220 - age.
- **Vigorous-intensity:** Conversation difficult. Challenging and hard-work. Examples: Running, swimming, and playing basketball.
    - Target heart rate between 77% and 93% of maximum heart rate

Adults should also do weight-training or resistance exercise ≥ 2 days weekly.

Note: Additional health benefits are gained by engaging in physical activity beyond 300 minutes of weekly moderate-intensity exercise.

Reference: Physical Activity Guidelines for Americans: 2nd Edition: https://health.gov/sites/default/files/2019-09/Physical_Activity_Guidelines_2nd_edition.pdf
Reference: CDC: Target Heart Rate and Estimated Maximum Heart Rate. https://www.cdc.gov/physicalactivity/basics/measuring/heartrate.htm

118. (Content: III-F-5c) A general surgeon is discussing one potential bariatric surgical option with a patient in which 80% of the greater curvature of the stomach is resected laparoscopically, allowing for 2-3 ounces (60-90 mL) of volume intake. Which of the following is true regarding the described procedure?

A. Dumping syndrome is a common complaint
B. It is the second most common bariatric procedure
C. The procedure does not affect hunger hormones
D. Patients are prone to experience vitamin B$_{12}$ deficiency
E. This surgery is most effective for treating diabetes

(D) Sleeve gastrectomy is the most common bariatric procedure performed worldwide. Due to the removal of 80% of the stomach **1**, many gastric parietal cells (which make intrinsic factor and ghrelin) are removed, thus making patients **more prone to B$_{12}$ deficiency.** Importantly, the pylorus remains intact **2** without concerns of gastric motility issues.

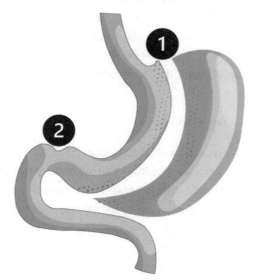

Note: Patients who underwent a Roux-en-Y gastric bypass had more significant weight loss, slightly higher diabetes remission with decreased relapse, and better long-term glycemic control compared to sleeve gastrectomy[1].

Image citation: Image created by Charu G. Copyright owned by Kevin Smith, DO
[1]**Reference:** McTigue KM, Wellman R, Nauman E, et al. Comparing the 5-Year Diabetes Outcomes of Sleeve Gastrectomy and Gastric Bypass: The National Patient-Centered Clinical Research Network (PCORNet) Bariatric Study. JAMA Surg. Published online March 04, 2020. doi:10.1001/jamasurg.2020.0087

119. (Content: III-F-3) A 39-year-old female with a history of type 2 diabetes and sleep apnea is presenting to her general surgeon after undergoing a Roux-en-Y gastric bypass six months ago. She has noted a weight loss of 47 lbs (21.3 kg) and is happy with the results. She regularly meets with her dietician and the weight loss clinic. Her only complaint is that after she eats certain meals, she experiences facial flushing and lightheadedness. Given the most likely etiology of these symptoms, what other associated finding is she likely to encounter?

A. Intermittent constipation
B. Excessive belching
C. Wheezing
D. **Reactive hypoglycemia**
E. Bacterial overgrowth

(D) Dumping syndrome is a complication most commonly seen after Roux-en-Y gastric bypass (typically within 18 months postoperatively), as the pyloric mechanism is bypassed. Thus, high carbohydrate loads can rapidly empty into the small bowel, leading to symptoms of abdominal pain, cramping, tachycardia, diarrhea, and facial flushing. Although rapid glucose absorption initially leads to hyperglycemia, the subsequent **exaggerated insulin release can cause symptomatic hypoglycemia.** It can be prevented by avoiding excess simple carbohydrates.

Other complications of Roux-en-Y include:

- **Internal hernia:** A small bowel obstruction (SBO) can be caused by a mesenteric defect. Prior to an SBO, intermittent symptoms can be seen in the absence of computed tomography abnormalities.
- **SIBO:** Small intestine bacterial overgrowth can occur due to a blind loop that allows excess bacteria to grow, causing abdominal pain, bloating, diarrhea, and D-lactic acidosis.
- **Gallstone complications:** This can occur with any rapid weight loss. Prophylactic cholecystectomy during Roux-en-Y surgery is not recommended, although 8% will require it at some point after surgery.

Reference: Up to Date: "Laparoscopic Roux-en-Y gastric bypass"

120. (Content: III-F-3) A rapid response is called on a 33-year-old female 12 hours after undergoing a Roux-en-Y gastric bypass. She complains of progressively worsening mid-epigastric pain with radiation to her left chest and mild dyspnea. Vital signs reveal a heart rate of 120 BPM, respirations 24/min, and oxygen saturation of 99% on room air. A portable chest x-ray shows a new left-sided pleural effusion. A complete blood count reveals a white blood cell count of 13.4 x 10^3/mcL (reference range: 4.8-10.8 x 10^3/mcL). What is the next best step in management?

    A.   Start empiric ceftriaxone and azithromycin
    B.   Order a stat CTA of the chest
    C.   Administer 1 mg/kg low molecular weight heparin
    D.   Contact the attending surgeon
    E.   Order an electrocardiogram

(D) This patient has concerning findings for an anastomotic leak causing a reactive pleural effusion and leukocytosis. Therefore, the best next step would be **to contact the surgeon for further evaluation** and possibly return to the operating room (if the leak is not contained).

Note: Tachycardia after bariatric surgery is concerning you for an anastomotic leak or a pulmonary embolism.

Anastomotic leaks usually occur within the first few days of surgery, becoming increasingly rare beyond two weeks. It more commonly occurs at the gastrojejunostomy anastomosis and presents as fever, worsening abdominal or chest pain, tachycardia, and leukocytosis.

Complications with Roux-en-Y Gastric Bypass	
Short-Term (30 days)	**Long-Term**
-Death (1:500)	-Peptic ulcer (3-5%)
-Anastomotic leak (1%)	-Small bowel obstruction (1%)
-Infection (2%)	-Internal (1-2%) hernia
-DVT/PE (1-2%)	-Incisional (0.8%) hernia
-Dehydration (2%)	-Stenosis/stricture (2%)
-Mesenteric thrombosis (0.3%)	-Malnutrition (15-40%)

DVT: Deep venous thrombosis; **PE:** Pulmonary embolism

Reference: Obesity medicine association: Obesity Algorithm (2021)

121. (Content: III-D-5) A 39-year-old female presents to the clinic due to nausea, vomiting, and increased fatigue over the past three weeks. Past medical history includes class II obesity, migraines, and polycystic ovarian syndrome (PCOS). She is on oral combined birth control and phentermine/topiramate ER. She has lost 19 lbs (8.6 kg) over the past 4 months but has recently started to regain some weight over the past month. Which of the following could have prevented the underlying cause of her symptoms?

A. **Adhering to the Risk Evaluation and Mitigation Strategy program**
B. Referral to a dietician to discuss a low-carbohydrate diet
C. Prophylactic ondansetron to take before anti-obesity medication
D. Cognitive behavioral therapy to prevent anxiety from phentermine
E. Adding metformin to treat the current PCOS symptoms

(A) This patient presents with pregnancy symptoms, including nausea, vomiting, fatigue, and weight gain. Topiramate can increase the metabolism of oral contraceptive birth control, leading to decreased effectiveness and an increased risk of pregnancy. The **FDA created the Risk Evaluation and Mitigation Strategy (REMS) program** to promote the safe use of medications that carry high safety risks, including those that may cause serious birth defects.

Phentermine/topiramate ER (Qsymia®) is included as part of the REMS program due to the increased risk of cleft lips and palate if pregnancy occurs while taking this medication (topiramate). The REMS program recommends specific forms of birth control and monitoring to reduce pregnancy risk.

- Pregnancy test before starting medication and monthly after that
- Effective birth control:
  - Used alone: Tubal ligation, intrauterine device, progestin implant, or male partner vasectomy
  - Barrier addition: Any other hormonal birth control, including progestin injection, OCP, and the transdermal patch, requires an additional barrier method to be considered adequate

Notably, the REMS training program is currently not required to prescribe Qsymia® (as of 3/2022), but these recommendations still stand.

Reference: Risk Evaluation and Mitigation Strategy (REMS) | Qsymia®: https://qsymiarems.com

122. (Content: III-G-3) A 39-year-old male presents to the obesity clinic for a 2-month follow-up appointment. He was started on semaglutide six months ago, and has maintained exercise of 200 minutes weekly. He states he feels well and plans to continue his current treatment regimen. Vital signs are within normal limits. Over the past year, he has lost 34 lbs (15.4 kg), accounting for an 8% total body weight loss. He is now at his lowest weight since being seen at the clinic. If he maintains his current regimen, what can you predict about his weight loss in the future?

A. He will continue to lose weight but at a slower pace
B. **Eventually he will plateau and regain weight**
C. He will lose weight until he plateaus at his ideal body weight
D. Eventually he will relapse to his previous weight

(B) Patients who lose weight are often disheartened when they eventually **plateau and experience some weight gain** if their treatment regimen isn't adjusted. This should be discussed early in treatment to prevent frustration, with pre-emptive plans to adapt and intensify their regimen accordingly.

Importantly, patients who lose weight will likely plateau and regain weight to some extent. This is related to decreased caloric utilization at a reduced weight (a 300 lb person burns more calories than a 200 lb person doing the same task) and hormonally-mediated etiologies.

The national weight control registry looks at patients who have successfully maintained weight loss for extended periods. Common traits shared amongst participants include:

- Maintaining high levels of physical activity by exercising an average of 1 hour daily (90%)
- Eating breakfast every day (78%)
- Watching < 10 hours of TV weekly (62%)
- Weighing themselves at least once weekly (75%)

Reference: The National Weight Control Registry Brown Medical School/The Miriam Hospital. Weight Control & Diabetes Research Center

123. (Content: III-F-3) A 44-year-old male is being evaluated in the intensive care unit after a biliopancreatic diversion with duodenal switch. The surgery was particularly time-consuming due to anatomic variation and significant scar tissue from prior abdominal surgeries. The nurse is concerned as his urine has darkened, and the urine output has decreased to < 40 mL per hour despite adequate fluid hydration. His abdomen is soft, with no bowel sounds appreciated. Which of the following tests will most likely be abnormal?

A. **Urinalysis hemoglobin**
B. Renal parenchymal ultrasound
C. Renal vasculature doppler
D. Urine eosinophil count
E. Urine microscopy

(A) This patient who is presenting with darkening urine and decreased urine output in the setting of a prolonged surgery has findings concerning for rhabdomyolysis causing an acute kidney injury. Because urinalysis (dipstick) hemoglobin cannot differentiate between myoglobin, hemoglobin, and red blood cells, **the urinalysis hemoglobin is likely to be positive**. Because it is myoglobin and not red blood cells, urine microscopy would be normal.

Rhabdomyolysis can occur in the setting of prolonged surgery, with severe obesity being a risk factor. Muscle breakdown can occur as the patient's body lies on the minimally padded operating room table.

Diagnosis is confirmed with serum creatine phosphokinase (CPK) levels. In order to affect kidney function, levels typically need to be greater than 10,000 IU/L, with decreased urine output being one of the initial findings. Myoglobin can turn the urine dark, as seen in this patient.

Treatment includes supportive care with significant intravenous fluids.

Reference: Up to Date: "Clinical manifestations and diagnosis of rhabdomyolysis"

124. (Content: III-D-5) A 62-year-old female is presenting to her primary care physician's office to discuss semaglutide (Wegovy®) for weight loss and diabetes. Her medical comorbidities include diabetes type II and hypertension. She is currently taking metformin, rosuvastatin, sitagliptin, and chlorthalidone. She drinks two alcoholic beverages nightly and quit tobacco products six years ago. Which of the following is the most appropriate action before starting semaglutide?

A. Obtain baseline lipase levels
B. Discontinue one of her current medications
C. Inquire about a family history of MEN 1 syndrome
D. Require alcohol cessation due to interactions
E. Obtain triglyceride levels

(B) This patient is being evaluated for the appropriateness of semaglutide, which was approved in 2021 for chronic weight management. DDP-4 inhibitors **(i.e., sitagliptin) should be discontinued** when GLP-1 agonists are initiated, as there is no additional benefit, and it is not cost-effective.

Summary: If starting a GLP-1, discontinue DDP-4 inhibitors.

Semaglutide (Wegovy®)	
Dose	Inject 0.25 mg subcutaneously weekly for one month. Increase the weekly dose to 0.5 mg, 1.0 mg, 1.7mg, and 2.4 mg at one-month intervals.
Mechanism	Glucagon-like peptide 1 receptor agonists activate the hypothalamus, reducing food intake, increasing satiety, decreasing caloric intake, and improving glucose metabolism (incretin).
Contraindications	Prior hypersensitivity to GLP-1 agonists, history of or family history of medullary thyroid carcinoma (black box warning), patients with multiple endocrine neoplasia type 2, and pregnancy. *Relative contraindication: Severe gastroparesis and increased risk of pancreatitis[1]
Side Effects	Gastrointestinal distress (abdominal pain, nausea, vomiting, constipation), dizziness, hypoglycemia, increased lipase (increased risk of pancreatitis) [1]

[1]Meta-analysis has shown no increased risk of pancreatitis or pancreatic cancer with GLP-1 use.

Reference: Semaglutide and sitagliptan package inserts.

125. (Content: III-F-3) A 42-year-old female presents with chronic diarrhea, abdominal pain, and bloating for six months. She underwent a duodenal switch approximately eight years ago and has had minimal follow-up due to losing insurance. She admits to now feeling weak and lightheaded with exertion. Laboratory examination reveals macrocytic anemia with increased folate levels. Which of the following tests is most appropriate at this time?

A. Urea breath test
B. Carbohydrate breath test
C. Hydrogen breath test
D. Stool cultures
E. Endoscopic evaluation

(B) Patients with small intestinal bacterial overgrowth (SIBO) often present with bloating, abdominal pain, watery diarrhea, B_{12} deficiency (due to competitive absorption with the host), and folate excess (over-synthesized by the excessive bacteria). Diagnosis of SIBO is made by a **carbohydrate breath test.**

Normal defense mechanisms to prevent excessive overgrowth of colonized bacteria in the small intestines aim to destroy excess bacteria through digestive or proteolytic enzymes, including gastric acid and bile salts. If these mechanisms are altered, bacterial overgrowth is more prone to occur. In the setting of a gastric bypass or a duodenal switch, a blind intestinal loop may allow for uncontested microbiota growth.

Overgrowth of bacteria may lead to enterocyte damage, leading to:
- **Decreased absorption of carbohydrates:** This causes fermentation of unabsorbed carbohydrates and subsequent release of carbon dioxide, methane, and hydrogen. This leads to abdominal distention, bloating, and flatulence.
- **Fat malabsorption:** In addition to fat malabsorption causing steatorrhea, fat-soluble vitamin deficiency may occur.
- **Neurologic findings:** The production of toxins such as D-lactic acidosis may cause neurologic changes such as confusion, ataxia, and seizures.

Reference: Up to Date: "Small intestinal bacterial overgrowth: Clinical manifestations and diagnosis"
Reference: Up to Date: "Small intestinal bacterial overgrowth: Etiology and pathogenesis"

126. (Content: III-D-9) A 37-year-old male with type 1 diabetes presents to his primary care practitioner to discuss anti-obesity medication. In particular, he would like to start semaglutide. His last HbA1c was 7.4% (reference range: <5.7%) and he is on 18 units of glargine nightly and dosing the aspart based on carbohydrate counting. His current BMI is 31 kg/m^2, which has increased from 27 kg/m^2 since last year. Which of the following is the most accurate statement regarding his inquiry?

A. Semaglutide is contraindicated in patients with type 1 diabetes
B. I will discuss this with your endocrinologist
C. You do not meet the criteria for anti-obesity medications
D. Tirzepatide would be a safer alternative
E. I would like to discuss intermittent fasting or a ketogenic diet today

(B) Certain glucagon-like peptide 1 receptor agonists (GLP-1 RA), such as semaglutide and liraglutide, are approved for both weight loss and diabetes mellitus type II. Although GLP-1 RA are not approved to treat diabetes type 1 (DMT1), they can be used to treat obesity in those with DMT1, although this needs to be done cautiously. Patients may benefit from continuous glucose monitoring due to the need for less insulin. A recent study showed improved weight, less insulin requirements, and no significant increase in hypoglycemia risks. Regardless, this should be orchestrated with the patient's **endocrinologist.**

In diabetes, GLP-1 RA work via an incretin effect, increasing pancreatic insulin secretion in the setting of carbohydrate ingestion. However, the central effects of GLP-1 RA provide additional weight loss benefits via activation of the POMC/CART pathway leading to increased satiety and energy expenditure. These latter benefits occur independently of diabetes leading to weight loss. In a patient with T1DM in which the pancreas has undergone auto-immune destruction, patients with excess weight can still have weight improvements with this class of medications.

Importantly, ketogenic diets and intermittent fasting may increase the risk of diabetic ketoacidosis and are generally avoided in those with T1DM or insulin-dependent diabetes type 2, as well as those on SGLT-2 inhibitors.

Reference: Guyton J, Jeon M, Brooks A. Glucagon-like peptide 1 receptor agonists in type 1 diabetes mellitus. Am J Health Syst Pharm. 2019 Oct 15;76(21):1739-1748. doi: 10.1093/ajhp/zxz179. PMID: 31612934.

127. (Content: III-A-2) A 9-year-old female presents to her pediatrician's office after her mother has concerns about her weight. Her mother states that the patient snores loudly and has episodes where she appears to hold her breath. Compared to other kids her age, the mother states her daughter seems much larger. She is at the 100th percentile for her weight and 56th percentile for height. Her weight is 174 pounds (78.9 kg). Which of the following is the recommended initial course of action with this patient?

A. **Monitor dietary intake**
B. Perform overnight pulse-oximetry
C. Discuss pharmacologic therapy
D. Initiate meal replacement
E. Provide reassurance

(A) **Self-monitoring** is part of cognitive-behavioral therapy (CBT), the treatment of choice for prepubescent children for obesity. This focuses on changing behaviors through cognitive restructuring to reinforce good behaviors and extinguish undesirable ones.

Note: Self-monitoring, in particular, can be accomplished through dietary, weight, and exercise logs through the internet or phone-based applications.

CBT is the treatment of choice for many eating disorders (i.e., binge eating disorder, bulimia nervosa, etc.) and is a crucial component in weight loss therapy.

The components of CBT are discussed below.

Components of Cognitive Behavioral Therapy	
Self-monitoring	Enlisting social support
Stimulus control	Relapsing prevention training
Problem-solving	Stress management
Goal setting	Rewards
Contingency management	Ongoing contact

Reference: Dalle Grave R, Centis E, Marzocchi R, El Ghoch M, Marchesini G. Major factors for facilitating change in behavioral strategies to reduce obesity. Psychol Res Behav Manag. 2013;6:101-110. Published 2013 Oct 3. doi:10.2147/PRBM.S40460

128. (Content: III-G-1) A geriatrician notices that many of his patients have lost muscle mass with debility or reduced physical activity, but continue to gain excess fat mass. Although some of these patients have certain conditions predisposing them to muscle wasting, including malignancy, fractures, and neurodegenerative conditions, the majority experience frailty independent of any underlying diseases. Which of the following would be an important part of the multidisciplinary treatment plan in regard to preventing sarcopenia and subsequent frailty?

  A. Prescribe megestrol acetate
  B. Encourage resistance training
  C. Target protein intake of 0.8 g/kg/day
  D. Consider testosterone supplements (males)
  E. Encourage water aerobics

(B) Sarcopenia, or muscle loss, is a predisposing condition to eventual frailty, which is characterized by weight loss (often lean body mass), weakness, and reduced physical activity levels. Both of these conditions are related to aging and are treated with the following:

- Adequate protein intake (1-1.5 g/kg/day)
- **Resistance exercise training**
- Adequate vitamin and mineral supplementation

Water aerobics, or non-weight-bearing exercise, has less effect on muscle mass gain and nearly no impact on bone health.

Importantly, patients can increase their weight, without increasing muscle mass, by adding adipose tissue (i.e., sarcopenic obesity). Similarly, weight loss in the setting of malnutrition or debility often reduces lean body mass, including muscle mass, which is disproportionately more difficult to regain. Therefore, in those who are elderly, extra caution should be taken to target the loss of fat mass, not lean body mass.

Reference: Morley JE. Treatment of sarcopenia: the road to the future. J Cachexia Sarcopenia Muscle. 2018;9(7):1196-1199. doi:10.1002/jcsm.12386

129. (Content: III-F-5b) A 26-year-old female presents to the emergency department with a laceration above her right eye from a fall. She underwent a single anastomosis duodeno-ileal bypass with sleeve gastrectomy (SADI-S) six months prior and has not followed up with any providers since the surgery. She states she felt light-headed when getting up to go to the restroom and "passed-out" in the bathroom. Her skin turgor is normal. Which of the following questions will assist in preventing future similar hospital admissions?

A. Have you been drinking sufficient fluids?
B. Are you taking your daily vitamins?
C. Have you discontinued your sitagliptin post-operatively?
D. Did you have any alcohol before the fall?
E. **Are you still taking blood pressure medication?**

(E) This patient likely experienced a fall from orthostatic hypotension, given her light-headedness with standing. After bariatric and metabolic surgery with significant weight loss, frequent follow-up is necessary to adjust medications. Due to the patient's lack of follow-up, she may still be taking the same dose of blood pressure medications, causing hypotension. Therefore, **asking about blood pressure medication** would be most appropriate. Other reasons for an increased risk of falls post-operatively include:

- Dehydration (patient had normal skin turgor)
- Thiamine deficiency causing ataxia or neuropathy (would not be transient or cause pre-syncope as seen in this patient)
- Hypoglycemic agents, with insulin and sulfonylureas being the most common (sitagliptin is an incretin that does not cause hypoglycemia).
- Alcohol is more readily absorbed after bariatric surgery, leading to more rapid intoxication.

At each post-operative follow-up visit, recommendations include reviewing vital signs, medication adjustment, monitoring dietary adherence (including avoiding NSAIDs, alcohol, and taking vitamins), evaluating for complications of weight loss (gallstones or gout), and ordering labs as appropriate. Body contouring surgery and bone density scans are addressed approx. 2 years post operatively.

Reference: Kim TY, Kim S, Schafer AL. Medical Management of the Postoperative Bariatric Surgery Patient. [Updated 2020 Aug 24]. In: Feingold KR, Anawalt B, Boyce A, et al., editors. Endotext [Internet]. South Dartmouth (MA): MDText.com, Inc.; 2000-. Available from: https://www.ncbi.nlm.nih.gov/books/NBK481901/

130. (Content: III-H-1) A 9-year-old male is presenting for follow-up regarding elevated blood pressures. Both of his parents have concerns about his sedentary lifestyle and picky eating habits that often cause him to snack throughout the day. His BMI is in the 80th percentile for age and gender, and his height has maintained the 60-65th percentile. He undergoes 24-hour ambulatory blood pressure monitoring, which shows normal blood pressure levels. Which is the most appropriate treatment modality for his current weight?

A. **Prevention**
B. Stage 1: Prevention plus
C. Stage 2: Structured weight management
D. Stage 3: Comprehensive multidisciplinary intervention
E. Stage 4: Tertiary care intervention

(A) According to the 2007 expert committee recommendations, this patient does not yet meet the criteria for the 4-tiered intervention and can instead continue focusing on **preventing obesity** through healthy eating and activity.

- **BMI 5th- 84th percentile:** Target problem behaviors and praise good practices (i.e., prevention[1]).
- **BMI 85th-94th percentile:** If there is no evidence of health risks, it is safe to do prevention (above). If health risks, then start 4-tiered system.
- **BMI ≥ 95th percentile:** Start 4-tiered system.

Stage	Name	Location of Intervention	Follow-up
4-Tiered Approach for Management of Pediatric Obesity			
Stage 1	Prevention plus	Primary care office	Monthly
Stage 2	Structured weight management	Primary care office with support	Monthly
Stage 3	Comprehensive multidisciplinary intervention	Pediatric weight management center	Weekly
Stage 4	Tertiary care intervention	Tertiary care center	Weekly

[1]**Note:** Prevention of obesity includes: limit screen time to 2 hours daily, encourage sleeping ≥ 9 hours nightly, ≥ 5 servings of fruits and vegetables daily, eliminate sugar-sweetened beverages, prepare meals at home when possible, eat at the table with family ≥ 5 times weekly, consume a healthy breakfast every morning, perform at least 60 minutes of physical activity daily.

Reference: Expert Committee Recommendations Regarding the Prevention, Assessment, and Treatment of Child and Adolescent Overweight and Obesity: Summary Report. Sarah E. Barlow. Pediatrics Dec 2007, 120 (Supplement 4) S164-S192; DOI: 10.1542/peds.2007-2329C

131. (Content: III-E) A patient presents to her nutritionist to discuss an article she read on the internet. It discussed making dietary changes by adding nutrients that have potentially favorable effects beyond basic nutrition. She most likely read an article on which of the following topics?

    A. Supplements
    B. Over-the-counter medications
    C. Functional foods
    D. Prescription medications
    E. Herbal remedies

(C) **Functional foods** are nutrients that have potentially favorable effects beyond basic nutrition, such as oatmeal having positive effects on cholesterol. Other examples are discussed below:

- **Dietary fiber:** This may increase the sense of fullness and marginally decrease percent body fat.
- **Prebiotics:** Indigestible oligosaccharides may stimulate intestinal growth, promoting a microbiome conducive to weight loss.
- **Probiotics:** Bacteria (i.e., lactobacilli) in yogurt etc., may protect against unfavorable yeast/bacterial overgrowth.
- **Caffeine or green tea** (not extracts): May reduce appetite, increase fat oxidation, and provide antioxidants.

In contrast to functional foods, supplements are substances taken in addition to dietary intake (i.e., herbs, vitamins, etc.), are not approved by the FDA (considered food, not a drug), and cannot be marketed to treat, prevent, or cure disease.

Finally, the FDA considers over-the-counter medications safe and effective but they do not require a prescription.

Reference: Obesity medicine association: Obesity Algorithm (2021)

132. (Content: III-D-2) A 28-year-old healthy male presents to his primary care physician after frustration with his inability to lose a significant amount of weight. For the past six months, he has changed to a vegan diet and exercises 30 minutes daily. Although he has lost 8 lbs (3.6 kg), he feels he should have lost more. His current BMI is 31 kg/m². After reviewing the side-effects of medications, he chooses one that he feels will be a safe option. After two months, he returns with no significant weight loss. Which of the following anti-obesity medication was he most likely prescribed?

    A. Phentermine/topiramate ER
    B. Orlistat
    C. Naltrexone/bupropion ER
    D. Liraglutide

(B) This patient has healthy eating habits and is a vegan. Therefore **orlistat,** which works by inhibiting gastrointestinal fat reabsorption, would be ineffective in a patient who does not intake fatty foods. The other options are more likely to have some weight-loss effect.

Note: Orlistat should not be taken within four hours of levothyroxine due to impaired absorption.

The table below summarizes important pharmacologic information.

Orlistat[1] (Alli®: Over the counter, Xenical® Prescription)	
Dose	-60 mg TID within 1 hour of a fatty meal (Alli®) -120 mg TID within 1 hour of a fatty meal (Xenical®)
Mechanism	-Pancreatic lipase inhibitor (inhibits the absorption of dietary fats by 30%)
Contraindications	Hypersensitivity to orlistat or formulary component, pregnancy, chronic malabsorption syndrome, and cholestasis *Avoid if a history of oxalate nephropathy
Side Effects	Headaches, oily rectal leakage, gastrointestinal pain

[1] Orlistat is approved for those ≥ 12 years old and is available at lower doses over-the-counter.

Reference: Orlistat package insert

133. (Content: III-F-3) A 24-year-old male is discussing his concerns about blood clots after his planned sleeve gastrectomy surgery next month. His father died from a pulmonary embolism (PE) one week after undergoing a total hip arthroplasty. The patient has no history of deep venous thrombosis, and besides his father, he knows of no other family history. He denies smoking. Which of the following would be the most appropriate statement regarding venous thromboembolism (VTE) in this patient?

A. Start VTE prophylaxis at least 24 hours after surgery
B. Low-molecular-weight heparin 40 mg twice daily is considered standard
C. **Failure to wean from ventilator support may indicate VTE**
D. He should be on extended chemoprophylaxis upon discharge
E. Given his family history, an IVC filter should be discussed

(C) Prophylaxis against venous thromboembolism is recommended for all patients after bariatric procedures. Prevention may include sequential compression devices in addition to pharmacotherapy, such as unfractionated heparin (UFH) or low-molecular-weight heparin (LMWH). Respiratory distress or **failure to wean from ventilator support postoperatively should prompt a work-up for a pulmonary embolism.**

Important points regarding VTE are discussed below:

- Extended chemoprophylaxis after hospital discharge should be considered in high-risk patients (history of VTE, known hypercoagulable condition, or those who have limited ambulation).
- The use of deep venous thrombosis risk calculators are recommended to guide the length of prophylaxis.
- All patients should be encouraged to ambulate early after surgery.
- IVC filters are associated with increased mortality and VTE risk.

Reference: AACE/TOS/ASMBS/OMA/ASA 2019 Guidelines: CLINICAL PRACTICE GUIDELINES FOR THE PERIOPERATIVE NUTRITION, METABOLIC, AND NONSURGICAL SUPPORT OF PATIENTS UNDERGOING BARIATRIC PROCEDURES – 2019 UPDATE. Recommendation 45, 46

134. (Content: III-G-7) A psychiatrist is evaluating a patient in a psychiatric hospital for a recent episode of mania. The patient has a diagnosis of bipolar type I. The patient states that she has stopped her lithium due to excessive weight gain, leading to this current episode. The patient would like to discuss alternative options that would not cause this adverse effect. Which option should be discussed with the patient?

A. Valproate
B. Sertraline
C. Divalproex
D. Gabapentin
E. **Lamotrigine**

(E) **Lamotrigine** is indicated for focal and general seizures, mood stabilization in those with bipolar, and trigeminal neuralgia prophylaxis. Of the options, it is the only weight neutral/negative medication used to treat her condition. Selective serotonin reuptake inhibitors such as sertraline should be avoided as monotherapy in the setting of bipolar disorder. All the other listed options are weight positive.

Lamotrigine is considered either weight-neutral or weight-negative. This variability may be dependent on dosing. Regardless, it is not considered weight positive.

Mood-Stabilizer Medications		
Weight Positive	**Weight Neutral**	**Weight Negative**
-Carbamazepine	-Oxcarbazepine	-Lamotrigine
-Divalproex		
-Lithium		
-Valproate		
-Gabapentin		

Weight effects are generalizations and may be based solely on observational trials and vary depending on dosing, treatment duration, and medication indications. Weight variability may be seen.
Note: Children/adolescents have more significant weight gain than adults with obesogenic medications

Reference: Obesity medicine association: Obesity Algorithm (2021)

135. (Content: III-B-1) A 48-year-old male presents for follow-up with the dietician. He has been doing research and wants to discuss some dietary plans. He has obesity class I without other obesity-related comorbidities and is currently taking no medications besides a daily multivitamin. He asks for an opinion related to frequently used dietary plans. Which of the following recommendations is most accurate?

A. Intermittent fasting allows for a time of restricted eating followed by unregulated calorie consumption
B. The Dietary Approach to Stopping Hypertension (DASH) diet plan provides significant weight loss with cardiovascular benefits
C. Low carbohydrate diets are more effective long-term for weight loss compared to low-fat dietary plans
D. **Eating low-density foods increases the sensation of fullness and thus promotes weight loss in comparison to high-density foods**

(D) **Intaking low-density, higher-weight foods, such as those high in fiber, including vegetables and fruits, promotes fullness, allowing patients to reduce their overall caloric intake and allowing them to obtain subsequent weight loss.** The volume discrepancy between high-density (often high-fat) foods compared to an equal caloric intake but with low-density foods can be staggering.

Newer dietary plans are always being developed and promoted, but often are 're-inventing the wheel' in terms of new names for similar macro-nutrient restrictions. Depending on their publicity, these fad diets may become very popular, while studies supporting their efficacy are lacking. Importantly, regardless of macronutrient content, a caloric deficit diet that is sustainable to the patient is most important for weight loss in the long term, while macronutrients may provide other benefits (cardiovascular risk reduction or diabetes control).

Several studies have focused on the efficacy of intermittent fasting. This dietary plan consists of fasting periods followed by eating periods. These periods can vary, ranging from 18 hours of fasting to 6 hours eating, to day-long periods of fasting/eating. Most importantly, the idea that completely unrestricted eating can occur during the eating period is not supported.

Reference: Stockman MC, Thomas D, Burke J, Apovian CM. Intermittent Fasting: Is the Wait Worth the Weight? Curr Obes Rep. 2018 Jun;7(2):172-185. doi: 10.1007/s13679-018-0308-9. PMID: 29700718; PMCID: PMC5959807.

136. (Content: III-F-1) A patient is meeting with a bariatric surgeon to discuss potential surgical options. Although she has done a lot of research, she still has not committed to one surgery. She asks about the estimated number of bariatric surgeries performed, including which are popular and which are becoming obsolete. Which of the following statements is accurate regarding bariatric surgery statistics over the past ten years?

A. The number of bariatric surgeries have declined in the past five years
B. Gastric banding has persistently made up 5% of bariatric surgeries
C. Roux-en-Y gastric bypass remains the most common surgery
D. Sleeve gastrectomy surgeries have nearly doubled in number
E. Intragastric balloons have been available since 2012

(D) Although bariatric surgeries have increased in the past ten years, there have been some interesting findings. **Sleeve gastrectomy has become the most common bariatric surgery performed (doubling)**, while Roux-en-Y gastric bypass has been cut in half. Also, biliopancreatic diversion with duodenal switch has never exceeded 2%, and laparoscopic bands have nose-dived in popularity.

The table below shows the estimated rates of bariatric surgery per American Society for Metabolic and Bariatric Surgery (ASMBS).

Bariatric Surgery Estimates (2012-2020)					
Year	2012	2014	2016	2018	2020[1]
Total	173,000	193,000	216,000	252,000	199,000
SG	33%	51.7%	58.1%	61.4%	61.3%
RYGB	37.5%	26.8%	18.7%	17%	20.6%
Band	20.2%	9.5%	3.4%	1.1%	1.2%
BPD/DS	1.0%	0.4%	0.6%	0.8%	1.7%
Revision	6%	11.5%	14%	15.4%	11.0%
Balloons	--	--	2.6%	2.0%	1.4%
SADI	--	--	--	--	0.2%
OAGB	--	--	--	--	0.7%

[1]Significant decrease in surgeries in 2020 related to covid pandemic
SG: Sleeve gastrectomy; **RYGB:** Roux-en-Y gastric bypass; **BPD/DS:** Biliopancreatic diversion with duodenal switch; **SADI:** Single anastomosis duodeno-ileal bypass; **OAGB:** One anastomosis gastric bypass

Reference: https://asmbs.org/resources/estimate-of-bariatric-surgery-numbers

137. (Content: III-D-2) A 29-year-old female with a past medical history of migraine headaches and pre-diabetes is presenting to a local weight-loss clinic frustrated about her lack of weight loss. She currently exercises 300 minutes/week, restricts her calories to 1200 kcal/day, and takes no medications. She has been working with a weight-loss coach for the past six months. She is interested in weight-loss surgery. Her BMI is 29 kg/m^2, and her vital signs and physical exam are otherwise unremarkable. Which of the following would be the most appropriate action to take now?

A. Further intensify lifestyle modifications
B. Begin weight-loss pharmacotherapy
C. Referral for bariatric surgery
D. Referral for dietician
E. Provide reassurance

(B) This patient, who has failed comprehensive and intensive lifestyle modifications with a BMI ≥ 27 kg/m^2, meets the criteria **for pharmacologic therapy.** Further intensifying her exercise or diet is unlikely to yield the results she desires, and she does not meet bariatric surgery criteria at this time.

All patients trying to lose weight should undergo comprehensive lifestyle interventions[1] before attempting adjunctive therapy or surgery. If unable to achieve or sustain weight loss, the following adjuvant treatments can be considered:

- **Pharmacotherapy:** In those with a BMI ≥ 30 kg/m^2 or ≥ 27 kg/m^2 with comorbidities
- **Bariatric surgery:** In those with a BMI ≥ 35 kg/m^2 or ≥ 30 kg/m^2 with metabolic disease (2022 ASBMS/IFSO update).

[1]High intensity comprehensive lifestyle changes consist of behavioral strategies, moderately reduced-calorie diet, and increased physical activity.

Reference: 2022 American Society for Metabolic and Bariatric Surgery (ASMBS) and International Federation for the Surgery of Obesity and Metabolic Disorders (IFSO): Indications for Metabolic and Bariatric Surgery. Published: October 20, 2022 DOI:https://doi.org/10.1016/j.soard.2022.08.013
Reference: 2013 AHA/ACC/TOS Guideline for the Management of Overweight and Obesity in Adults. A Report of the American College of Cardiology/American Heart Association Task Force on Practice Guidelines and The Obesity Society. Box 11-12.

138. (Content: III-A-1) You are discussing with a patient their interest in physical activity. After asking the patient to grade their motivation in readiness to initiate a workout plan, the patient states they are at a 6 out of 10. What is the most appropriate reply to their assessment?

A.   Why did you not select a number higher than that?
B.   Great- it seems like you are motivated
C.   **Why did you not select a 3?**
D.   What can I do to convince you to get it to a 10?
E.   It doesn't seem like you are quite ready yet

(C) 'Change talk' guides the patient to see the need for change. It can be helpful to have them rate their readiness or motivation to make a change. After rating, **asking why it is not a lower number** will allow them an opportunity to convince or reiterate to themselves their motivation. Asking why it is not a higher number, may create and reinforce barriers that may actually decrease their motivation. It is not up to you as a clinician during motivation interviewing to convince them to change, but rather help them channel their motivation and desire to change.

Importantly, once you have helped evoke the change, it is helpful to know their barriers to assist with planning, but doing so in a way that allows them to overcome the barriers, such as "if you have had difficulty getting transportation to the gym in the past, what are ways we can ensure reliable transportation this time?"

Motivational interviewing is all about allowing the patient to come up with solutions to barriers and assisting their internal motivation to move them forward. On board exams, look for the answer that promotes this internal change or revelation.

Reference: Obesity medicine association: Obesity Algorithm (2021)

139. (Content: III-F-5c) A patient is six months post biliopancreatic diversion with duodenal switch and has been happy with her weight loss thus far. However, she has noticed that her hair has grown slower and started to fall out. This is very concerning to her. She admits to taking one prenatal vitamin daily and following all food restrictions. Recent thyroid levels and complete metabolic panel were normal. Given these findings, what micro deficiency is the most likely explanation for her symptoms?

- A. Selenium
- **B. Zinc**
- C. Copper
- D. Vitamin K
- E. Vitamin A

(B) Micronutrient deficiencies occur most commonly in malabsorptive procedures. **Zinc deficiency** can cause alopecia, anosmia, brittle nails, and chronic diarrhea. In males, it can also cause hypogonadism or erectile dysfunction. Importantly, telogen effluvium is common with rapid weight loss and should be considered in the absence of micronutrient deficiencies.

The table below summarizes high-yield deficiencies and their symptoms.

Micronutrient Deficiencies after Malabsorptive Procedures	
Nutrient	**Symptoms of Deficiency**
Vitamin A	Night blindness, follicular hyperkeratosis
Vitamin E	Hemolytic anemia, neuromuscular, or ophthalmologic findings
Vitamin K	Excessive bleeding or bruising
Selenium	Unexplained anemia, fatigue, persistent diarrhea, cardiomyopathy, or metabolic bone disorder
Zinc	Chronic diarrhea, alopecia, pica, dysgeusia, anosmia, hypogonadism or erectile dysfunction (males)
Copper	Anemia, neutropenia, myeloneuropathy, or impaired wound healing
Biotin[1]	Seborrheic dermatitis, alopecia, neurologic manifestations

[1]Can be caused by a large consumption of raw eggs.
Note: Nutritional anemias can occur from Vitamin B12, folate, protein, copper, selenium, zinc, or iron deficiency

Reference: AACE/TOS/ASMBS/OMA/ASA 2019 Guidelines: CLINICAL PRACTICE GUIDELINES FOR THE PERIOPERATIVE NUTRITION, METABOLIC, AND NONSURGICAL SUPPORT OF PATIENTS UNDERGOING BARIATRIC PROCEDURES – 2019 UPDATE. Recommendation 57, 62, 63-65

140. (Content: III-F-2) A family practice physician sees multiple patients during her dedicated bariatric clinic session. A number of them have approached her regarding evaluation for bariatric surgery. Which of the following patients would be the best current candidate for weight-loss surgery?

A. 29-year-old male (BMI 36 kg/m²) who is a current tobacco user with a history of hypertension and obstructive sleep apnea
B. 34-year-old female (BMI 41 kg/m²) with a history of cervical cancer status post hysterectomy with clean margins
C. 52-year-old female (BMI 55 kg/m²) with a history of hypertension, refusing to undergo mammography and colonoscopy
D. **60-year-old male (BMI 34 kg/m²) with a history of osteoarthritis, hyperlipidemia, diabetes type 2, and chronic kidney disease stage 2**

(D) Although it is still recommended to trial medication management initially in those with obesity class I, new metabolic and bariatric surgery criteria (2022) include patients with a **BMI ≥ 30 kg/m² with metabolic disease** (type 2 diabetes, prediabetes, metabolic syndrome, hypertension, metabolic associated fatty liver disease/metabolic associated steatohepatitis, obstructive sleep apnea, polycystic ovarian syndrome, etc). Bariatric surgery is also recommended in those with a BMI ≥ 35 kg/m² regardless of comorbidity.

Other valuable perioperative recommendations are discussed below:

- Age is not a contraindication, although perceived long-term benefits should be considered.
- Patients must quit nicotine products 6-8 weeks before surgery.
- Patients should be up to date on all preventative cancer screenings.
- Avoid pregnancy before surgery and 12-18 months postoperatively.
- Estrogen should be stopped for one cycle of oral contraceptives (premenopausal) or three weeks of hormone replacement therapy (postmenopausal) to reduce the risk of post-procedure thrombosis.

Reference: 2022 American Society for Metabolic and Bariatric Surgery (ASMBS) and International Federation for the Surgery of Obesity and Metabolic Disorders (IFSO): Indications for Metabolic and Bariatric Surgery. Published: October 20, 2022 DOI:https://doi.org/10.1016/j.soard.2022.08.013
Reference: AACE/TOS/ASMBS/OMA/ASA 2019 Guidelines: CLINICAL PRACTICE GUIDELINES FOR THE PERIOPERATIVE NUTRITION, METABOLIC, AND NONSURGICAL SUPPORT OF PATIENTS UNDERGOING BARIATRIC PROCEDURES – 2019 UPDATE. Recommendation 2, 17, 18, 23, 33

141. (Content: III-B-4) A 48-year-old female with the disease of obesity presents as a follow-up appointment regarding increased liver enzymes. She recently completed a right upper quadrant ultrasound that revealed fatty liver infiltration. She denies any significant alcohol use. Which of the following diets should be recommended to her at this time?

    A. **Mediterranean-style**
    B. DASH diet
    C. Low glycemic index
    D. Low fat
    E. High protein

(A) Although reducing total calories should be the main component of weight loss intervention, specific dietary compositions may be preferred in certain patient populations. **A Mediterranean-style diet is beneficial, independent of weight loss, in hepatic steatosis.**

Diet	Potential Benefits
Mediterranean-style	- Decreases certain cancer risks - Improves hepatic steatosis - Reduces cardio-metabolic risk - Improves renal function
Low glycemic index	- Decreases adipocyte diameter - Decreases glycemic variability
DASH diet[1]	- Improves blood pressure - Not necessarily designed for weight loss
High protein[2]	- Improves cardio-metabolic risks - Decreases adipocyte diameter - Less relative loss of muscle mass - Prolongs benefit on waist circumference and percent of fat reduction
Low fat	- Beneficial effect on lipids - Improves renal function

[1]Every 1 lb decrease in weight corresponds to the reduction of systolic and diastolic BP by 1 mmHg
[2]Animal proteins (not plant) are associated with increased inflammation

Reference: AACE/ACE Guidelines: AMERICAN ASSOCIATION OF CLINICAL ENDOCRINOLOGISTS AND AMERICAN COLLEGE OF ENDOCRINOLOGY COMPREHENSIVE CLINICAL PRACTICE GUIDELINES FOR MEDICAL CARE OF PATIENTS WITH OBESITY (2016): Recommendation 47, 65-66.

142. (Content: III-B-3) A 42-year-old male presents to a dietary clinic for his initial consultation. He admits that his work schedule is hectic, requiring him to travel frequently, and thus, he feels his weight gain is most likely due to his fast-food intake. He is not interested in calorie counting. His weight loss goals include losing approximately 10% of his weight within the next year, based on mostly diet changes, as he already exercises every morning. His BMI is 37 kg/m^2, and he has no prior medical history. Given these preferences, which would be the best fit regarding weight-loss management?

A. Mediterranean diet
B. Paleo diet
C. Bariatric surgery
D. **Meal replacement**
E. Pharmacotherapy

(D) This patient who wants significant weight loss, but has time constraints and travels frequently, would be a great candidate for **meal replacement therapy.** Pharmacotherapy would not be a great option, as it doesn't change his poor diet. Also, bariatric surgery requires significant commitment and diet monitoring, which he does not appear to be able to commit to at this time.

Meal replacements are a convenient option that can be taken on trips, as they require no cooking or significant preparation. Preferably, it provides a predictable amount of reduced calories (< 200 calories), high-protein (15-30 g) to suppress appetite, and low carbohydrates (< 10 g) to prevent weight gain. Also, they can be added to any diet and contain appropriate macro and micronutrients.

Note: Meal replacements are commonly used as a meal substitute twice daily for weight loss and once daily for weight maintenance. The Look Ahead trial showed increased use of meal replacement of approximately 2 per day were associated with higher levels of weight loss (11.9%) compared to a lower use of 2 per week (5.9%).

Reference: One-year Weight Losses in the Look AHEAD Study: Factors Associated With Success. Thomas A. Wadden Delia S. West Rebecca H. Neiberg Rena R. Wing Donna H. Ryan Karen C. Johnson John P. Foreyt James O. Hill Dace L. Trence Mara Z. Vitolins. Look AHEAD Research Group. First published: 06 September 2012 https://doi.org/10.1038/oby.2008.637

143. (Content: III-D-2) A 52-year-old male presents for follow-up at the transplant center. He was diagnosed with cirrhosis secondary to long-standing metabolic-associated fatty liver disease. He has minimal ascites and his last hospitalization was three months ago for hepatic encephalopathy. His BMI is currently 38 kg/m², and he must lose 25 lbs (11.3 kg) before being placed on the liver transplant list. Which of the following anti-obesity medications is contraindicated in this patient?

A. Setmelanotide
B. **Naltrexone/bupropion ER**
C. Semaglutide
D. Orlistat
E. Cellulose and citric acid hydrogel

(B) Levels of naltrexone can increase 5 to 10-fold in those with cirrhosis and, therefore, should be avoided. Of the FDA-approved anti-obesity medications, both phentermine/topiramate ER and **naltrexone/bupropion ER**

should be reduced in moderate hepatic impairment (Child-Pugh class B) and avoided in severe impairment/cirrhosis (Child-Pugh class C).

Anti-obesity medications (AOM) can be a great tool to assist those pursuing weight loss to be placed on a transplant list. Knowing which AOM to avoid in the setting of liver or renal impairment is testable.

Anti-Obesity Medication Adjustments in Liver Disease			
Level of Impairment (Child-Pugh class)	Mild (Class A)	Moderate (Class B)	Severe/Cirrhosis (Class C)
Phentermine/topiramate ER	--	Reduce[1]	AVOID
Naltrexone/bupropion ER	--	Reduce[2]	AVOID
Semaglutide and liraglutide	--	--	--
Orlistat	--	--	--
Cellulose and citric acid hydrogel	--	--	--

[1]Max dose: Phentermine 7.5 mg/topiramate 46 mg once daily
[2]Max dose: Naltrexone 8 mg/bupropion 90 mg twice daily
-- indicates no dosage adjustment necessary

Reference: Package inserts for medications listed

144. (Content: III-D-1) A patient returns to the office extremely concerned because she recently found out her grandfather had medullary thyroid carcinoma (MTC). She started on semaglutide at her prior appointment to help with weight loss. Which of the following is the best advice to provide the patient?

A. "It is fine to continue the medication, as MTC is not associated with this class of medications."
B. **"The associated risk of MTC has only been shown in animal studies, not in human trials."**
C. "We must monitor calcitonin levels and order a RET oncogene test while on this medication."
D. "Unfortunately, the risk of developing MTC has increased significantly, given your family history."

(B) Although there is a contraindication to any GLP-1 receptor agonist if there is a family history of medullary thyroid cancer or multiple endocrine neoplasia syndrome type 2 (MEN 2) syndromes, the increased risk of MTC has only been shown in rat studies (duration and dose-dependent), and the risk to humans is unknown. This patient was likely started on a lower initial starting dose and has not been on the medication for long. The best course of action is to discontinue this medication immediately, but provide reassurance that this **medication has only shown an increased risk of MTC in animal studies**.

GLP-1 receptor agonists, including dual incretins such as tirzepatide, carry a black-box warning against use in those with a family history of MTC or MEN 2 syndromes. The recommendation from the manufacture is to:

- Discuss this risk with patients
- Discuss symptoms of thyroid cancer, including dysphagia, voice hoarseness, dyspnea, or a neck mass
- Routine monitoring (calcitonin, a tumor marker for MTC, or thyroid ultrasound) has no current evidence to support its use

GLP-1 receptor agonists have also been associated with pancreatitis, which through a metanalysis has been shown to unlikely be a true association, although this remains listed in the package insert.

Reference: Cao C, Yang S, Zhou Z. GLP-1 receptor agonists and pancreatic safety concerns in type 2 diabetic patients: data from cardiovascular outcome trials. Endocrine. 2020 Jun;68(3):518-525. doi: 10.1007/s12020-020-02223-6. Epub 2020 Feb 26. PMID: 32103407.
Reference: Semaglutide package insert.

145. (Content: III-F-1) A 37-year-old male presents to discuss bariatric surgical options. He had a friend that underwent a single anastomosis duodeno-ileostomy with sleeve gastrectomy (SADI-S) and has done well. He is wondering about the benefits and risks of this procedure compared to a Roux-en-Y gastric bypass. What is the best advice to provide?

A. The SADI-S has more anastomotic sites than the RYGB
B. The SADI-S reduces ghrelin significantly more than RYGB
C. A RYGB requires more frequent monitoring of vitamin levels
D. The RYGB leads to increased remission rates of diabetes mellitus
E. The SADI-S is done through an open abdominal procedure

(B) The SADI-S, used interchangeably with the Stomach Intestinal Pylorus Sparing Surgery (SIPSS), is a malabsorptive procedure that includes performing a concurrent sleeve gastrectomy, **thus reducing ghrelin levels significantly**, as this orexigenic hormone is produced in the gastric fundus.

A SADI-S may be preferred over RYGB in certain patients, including those with a BMI > 50 kg/m². Malabsorptive procedures such as the SADI-S and duodenal switch provide 15% more weight loss than a RYGB, and higher resolution of diabetes. Compared to the duodenal switch, the SADI-S has fewer anastomotic sites, less malabsorption, and fewer overall complications, thus increasing its popularity. Like the duodenal switch, the SADI-S may be used as a revision of a prior surgery or staged procedure in high surgical risk patients.

Comparison of Malabsorptive Procedures			
Surgery	SADI-S	BPD/DS	RYGB
Malabsorptive	++	+++	+
Sleeve gastrectomy	Yes	Yes	No
Common channel	300 cm	75-150 cm	Variable
% intestine bypassed	50%	80%	--
Excess weight loss	75-95%	75-95%	65-80%
Anastomosis sites	1	2	2

SADI-S: Single Anastomosis Duodeno-ileostomy with Sleeve; **BPD/DS:** Biliopancreatic diversion with a duodenal switch; **RYGB:** Roux-en-Y gastric bypass

Reference: Sánchez-Pernaute A, Herrera MÁR, Ferré NP, Rodríguez CS, Marcuello C, Pañella C, Antoñanzas LL, Torres A, Pérez-Aguirre E. Long-Term Results of Single-Anastomosis Duodeno-ileal Bypass with Sleeve Gastrectomy (SADI-S). Obes Surg. 2022 Mar;32(3):682-689. doi: 10.1007/s11695-021-05879-9. Epub 2022 Jan 15. PMID: 35032311; PMCID: PMC8760573.

146. (Content: III-D-7) A recently graduated advanced practice nurse is prescribing pharmacologic therapy in the clinic. Although she has received her national provider identifier (NPI) number, she currently does not have her drug enforcement agency (DEA) license. Because of this limitation, which of the following medications is she able to prescribe?

    A. Diethylpropion
    B. Phentermine/topiramate ER
    C. Phendimetrazine
    D. Naltrexone/bupropion ER

(D) Of the options above, only **naltrexone/bupropion ER** is not a controlled substance and does not require a DEA license for prescribing. The other FDA-approved long-term medications, including liraglutide, semaglutide, and orlistat, are not controlled drugs.

Despite the lack of evidence in well-controlled animal or human studies that phentermine and other sympathetic amines cause physical dependence (as evidenced by abuse and withdrawals), their structural similarities to other classes of medication (i.e., amphetamines) cause certain medications to be classified as controlled substances.

This includes the following:

- Long-term use (2)
  - Lorcaserin (removed from market 2/2020) (Class IV)
  - Phentermine/topiramate ER (Class IV)
- Short-term use (4)
  - Diethylpropion (Class IV)
  - Phentermine (Class IV)
  - Benzphetamine (Class III)
  - Phendimetrazine (Class III)

Note: Most obesity medications are approved for adults only. The exceptions are phentermine for those ≥ 16 years old, and phentermine/topiramate ER (Qsymia®), orlistat, and liraglutide (Saxenda®) for those ≥ 12 years old. Criteria includes class I obesity with weight comorbidities or class 2 obesity or greater. Semaglutide is expected to be approved in those ≥ 12 years old soon.

Reference: Up to Date: "Overweight and obesity in adults: Health consequences"

147. (Content: III-A-1) A 29-year-old female affected by obesity is presenting for help with losing and maintaining weight. During discussions, the importance of losing 5-10% of her baseline weight related to her health is reiterated, specifically related to improving current medical conditions and preventing future issues. This discussion falls into which of the following categories of the "5 A's of obesity management"?

A. Ask
B. Assess
C. Advise
D. Agree
E. Arrange/assist

(C) This patient is being **advised on the benefits** of modest weight loss related to her health. Advisement can incorporate the health risks, benefits, and the need for treatments, as well as potential long-term options.

The 5 A's of motivational interviewing is a memory aid and technique not limited to obesity medicine but is commonly implemented in obesity practice. The five components are summarized in the table below.

The 5 A's Of Obesity Management	
Ask	-Ask for permission to discuss body weight -Explore readiness to change
Assess	-Assess BMI and waist circumference -Explore obstacles and complications of excess weight
Advise	-Advise about the health risks of obesity -Discuss the benefits of weight loss (even modest amounts) -Present the importance of a long-term strategy -Provide potential treatment options
Agree	-Agree on realistic weight-loss goals and expectations -Document specific details of the agreed-upon treatment plan
Arrange/ Assist	-Assist in identifying barriers to weight loss -Provide resources, including consultations with providers -Arrange regular follow-up

Reference: Obesity medicine association: Obesity Algorithm (2021)

148. (Content: III-B-4) A 67-year-old male presents for lifestyle modification education after recently having a cardiac stent placed for unstable angina. In particular, he is wondering about "good fats" that his wife has talked about. Which of the following is the most accurate statement?

    A. Saturated fats are unlikely to be absorbed and thus preferred
    B. Trans fats should only be consumed in moderation
    C. **Increasing polyunsaturated fats reduces cardiac risk factors**
    D. Coconut oil is preferred instead of vegetable oil
    E. Tilapia is a cheaper alternative to salmon with similar benefits

(C) Polyunsaturated fatty acids include omega-3, which has anti-inflammatory effects, thus having cardiovascular benefits and may help prevent/treat atherosclerosis. In contrast, saturated fats should be limited and trans fats have been removed from the market due to adverse cardiac effects. A good rule of thumb is that fats that are solid at room temperature (coconut oil, butter, etc.) contain higher amounts of saturated fats and should be avoided. This contrasts with polyunsaturated fats such as vegetable and olive oil.

Replacing saturated fats with polyunsaturated fats has been shown by the American College of Cardiology to reduce the risk of cardiovascular disease by 30%, having a similar quantitative effect as statin use.

Alpha-linoleic acid is a form of omega-3 polyunsaturated fatty acids that reduces the risk of fatal coronary heart disease and is recommended by the American Heart Association (AHA). This form can be found in fattier fish such as cod, sardines, tuna, salmon, herring, and lake trout. Other sources include avocados, vegetable oil, flax seed oil, walnuts, soy, spinach, and kale.

Importantly, alpha-linoleic acid is involved with neurologic development in children and to some degree is converted to eicosatetraenoic acid (EPA) and docosahexaenoic acid (DHA). It is preferred to obtain these nutrients through food rather than supplementation if possible.

Reference: Dietary Fats and Cardiovascular Disease: A Presidential Advisory from the American Heart Association. Circulation 2017;Jun 15:
Reference: Up to Date: "Dietary fat"

149. (Content: III-F-5 and III-D-3) A 52-year-old female presents to the emergency room by ambulance after a witnessed seizure. The patient is not on any current medications. She underwent a successful Roux-en-Y gastric bypass nearly 2 years ago, with hypertension currently in remission. Her husband states she has complained of lightheadedness and fatigue 1-2 hours after meals for the past few months. However, this is the first time she has had a seizure. Point of care glucose on arrival is 23 mg/dL (reference range: 74-106 mg/dL). Which of the following daily medications may have prevented her seizure?

A. Semaglutide
B. Metformin
C. Metoprolol
D. Acabrose
E. Sitagliptan

(D) This patient presents with post-prandial hypoglycemia symptoms more than one year after Roux-en-Y gastric bypass, consistent with post-gastric bypass hypoglycemia (PGBH). Besides **acarbose,** all of the options above may worsen symptoms (or, as with metoprolol, may initially mask symptoms).

Initial treatment of PGBH should focus on dietary modifications with a low carbohydrate, mixed diet. If these conservative measures are ineffective, pharmacotherapy can be considered:

- Acarbose: This complex disaccharide delays the digestion of carbohydrates, resulting in delayed/diminished insulin release.
- Octreotide: This somatostatin analog is a potent insulin inhibitor
- Calcium channel blockers: This class of medications acts directly on the β-cells to inhibit glucose-dependent insulin release.
- Diazoxide: Suppresses insulin secretion via β-cell channels.

In severe cases where the above therapies are ineffective, reversal of the RYGB or conversion to a gastric sleeve should be considered.

Note: Late dumping syndrome may present similar in timeframe as PGBH but will not cause neuroglycopenia and will respond to dietary changes alone.

Reference: Malik S, Mitchell JE, Steffen K, Engel S, Wiisanen R, Garcia L, Malik SA. Recognition and management of hyperinsulinemic hypoglycemia after bariatric surgery. Obes Res Clin Pract. 2016 Jan-Feb;10(1):1-14. doi: 10.1016/j.orcp.2015.07.003. Epub 2015 Oct 27. PMID: 26522879; PMCID: PMC5688875.

150. (Content: III-F-1 and 2) A 28-year-old female with a history of rheumatoid arthritis and epilepsy presents to a multidisciplinary weight loss clinic after not meeting weight loss goals with lifestyle modifications. Her BMI is 36.2 kg/m². She is interested in long-term weight loss options in combination with behavioral therapy. Which of the following would be the most appropriate option for her?

    A. Gastric balloon
    B. Naltrexone/bupropion ER
    C. Open sleeve gastrectomy
    D. Aspiration device
    E. TransPyloric shuttle

(D) The **AspireAssist®** is an FDA-approved, long-term weight loss device for adults aged ≥22 years old with a BMI of 35-55 kg/m². A percutaneous endoscopic gastrostomy tube with an accessible skin port is connected to a companion device to allow for the aspiration of 25-30% of consumed calories 20-30 minutes after meal consumption.

Note: Gastric balloons (<6 months) and the TransPyloric shuttle® (<12 months) are short-term options, while bariatric should be laparoscopic, not open. Bupropion is contraindicated with a history of seizure disorders.

A lanyard ❹ carries the companion device ❺. When used, gastric contents ❶ are removed through gravity, not active suctioning, and drained into the toilet ❷. The reservoir bag ❸ is filled with water and can be squeezed to flush the port.

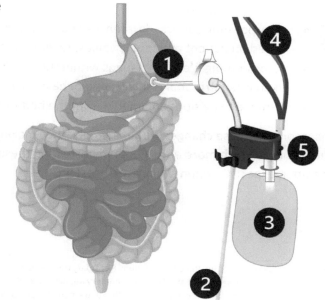

151. (Content: III-H-4) An 8-year-old male with excess weight presents to his pediatrician, accompanied by his mother. The patient appears happy and has no other medical conditions and takes no medications. The mother states the school year has been busy with music lessons and chess tournaments, which he prefers over sports. She says he is physically inactive but has eliminated soda from his diet. Given the mother's work schedule, they often pick up food from restaurants in the evening. Which of the following would be the most effective method to promote weight loss in this patient?

A. Initiate pharmacotherapy
B. Wake patient up early to exercise
C. Restrict dinner portion sizes
D. Sign the patient up for soccer
E. **Involve the family in weight loss**

(E) Pediatric patients tend to have more favorable outcomes **when the family is integrated into the obesity treatment plan**. This is one of the most important steps in treating childhood obesity so the child does not feel singled out.

There are many opportunities for family involvement, including:

- Family recognition of the problem (first step!)
- Increasing the number of family meals together at home
- Limiting eating out
- Incorporating cultural differences and adapting recommendations based on patient and family values, religion, etc.
- Incorporating lifestyle changes within the family unit, including exercise, nutritional changes, and behavioral modification
- Remove televisions and media from the bedrooms and kitchen

Incorporating these changes within a family, thus making it a "new normal" for the family, is much more effective than bestowing these changes on one family member, especially when siblings are present.

Reference: Expert Committee Recommendations Regarding the Prevention, Assessment, and Treatment of Child and Adolescent Overweight and Obesity: Summary Report and APPENDIX. Sarah E. Barlow and the Expert Committee; Pediatrics December 2007, 120 (Supplement 4) S164-S192; DOI: https://doi.org/10.1542/peds.2007-2329C.

152. (Content: III-D-1) A 31-year-old female with a body mass index of 36 kg/m² presents to her primary care physician after discussing weight loss medications with her friend. She is interested in starting a medication but is unsure of the best option. She denies any tobacco or alcohol abuse. Past medical history reveals a history of recurrent nephrolithiasis and epilepsy. Physical exam reveals truncal obesity with a small and reducible umbilical hernia with minimal abdominal striae. Of the options below, which would be her best long-term option?

    A. Phentermine/topiramate ER
    B. Phentermine monotherapy
    C. Liraglutide
    D. Naltrexone/bupropion ER
    E. Orlistat

(C) In patients with or at risk of oxalate nephropathy or nephrolithiasis, topiramate and orlistat should be avoided. Bupropion is contraindicated in epilepsy, seizure disorders, or those at risk for seizures (i.e., alcohol use disorder or eating disorders). Although often used long-term with close monitoring, phentermine is less effective than **liraglutide,** which has an FDA approval for long-term weight management and diabetes.

Note: Although liraglutide is safe in a patient with nephrolithiasis or oxalate nephropathy, a relatively common side-effect is gastrointestinal distress. Therefore, liraglutide should be discontinued if nausea, vomiting, and diarrhea cause hypovolemia or volume contraction, as hypovolemia can increase the risk of nephrolithiasis.

Note: Although phentermine/topiramate ER can be used in those with a history of seizures, all patients should be slowly tapered off this medication if discontinued, especially at higher doses, to decrease the risk of seizures.

Reference: AACE/ACE Guidelines: AMERICAN ASSOCIATION OF CLINICAL ENDOCRINOLOGISTS AND AMERICAN COLLEGE OF ENDOCRINOLOGY COMPREHENSIVE CLINICAL PRACTICE GUIDELINES FOR MEDICAL CARE OF PATIENTS WITH OBESITY (2016). Recommendation 86 and 87.

153. (Content: III-A-1) A 59-year-old female presents to an obesity medicine specialist. She has tried numerous dietary plans and becomes frustrated with the associated restrictions and rules. Since the beginning of the covid pandemic, she has worked from home, exercises 200-300 minutes weekly, and does resistance training twice weekly. She is interested in anti-obesity medications but also wants to continue working on lifestyle modifications. Which of the following recommendations would be most useful for her?

A. Recommend increasing her weekly physical activity
B. Provide resources on mindful eating
C. Discuss phone-based applications to count calories and macronutrients
D. Initiate medications and put lifestyle changes on hold
E. Begin sertraline to help with depression and improve motivation

(B) This motivated patient exercises regularly but struggles with the constraints of dietary plans. Therefore, in addition to continuing her physical activity and discussing anti-obesity medications, a discussion on **mindful eating** may be a great individualized option for her.

Mindful eating is not a dietary plan but an approach to eating that can be applied to any dietary plan or even by itself. The tenants of this approach are being mentally present when eating and focusing on the eating experience including the thoughts and feelings about what you are eating without concern of judgment. Although this approach sounds like it could encourage unhealthy eating, it often leads to the opposite. Some key points are below:

- It promotes knowing your personal hunger signals. In other words, do not eat unless you feel hungry (i.e., homeostatic hunger).
- Paying attention to the food is important, selecting foods they enjoy, but also foods that are consistent with their desired health benefits. They are encouraged to examine the food, smell it, focus on the taste, etc. Instead of eating a large bite (or a handful of items), they eat small bites or individual items and enjoy each one.
- It helps avoid stringent rules or calorie counting, which many patients with a history of eating disorders or obsessive-compulsive disorder may struggle with.

Reference: Nelson JB. Mindful Eating: The Art of Presence While You Eat. Diabetes Spectr. 2017 Aug;30(3):171-174. doi: 10.2337/ds17-0015. PMID: 28848310; PMCID: PMC5556586.

154. (Content: III-F-3) A 37-year-old female is following up with her bariatric surgeon after undergoing a successful Roux-en-Y gastric bypass procedure three weeks prior. Overall she is doing well, however, she points to her mid-epigastric region as having increased constant pain, which is not relieved with famotidine. Also, yesterday she noticed nausea, and today she has had two bouts of emesis. She does admit to starting smoking again, but only 4-5 cigarettes daily. Her last bowel movement was three days ago. Which of the following is the most likely diagnosis?

    A.   Internal hernia
    B.   Gastric outlet obstruction
    C.   Mesenteric ischemia
    D.   Anastomotic stricture
    E.   Marginal ulcer

(E) **Anastomotic or marginal ulcers** are relatively common in gastric bypass, occurring in up to 10% of patients. Patients will classically complain of localized abdominal pain, without alarming abdominal exam findings, with patients often complaining of nausea and vomiting. Smoking, as seen in this patient, is a strong risk factor.

The table below compares two common postoperative complications:

Anastomotic Ulcer versus Stricture		
Complication	Ulcer	Stricture/Stenosis
Prevalence	Approximately 10%	Approximately 25%
Symptoms	Localized abdominal pain, nausea, vomiting	Dysphagia, solid food intolerance, weight loss
Complications	Perforation, bleeding	Malnutrition, dehydration
Risk factors	NSAIDs, smoking, steroids, H. pylori, ischemia	Surgical technique, ischemia, inflammation
Diagnosis	EGD	Upper GI barium, EGD
Treatment	PPI, sucralfate, risk factor reduction (i.e., smoking)	Balloon dilation. Rarely surgical intervention

NSAIDs: non-steroidal anti-inflammatory drugs; **EGD:** esophagogastroduodenoscopy; **GI:** gastrointestinal; **PPI:** Proton pump inhibitor

Reference: Obesity medicine association: Obesity Algorithm (2021)

155. (Content: III-C-1) A 31-year-old previously healthy male presents to his family care physician for evaluation of his chronic condition of obesity. He started seeing a dietician and is very happy with his progress regarding dietary changes and calorie counting. He has not begun to exercise but is interested. A history and physical is performed, with no limitations to exercise perceived. An exercise prescription is being written. Which of the following is directly part of this prescription?

    A. Patient safety
    B. Barriers to exercise
    C. Motivational interviewing
    D. Enjoyment of activity
    E. Physical limitations

(D) An exercise prescription should include the following, which can be remembered by the acronym FITTE:

- **Frequency:** The number of days or intervals (e.g., weekdays or every other day) necessary to achieve the total weekly physical activity time goals (listed below).
- **Intensity:** The patient's physical activity and safety should be considered, with moderate to vigorous-intensity exercise preferred.
- **Time:** 150-300 minutes per week of moderate-intensity (or 75-150 minutes of vigorous-intensity) exercise is recommended.
- **Type:** This typically focuses on aerobic/cardiorespiratory and strength/weight training. However, flexibility, functional and balance (safety), speed (competition), and core strengthening can be considered as well, based on goals.
- **Enjoyment:** An individualized exercise regimen based on patient preference (indoor versus outdoor, group classes versus trainer, water versus running) promotes consistent follow-through.

Example: Perform 30 minutes of brisk walking (moderate-intensity) around the park every weekday after dinner. In addition, perform resistance training twice weekly for 20-minute periods.

Reference: Physical Activity Guidelines for Americans: 2nd Edition: https://health.gov/sites/default/files/2019-09/Physical_Activity_Guidelines_2nd_edition.pdf

156. (Content: III-D-1) A 49-year-old female presents to her family practitioner with a complaint of weight gain. She was on fenfluramine in combination with phentermine in the distant past and would like to start on something similar, as it was very effective. She is started on phentermine 15 mg in the morning. What is the most common side effect this patient will likely experience?

A. **Xerostomia**
B. Nausea and vomiting
C. Diarrhea
D. Dysgeusia
E. Headaches

(A) **Xerostomia** (dry mouth) is one of the most common side effects of sympathetic amines like phentermine. Patients are encouraged to increase their water intake to prevent issues such as dental carries. In contrast, topiramate can cause dysgeusia (abnormal taste).

Fenfluramine in combination with phentermine, termed "fen-phen," was taken off the market in 1997 due to an increased risk of valvular heart defects caused by fenfluramine (serotonin 5-HT2B receptor agonist). Importantly, phentermine was never associated with these issues and has never been taken off the market (available since 1959). Lorcaserin (Belviq®), a serotonin 5-HT2C receptor agonist, was marketed to have similar weight loss given the similar serotonergic effects but without the valvular problems. It was removed from the market in February 2020 due to increased incidences of malignancy during a clinical trial.

Phentermine (Adipex®, Lomaira®)	
Formulary	-Capsule/Tabs: 15 to 37.5 mg once daily in morning -Lomaira®: 8 mg TID 30 minutes before meals
Mechanism	Sympathomimetic amines stimulate the hypothalamus to release norepinephrine, resulting in decreased appetite and increased energy expenditure.
Contraindications	Hypersensitivity to phentermine or other formulary components, concurrent MAOI use, hyperthyroidism, close-angled glaucoma, and pregnancy. Avoid in those with coronary artery disease, severe anxiety, or a history of substance use.
Side Effects	Insomnia, constipation, xerostomia, and tachycardia

Reference: Phentermine package insert

157. (Content: III-F-1) A 42-year-old female with a medical history of difficult to control diabetes mellitus type 2 and obesity class III presents for a bariatric seminar to learn more about surgical options. She is particularly interested in a more recently endorsed malabsorptive procedure. It is described as having a high diabetes remission rate and causing a significant reduction in hunger due to the removal of a portion of the stomach. Which surgical procedure is she referring to?

A. **Single anastomosis duodeno-ileostomy with sleeve gastrectomy**
B. Vertical sleeve gastrectomy
C. Roux-en-Y gastric bypass
D. Biliopancreatic diversion with a duodenal switch
E. One anastomosis gastric bypass

(A) **Single anastomosis duodeno-ileostomy with sleeve gastrectomy** (SADI-S), also referred to as a stomach intestinal pylorus sparing surgery (SIPSS), is a more recently endorsed metabolic and bariatric surgery.

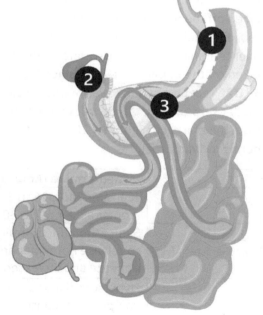

The SADI-S involves stapling and cutting the duodenum ❷ just distal to the pylorus (pylorus remains intact) and anastomosing a loop of the intestine to the stomach ❸. This procedure has less complications than the duodenal switch including less malabsorption and only one anastomosis. It has increased weight loss and diabetes remission when compared to the RYGB. In addition, a sleeve gastrectomy ❶ is performed, providing an additional restrictive and hormonal (decreased ghrelin) mechanism.

Image citation: Image created by Charu G. Copyright owned by Kevin Smith, DO
Reference: Eichelter J, Felsenreich DM, Bichler C, Gensthaler L, Gachabayov M, Richwien P, Nixdorf L, Jedamzik J, Mairinger M, Langer FB, Prager G. Surgical Technique of Single Anastomosis Duodeno-Ileal Bypass with Sleeve Gastrectomy (SADI-S). Surg Technol Int. 2022 May 27;41:sti41/1571. doi: 10.52198/22.STI.41.GS1571. Epub ahead of print. PMID: 35623034.

158. (Content: III-D-4) A 27-year-old female with a history of epilepsy is returning for a one month-follow up to her primary care physician's office. Three months ago, she was started on phentermine/topiramate ER after lifestyle changes failed to achieve her weight loss goals. Her current dose is 7.5/46 mg phentermine/ topiramate ER daily. She is tolerating the medication well but is unsure of its effectiveness. During the past three months, her weight has decreased from 220 lbs (100 kg) to 216 lbs (98 kg). Which option would be the most appropriate to initiate at this time?

    A. Monitor for weight loss for an additional month
    B. Take an additional phentermine/topiramate ER 3.75/23 mg tab at night
    C. Change the medication to naltrexone/bupropion ER
    D. Titrate up to phentermine/topiramate ER 15/92 mg daily
    E. Titrate off medication, then start liraglutide

(D) This patient, who is tolerating phentermine/topiramate ER, but is not seeing appropriate results (> 3% total body weight loss at 12 weeks), should **increase the dose to 11.25/69 mg x 14 days, then 15/92 mg daily (full strength) to evaluate for a response.** If weight loss is less than 5% of total body weight at the full strength dose, the medication should be discontinued, and alternatives may be trialed. Importantly, this patient has a history of epilepsy, making naltrexone/bupropion ER contraindicated.

Note: Phentermine/topiramate ER should be taken in the morning, as it can cause insomnia if taken later in the day or evening.

Reference: Phentermine/topiramate ER package insert

159. (Content: III-F-5b) A 31-year-old male presents for his initial 1-week post-bariatric surgery (sleeve gastrectomy) follow-up appointment with his dietician. He has continued on a liquid diet and has been taking crushed vitamin supplementation. His current vitamin intake includes the following:

- Two adult multivitamins
- Elemental calcium of 1200 mg daily
- 1000 international units of vitamin D
- 65 mg of iron taken on an empty stomach

Which of the following recommendations should be made to this patient?

A. Take iron with calcium for increased absorption
B. Avoid concentrated carbohydrates to prevent dumping syndrome
C. **Double the amount of vitamin D intake**
D. Decrease the multivitamin to one tablet daily
E. Ensure the multivitamins contain vitamin K

(C) Except for laparoscopic adjustable gastric banding, all patients status post-bariatric surgery should take two adult multivitamins containing folic acid, thiamine, and vitamin B_{12}. In addition, everyone should **take 2000-3000 international vitamin D units** with dosage titration to maintain dietary vitamin D levels > 30 ng/mL.

Minimum Daily Vitamin and Mineral Intake After Bariatric Surgery				
Procedure	SG	RYGB	BPD/DS & SADI-S	LAGB
Adult MV[1]	2	2	2	1
Calcium	1200-1500 mg		1800-2400 mg	1200-1500 mg
Vitamin D	2000-3000 IU			
Iron	18 mg (men)-60 mg (menstruating females)			

[1]Multivitamin should contain iron, folic acid, thiamine, and vitamin B_{12}
LAGB: Laparoscopic adjustable gastric banding; **SG** Sleeve gastrectomy; **RYGB** Roux-en-Y gastric bypass; **BPD/DS:** Biliopancreatic diversion with duodenal switch; **SADI-S:** Single anastomosis duodeno-ileal bypass with sleeve gastrectomy

Reference: AACE/TOS/ASMBS/OMA/ASA 2019 Guidelines: CLINICAL PRACTICE GUIDELINES FOR THE PERIOPERATIVE NUTRITION, METABOLIC, AND NONSURGICAL SUPPORT OF PATIENTS UNDERGOING BARIATRIC PROCEDURES – 2019 UPDATE. Recommendation 39.

160. (Content: III-F-5a) A 31-year-old female status post Roux-en-Y gastric bypass is being seen 4 hours postoperatively on the general medical floor by the hospitalist. There were no immediate surgical complications. The patient has type 2 diabetes mellitus and was previously on empagliflozin, tirzepatide, and metformin. She has tolerated a small amount of oral liquid intake. Point-of-care glucose testing reveals a current glucose level of 150 mg/dL. Of the following options, what is the most appropriate management of this patient's diabetes?

A. Decrease empagliflozin by 50%
B. Continue to monitor glucose levels
C. Initiate semaglutide
D. Change metformin to extended-release
E. Start insulin drip to maintain glucose levels of 140-180 mg/dL

(B) After bariatric surgery, patients with diabetes should maintain glucose levels between 140-180 mg/dL to prevent hypoglycemia yet minimize hyperglycemia, which can impair wound healing. Given the patient is in this range in the immediate postoperative period, it would be safe to **continue to monitor glucose levels**, while adding a subcutaneous insulin sliding scale as needed while inpatient. Other important post-bariatric surgery diabetes management include:

- Immediately postoperatively, insulin secretagogues (risk of hypoglycemia), sodium-glucose cotransporter-2 inhibitors (risk for dehydration), and thiazolidinediones should be discontinued.
- GLP-1 RA and tirzepatide could be continued post-operatively. Given the decreased gastric motility and longer half-life, there is a concern of aspiration due to food remnants in the setting of anesthesia and intubation. There are no formal guidelines yet on when to stop these pre-operatively, although some advocate for weeks before surgery.
- Incretin-based therapy and metformin can be continued, although metformin should be changed to immediate release.
- Subcutaneous insulin (non-ICU) and insulin drips (ICU) doses should be adjusted to minimize the hypoglycemic risk (goal 140-180 mg/dL).
- Consider an endocrinology consult if the patient with type 1 diabetes or type 2 diabetes has uncontrolled hyperglycemia.

Reference: AACE/TOS/ASMBS/OMA/ASA 2019 Guidelines: CLINICAL PRACTICE GUIDELINES FOR THE PERIOPERATIVE NUTRITION, METABOLIC, AND NONSURGICAL SUPPORT OF PATIENTS UNDERGOING BARIATRIC PROCEDURES – 2019 UPDATE. Recommendation 42

161. (Content: III-A-1) A 34-year-old male is presenting for a 2-week follow-up with his health coach. He had lost 3 lbs (1.4 kg) the first week but has regained that back. He states that work is busy, and he has difficulty avoiding eating fast food, which is convenient. The health coach agrees that losing weight does take effort and then states, "You are showing motivation to lose weight by coming to the office, but yet you continue to eat fast food frequently. How do those two go together?" What motivation interview principle did the coach display?

A. Empathy
B. Avoiding arguments
C. **Developing discrepancy**
D. Resolving ambivalence
E. Supporting self-efficacy

(C) This health coach uses the principle of developing discrepancy to show the mismatch between what the patient is currently doing and where the patient wants to be by comparing current eating habits to eventual weight loss.

Motivational interviewing uses several principles to explore, nurture, and strengthen the patient's motivation to target behavioral change:

- **Empathy:** Display understanding, collaboration, encouragement, and active listening
- **Avoiding arguments:** "Rolling with resistance" through reflection, shifting the focus, reframing, and siding with the negative
- **Developing discrepancy:** Explore the mismatch from where the patient is today to where they want to be in the future
- **Resolving ambivalence:** Amplify discrepancies and address the uncertainty for motivation to change
- **Supporting self-efficacy:** Affirm favorable results by focusing on patient successes, skills, and strengths

Reference: Obesity medicine association: Obesity Algorithm (2021)

162. (Content: III-D-3) A 24-year-old female presents for smoking cessation counseling. She has mild depression symptoms and increased weight gain since starting the night shift. The clinician starts her on a single medication that can treat all of these components. Which of the following parameters may increase once starting this medication?

A. LDL
B. Triglycerides
C. Glucose levels
D. **Blood pressure**
E. Heart rate

(D) Bupropion has several indications, including tobacco cessation, depression, attention deficit disorder, seasonal affective disorder, and the treatment of obesity. This medication is often combined with naltrexone for synergistic weight loss effects. Although this medication improves most cardiovascular parameters, **bupropion may increase blood pressure** and is contraindicated in the setting of uncontrolled hypertension.

Anti-obesity medications on the market improve all cardiovascular parameters via weight loss and weight-independent mechanisms. The exception to this is that bupropion can increase blood pressure despite weight loss, and therefore vital signs must be monitored closely while on this medication.

The table below summarizes the cardiovascular benefits of anti-obesity agents.

Cardiovascular Effects of Anti-Obesity Medications					
Medications	HDL	LDL	TG	HbA1c	BP
GLP-1 RA	↑	↓	↓	↓	↓
Bupropion SR/ Naltrexone	↑	↔	↓	↓	↑
Phentermine/ Topiramate ER	↑	↓	↓	↓	↓

HDL: High-density lipoprotein; LDL: Low-density lipoprotein; TG: Triglycerides; BP: Blood pressure (systolic); GLP-1 RA: Glucagon-like peptide 1 receptor agonist; SR/ER: Sustained/Extended release

Reference: Bupropion package insert
Reference: Vorsanger MH, Subramanyam P, Weintraub HS, Lamm SH, Underberg JA, Gianos E, Goldberg IJ, Schwartzbard AZ. Cardiovascular Effects of the New Weight Loss Agents. J Am Coll Cardiol. 2016 Aug 23;68(8):849-59. doi: 10.1016/j.jacc.2016.06.007. PMID: 27539178.

163. (Content: III-F-5b) A 35-year-old female is following up with her primary care physician two years after undergoing a Roux-en-Y gastric bypass. She has lost and maintained 65% of her excess body weight. Today, her vitamin D (OH-25) is 8 ng/mL (reference range > 30 ng/ml), her parathyroid hormone is slightly elevated, and her corrected calcium levels are normal. She undergoes a bone density scan, which is consistent with osteopenia. Which of the following is the most appropriate treatment at this time?

    A. Calcitriol
    B. Ergocalciferol
    C. Calcium oxalate
    D. Oral alendronate
    E. Intravenous zoledronic acid

(B) This patient is presenting with findings of severe vitamin D deficiency with secondary hyperparathyroidism and osteopenia. The first step should be to **treat the vitamin D deficiency**, which will normalize the parathyroid hormone and decrease bone reabsorption.

The following recommendations should be followed in post-bariatric surgery, especially malabsorptive procedures:

- Dual-energy x-ray absorptiometry may be indicated two years after surgery to monitor for osteoporosis.
- Baseline and annual vitamin D levels are recommended.
- Daily vitamin D supplementation should be taken after surgery to prevent secondary hyperparathyroidism.
- Antiresorptive agents (bisphosphonates or denosumab) should only be considered after bariatric procedures in those with osteoporosis who have normalized vitamin D and calcium levels.
- Use intravenous bisphosphonates only, as there is a risk of anastomotic ulceration and diminished absorption with oral formulations.

Reference: AACE/TOS/ASMBS/OMA/ASA 2019 Guidelines: CLINICAL PRACTICE GUIDELINES FOR THE PERIOPERATIVE NUTRITION, METABOLIC, AND NONSURGICAL SUPPORT OF PATIENTS UNDERGOING BARIATRIC PROCEDURES – 2019 UPDATE. Recommendation 53, 54, 55, Table 12

164. (Content: III-F-1) A 41-year-old male with a body mass index of 61 kg/m² presents for a surgery consultation regarding bariatric surgical options. Comorbidities include well-controlled obstructive sleep apnea, hypertension, and right knee osteoarthritis. Upon discussing goals, he states his primary goal is maximum weight loss. Given his prior medical history and weight loss goals, which of the following would be the most appropriate surgical option for him?

    A. Laparoscopic adjustable gastric banding (LAGB)
    B. Sleeve gastrectomy (SG)
    C. Roux-en-Y gastric bypass (RYGB)
    D. Biliopancreatic diversion with duodenal switch (BPD/DS)

(D) Given his maximum weight loss goals, a **BPD/DS would provide the most significant total body weight loss**. However, due to the difficulty of the surgery, it is not offered by every surgeon.

Procedure	Weight loss (% TBWL)	Positives	Negatives
		**Bariatric Surgery Options**	
LAGB	20-25%	-No anatomic alteration -Removable and adjustable	Erosion, high explant rates, slips
SG	25-30%	-Easy to perform/reproducible -Few long-term complications -No anastomosis -Metabolic effects	Leaks difficult to manage, little data beyond 5 years. GERD (20-30%)
RYGB	30-35%	-Strong metabolic effects - < 5% major complication risk -Effective for GERD -Can be used as 2nd stage	Marginal ulcers, internal hernias, long-term micro-nutritional deficits
BPD/DS	35-45%	-Powerful metabolic effects -Most pronounced weight loss -Effective for high BMI's -Can be used as 2nd stage	Malabsorptive, GERD, protein malnutrition, internal hernia, challenging, duodenal dissection
SADI-S	35-45%	-Similar to BPD/DS, however slightly less malabsorption risks and less complications. -Significant diabetes remission -Can be used as 2nd stage	Malabsorptive, GERD, micronutrient deficiencies

SG: Sleeve gastrectomy; **RYGB**: Roux-en-Y gastric bypass; **BPD/DS**: Biliopancreatic diversion with duodenal switch; **SADI-S**: Single anastomosis duodeno-ileal bypass with sleeve gastrectomy

Reference: AACE/TOS/ASMBS/OMA/ASA 2019 Guidelines: CLINICAL PRACTICE GUIDELINES FOR THE PERIOPERATIVE NUTRITION, METABOLIC, AND NONSURGICAL SUPPORT OF PATIENTS UNDERGOING BARIATRIC PROCEDURES – 2019 UPDATE. Table 6a.

165. (Content: III-D-8) A 43-year-old female presents to the office for increased weight since her last appointment. She was started on amlodipine for blood pressure and has noted a 2.2 lb (1 kg) weight gain despite no other changes to physical activity. What is the most likely explanation for this?

A. **Increased interstitial edema**
B. Increased appetite
C. Decreased energy expenditure
D. Activation of POMC/CART pathway
E. Placebo effect

(A) Amlodipine and nifedipine are dihydropyridine calcium channel blockers (CCBs) used to treat hypertension, vasospastic angina, and Raynaud's phenomenon. It may cause a slight weight gain due to adipose-independent mechanisms described below:

- **Edema:** CCBs cause smooth muscles in the vasculature to relax, leading to vasodilation. This vasodilation leads to an increase in intravascular hydrostatic pressure and therefore **increases gravity-dependent interstitial edema** in the lower extremities.
- **Constipation:** The other most common side effect of CCBs is constipation, leading to increased intestinal stool burden, which may also add minimal weight. Importantly, weight gain is not causing increased adipose tissue deposition.

Both of these common side effects are dose-dependent, with a higher prevalence in females. These effects are less pronounced in non-dihydropyridine CCBs such as verapamil or diltiazem.

In contrast to CCBs, some beta-blockers such as atenolol, propranolol, and metoprolol do increase adipose tissue, leading to increased weight. If patients require beta-blockers, carvedilol is the most weight-neutral option.

Note: Pioglitazone also increases total body weight by adipose-independent means by increasing water retention.

Reference: Amlodipine package insert

166. (Content: III-F-3) A 52-year-old female presents to her primary care physician with intermittent post-prandial fullness, nausea, and occasional vomiting. She underwent a laparoscopic Roux-en-Y gastric bypass two years prior and has been very happy with her weight loss. A barium swallow and subsequent EGD fail to explain her findings. The following week she goes to the emergency department for biliary emesis. The most likely cause of her symptoms is a(n)

A. mesenteric defect
B. small intestinal bowel overgrowth
C. H. pylori infection
D. marginal ulcer
E. anastomotic stricture

(A) This patient's intermittent abdominal pain and postprandial satiety is concerning for a **mesenteric defect causing an internal hernia.** These symptoms often occur before a small bowel obstruction. It is a difficult diagnosis, as the symptoms tend to be vague early in the course, and contrasted imaging studies are often normal without an acute obstruction.

Note: The most specific CT finding for an internal hernia is a "mesenteric swirl sign," although this may not always be evident.

Internal hernias are a late complication of laparoscopic bariatric and metabolic surgery, usually occurring > 1 year postoperatively after the patient has reduced their BMI by 15 kg/m^2. As the patient loses weight and the intraabdominal adipose tissue regresses, mesenteric defects become more amenable to bowel entrapment. Often this presents with intermittent symptoms initially.

A high clinical indication is necessary for this diagnosis, with colicky abdominal pain, nausea, and early satiety being the most specific findings.

Reference: Internal Hernia after Laparoscopic Gastric Bypass: A Review of the Literature; April 26, 2007 by Louis O. Jeansonne IV, MD; Craig B. Morgenthal, MD; Brent C. White, MD; and Edward Lin, DO

167. (Content: III-F-5b) A 41-year-old female presents to her primary care physician for concerns of diaphoresis, weakness, and tunnel vision approximately 2 hours after meals. She underwent a Roux-en-Y gastric bypass (RYGB) 3 years ago and subsequently lost 103 lbs (46.7 kg) with a current BMI of 26.1 kg/m². She denies ever having similar symptoms. She has decreased her carbohydrate intake, which helped minimally. Which of the following conditions most accurately describes her symptoms?

A. Dumping syndrome
B. Insulinoma
C. Post-gastric bypass hypoglycemia
D. Nesidioblastosis
E. Noninsulinoma pancreatogenous hypoglycemia syndrome

(C) This patient who is experiencing late (>1 hour) post-prandial neuroglycopenia years after a RYGB surgery is likely experiencing **post-gastric bypass hypoglycemia (PGBH).** This condition has a female predominance (92%) and can cause mild (lightheadedness, diaphoresis, flushing) to severe (confusion, blurry vision, seizures) transient symptoms.

The etiology of PGBH after RYGB is likely multifactorial but thought to be due to a persistent increase in incretins (GLP-1 and GIP) post-operatively, leading to hyperfunctioning/hypertrophied β-islet cells. This, along with improved insulin sensitivity with weight loss, may lead to symptoms.

Causes of Hypoglycemia (After RYGB)			
Condition:	PGBH	Dumping Syndrome[1]	Insulinoma
Hypoglycemia:	Post-prandial	Post-prandial. It may be euglycemic during initial symptoms.	Fasting and post-prandial
Timing:	>1 year post-op. 1-4 hours post-prandial	<1 year post-op. Within 15-30 minutes of a meal	Independent of surgery
Fasting C-peptide	Normal	Normal	Elevated

[1]Late dumping syndrome may present similarly to PGBH in timing but would not cause neuroglycopenia and corrects with dietary changes (minimizing simple sugars) alone.

Reference: Reference: Rariy CM, Rometo D, Korytkowski M. Post-Gastric Bypass Hypoglycemia. Curr Diab Rep. 2016 Feb;16(2):19. doi: 10.1007/s11892-015-0711-5. PMID: 26868861.
Reference: Up to Date: "Noninsulinoma pancreatogenous hypoglycemia syndrome"

168. (Content: III-G-7) A 39-year-old Caucasian female with a past medical history of obstructive sleep apnea adherent with CPAP and gout presents to her primary care office for follow-up regarding elevated blood pressures. Over the last three months, home and in-office blood pressures have ranged from 150-170/90-105 mmHg. Today her blood pressure is 164/98 mmHg with a BMI of 34 kg/m². Which of the following is the most appropriate medication to prescribe now?

A. **Losartan**
B. Naltrexone/bupropion ER
C. Chlorthalidone
D. Metoprolol

(A) Renin-angiotensin-aldosterone system (RAS) inhibition (either angiotensin receptor blockers or angiotensin-converting enzyme inhibitors), such as **losartan,** should be considered first-line anti-hypertensive medications to control blood pressure in patients with obesity. Beta-blockers can adversely affect metabolism (metoprolol is weight-positive), and diuretics such as chlorthalidone should be avoided in a patient with gout.

RAAS activation seems to be a primary mediator in hypertension in patients with obesity (especially in children). This is because pro-inflammatory adipokines released by excessive adipose tissue activate the sympathetic nervous system, ultimately activating RAAS, leading to aldosterone-mediated sodium and water absorption within the kidney.

Although weight-loss ultimately will help improve chronic diseases (i.e., diabetes, hypertension, sleep apnea, etc.), medications should be prescribed to control comorbidities and then decreased as able once weight-loss is achieved.

Importantly, naltrexone/bupropion ER should be avoided, as this combination drug is contraindicated in uncontrolled hypertension and should be avoided if other weight-loss medications can be used in the setting of hypertension.

Reference: AACE/ACE Guidelines: AMERICAN ASSOCIATION OF CLINICAL ENDOCRINOLOGISTS AND AMERICAN COLLEGE OF ENDOCRINOLOGY COMPREHENSIVE CLINICAL PRACTICE GUIDELINES FOR MEDICAL CARE OF PATIENTS WITH OBESITY (2016). Recommendation 91-94.

169. (Content: III-H-1) An 8-year-old female affected by obesity is returning for a follow-up visit regarding weight. Over the past five months, she has met biweekly with either a dietician, physician, or psychiatrist for behavioral therapy to address her weight. During this time, she has continued to gain weight despite following recommendations. She has increased from the 97th percentile for BMI to the 99th percentile. Which of the following is the most appropriate recommendation at this time?

    A. Send the patient to a tertiary weight loss center
    B. Maintain current weight with continued growth
    C. Initiate pharmacotherapy
    D. Target a 2-pound weekly weight loss
    E. Limit screen time to 2 hours daily

(D) This patient undergoing intervention for weight loss has not responded to structured weight management (stage 2 of the four-tiered approach to managing obesity) and should move on to stage 3. This stage includes incorporating a comprehensive multidisciplinary intervention and meeting at increased frequencies (weekly). Goals include **targeting a 2-pound weekly weight loss** through a negative-energy balanced diet and meal replacements.

Note: Patients should progress through the 4 tiers based on if they fail to have improvements within 3-6 months on their current stage. Weight and health severity should also be considered.

Goals with 4-Tiered Approach to Pediatric Obesity (Stage 1-3)			
Stage	Weight Target[1]	Physical Activity	Screen Time
1	Maintain weight	≥ 60 mins/day	≤ 2 hours/day
2	Age 2-11: ≤ 1 lb/month Age > 11: 2 lbs/weekly	≥ 60 mins/day[2]	≤ 1 hour/day
3	Age 2-5: ≤ 1 lb/month Age > 5: 2 lbs/weekly	≥ 60 mins/day[2]	≤ 1 hour/day

[1]Weight maintenance or loss to achieve BMI < 85%
[2]Must be supervised active play

Reference: Expert Committee Recommendations Regarding the Prevention, Assessment, and Treatment of Child and Adolescent Overweight and Obesity: Summary Report and APPENDIX. Sarah E. Barlow and the Expert Committee; Pediatrics December 2007, 120 (Supplement 4) S164-S192; DOI: https://doi.org/10.1542/peds.2007-2329C.

170. (Content: III-F-4) A 51-year-old female is presenting to her primary care physician with plans to undergo a sleeve gastrectomy. She has a prior diagnosis of polycystic ovarian syndrome and hypertension, for which she is taking metformin and lisinopril. Overall she states she feels well. Her physical activity consists of briskly walking (5 metabolic equivalents) for 45 minutes daily. Physical examination is unrevealing. Her STOP-BANG score is 1. Which would be the most appropriate test to perform before surgery?

    A. Pharmacologic stress test
    B. Fasting lipid panel
    C. Thyroid-stimulating hormone
    D. Dexamethasone suppression test
    E. Overnight polysomnography

(B) A **fasting lipid panel** should be obtained in all patients with obesity, with treatment initiated based on current practice guidelines. A patient that is asymptomatic or lacks suggestive physical exam findings should not be routinely tested for secondary causes of obesity, including hypothyroidism. Also, this patient's STOP-BANG score is low-risk, negating the need for polysomnography, and her ability to perform > 4 METS does not warrant further formal stress testing.

Importantly, cardiac evaluation should be completed during the history and physical exam, with subsequent testing based on the ACC/AHA perioperative guidelines, similar to other abdominal surgeries. A formal cardiac preoperative consultation is recommended if the patient <u>has</u> cardiac disease.

Note: Those <u>at risk</u> for heart disease should undergo evaluation for peri-procedure beta-adrenergic blockade.

Finally, routine screening for primary hypothyroidism in the absence of clinical findings suggestive of the condition is not recommended (although insurance may require this preoperatively).

Reference: AACE/TOS/ASMBS/OMA/ASA 2019 Guidelines: CLINICAL PRACTICE GUIDELINES FOR THE PERIOPERATIVE NUTRITION, METABOLIC, AND NONSURGICAL SUPPORT OF PATIENTS UNDERGOING BARIATRIC PROCEDURES – 2019 UPDATE. Recommendation 15, 16, 20, 21

171. (Content: III-F-1) A patient is researching different bariatric procedures and is considering a duodenal switch. In discussing this procedure with the patient, which of the following most accurately describes this procedure?

    A. It is preferred in those with a BMI < 45 kg/m²
    B. The common channel is less than 20 cm in length
    C. Digestive enzymes enter the digestive loop
    D. A portion of the stomach is removed

(D) A duodenal switch is a malabsorptive procedure in which the **stomach is made into a tubular pouch** (4-8 oz), and a surgical "duodenal switch" delays the combination of the food (digestive loop) with the digestive enzymes (biliopancreatic loop), until 75-150 cm before the large intestine (common channel). It has the best long-term weight loss but carries a higher mortality and complication risk and therefore is typically reserved for those with the most elevated BMIs.

In a duodenal switch, there is a sleeve gastrectomy performed ❶. The intestine just distal to the stomach is cut and stapled ❸ and a portion of the small intestine is brought up and and creates an anastomosis with the stomach ❷. The portion of the intestine that contains the digestive enzymes is connected to the alimentary tract, thus making a common channel ❹ that eventually drains into the large intestines.

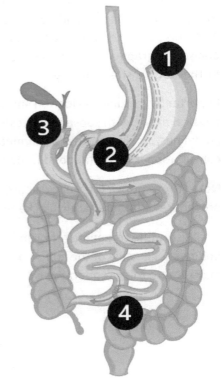

Reference: Image created by Charu G. Copyright owned by Kevin Smith, DO
Reference: Up to Date: "Bariatric procedures for the management of severe obesity: Descriptions"

172. (Content: III-E) A clinical trial is evaluating an oxyntomodulin analog, which is a potential investigational obesity therapy that has shown promising effects in animal studies. It is theorized that this medication will increase satiety, decrease food intake, and potentially have beneficial glucose effects in patients with type 2 diabetes mellitus. The beneficial effects of this intravenous peptide most likely occur as a result of which of the following mechanisms?

A. **GLP-1 receptor agonist**
B. Glucagon receptor antagonism
C. NPY/AgRP direct antagonist
D. Increase in central serotonin levels
E. Ghrelin binding and inactivation

(A) Oxyntomodulin is a peptide hormone released endogenously in post-prandial states. It reduces food intake (increases satiety) and increases energy expenditure, thus promoting weight loss. It has two primary effects, **including glucagon-like peptide 1 (GLP-1) and glucagon receptor agonism,** with subsequent results discussed below:

- **GLP-1 receptor agonist:** Similar to currently available exogenous GLP-1 receptor agonists, this hormone has an incretin effect, slowing down gastric emptying and activating the POMC/CART pathway.
- **Glucagon receptor agonist:** This effect is undesirable, as glucagon works to counter insulin secretion and increase circulating glucose levels. However, the more pronounced GLP-1 effects discussed above counterbalance this deleterious effect and thus maintain a net positive impact.

Reference: Pocai A. Action and therapeutic potential of oxyntomodulin. Mol Metab. 2013;3(3):241-251. Published 2013 Dec 14. doi:10.1016/j.molmet.2013.12.001
Reference: Obesity Medical Association: Obesity Algorithm 2021

173. (Content: III-F-5c) A 52-year-old male presents to a gastroenterologist for evaluation of esophageal dysphagia. He underwent an open Roux-en-Y gastric bypass 15 years prior. Although he has maintained significant weight loss, he has not been adherent to physical activity or taking vitamins. An image from the upper gastrointestinal series is shown below.

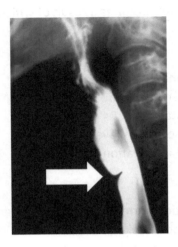

Given this finding, which other feature is likely found on physical examination?

A. **Koilonychia**
B. Hepatomegaly
C. Dermatitis
D. External hemorrhoids
E. Actinic cheilitis

(A) Chronic iron deficiency can lead to a condition called Plummer-Vinson syndrome, which is characterized by significant microcytic anemia and esophageal webs (arrow in image). This is particularly prevalent in Roux-en-Y gastric bypass surgery, as the duodenum, which is the location for iron absorption, is bypassed. Other findings associated with iron deficiency include **koilonychia** (also called "spoon nails" in which the fingernails lose convexity), pica, glossitis, cheilosis, and restless leg syndrome.

174. (Content: III-B-1 and 4) A 29-year-old female presents to the clinic with concerns about an abnormal fasting lipid panel on screening blood work for life insurance.

Test	Value	Reference Range
Total cholesterol	287 mg/dL	< 200 mg/dL
LDL	188 mg/dL	< 130 mg/dL
HDL	31 mg/dL	> 40 mg/dL
Triglycerides (TG)	388 mg/dL	< 150 mg/dL

In discussing a carbohydrate versus fat-restricted diet, which of the following would be an accurate statement to provide to this patient?

A. A ketogenic diet is preferred to improve the LDL value
B. A diet consisting of < 30% fats will preferentially improve HDL
C. Genetic hypercholesterolemia responds to carbohydrate restriction
D. Low-fat diets do not affect insulin resistance or glucose levels
E. Carbohydrate-restricted diets would have a greater effect on TG

(E) Carbohydrate and fat-restricted diets each have their benefits in regard to the cholesterol panel. In general, **low carbohydrate diets have more significant improvements in HDL and TG,** whereas fat restriction improves LDL.

- *Low carbohydrate diets:*
  - More significant increase in HDL and decrease in triglycerides
  - May increase LDL, which may be very significant in those with genetic hypercholesterolemia
  - A ketogenic diet is associated with moderately increased LDL and total cholesterol, as carbohydrates are often exchanged for foods higher in cholesterol and saturated fats.
  - Improvements in insulin resistance, glucose levels, and HbA1c occur irrespective of weight loss
- *Low-fat diets:*
  - A greater decrease in LDL. It may also decrease HDL levels.
  - Improvements in insulin resistance, glucose levels, and HbA1c are only apparent with associated weight loss

Reference: Obesity medicine association: Obesity Algorithm (2021)

175. (Content: III-G-7) A 42-year-old female presents for her 3-month follow-up appointment with her diabetes specialist. The patient has noticed increased polyuria over the past month and admits to having some "slip-ups" following her carbohydrate-restricted diet. Medical history includes type 2 diabetes, heart failure with preserved ejection fraction, and mild diabetic nephropathy. Medications include metformin 2000 mg daily, lisinopril 10 mg daily, and hydrochlorothiazide 25 mg. Body mass index is 34 kg/m^2, whereas vital signs and physical examination are otherwise normal. Her most recent HbA1c is 8.6% (reference range: < 5.7%), an increase of 0.5% since her prior appointment. Which of the following is the most appropriate management change at this time?

    A. Increase metformin
    B. Initiate basal insulin
    C. Start a DPP-4 inhibitor
    D. Prescribe an SGLT-2 inhibitor
    E. Lifestyle changes only

(D) This patient, who is already on a maximum dose of metformin yet has uncontrolled diabetes, should be started on a second anti-diabetic agent (preferably a weight-neutral or weight-negative pharmacologic option). Preferred options would include a GLP-1 agonist or an SGLT-2 inhibitor. Given the concurrent diastolic heart failure, **an SGLT-2 would be preferred.**

Diabetes Medication and Weight Effects		
Weight Positive	**Weight Neutral**	**Weight Negative**
-Insulin[1]	-DPP-IV inhibitors	-GLP-1 agonists[2]
-Thiazolidinediones	-Alpha glucosidase	-SGLT-2 inhibitors[3]
-Meglitinides	inhibitors	-Biguanides[4]
-Sulfonylureas		-Amylin analogs

Weight effects are generalizations and may be based solely on observational trials and vary depending on dosing, duration of treatment, and indications of medication. Weight variability may be seen.
Note: Children/adolescents have more significant weight gain than adults with obesogenic medications
[1]Insulin: Initiate early if HbA1c is ≥ 10%
[2]GLP-1 agonist: Preferred if atherosclerosis or kidney disease is present
[3]SGLT-2 inhibitors: Preferred if kidney disease, heart failure, or atherosclerosis is present
[4]Metformin: Preferred initial pharmacologic agent for T2DM

Reference: American Diabetes Association: Standards of Medical Care in Diabetes—2020 Abridged for Primary Care Providers; Clinical Diabetes 2020 Jan; 38(1): 10-38. https://doi.org/10.2337/cd20-as01

176. (Content: III-F-2) A patient presents to a bariatric seminar, as he is interested in undergoing surgery for weight loss. He has struggled with weight his entire life, and despite recommended dietary and physical activity changes, his body mass index is still > 60 kg/m². At the end of the seminar, he discusses with the surgeon an option that he has read about, but was not presented by the surgeon, which included placing a balloon into the stomach for weight loss. Which of the following is a true statement regarding this procedure for weight loss?

A. This device is not FDA-approved for use in the United States
B. Intragastric balloons account for 10% of bariatric procedures
C. **Indications includes a BMI between 30-40 kg/m² with comorbidities**
D. Intragastric balloons have been proven ineffective for weight loss
E. The balloons are placed for 12 months, then removed

(C) Intragastric balloons, accounting for 2% of bariatric procedures, are a short-term option (6 months maximum) in adults with a body mass index of **30-40 kg/m² and one or more obesity-related comorbidity** in those who failed lifestyle modifications. There are FDA-approved options including the endoscopically-placed ReShape® (dual balloon system, as shown in the image below) and Obera® (single balloon system), as well as the swallowed capsule (Obalon®). Important information is summarized below:

- Intragastric balloons have proven short-term effectiveness, ranging from a 6.8%-10.2% decrease in body weight.
- They should not remain in place for longer than six months due to the risk of balloon deflation and subsequent intestinal obstruction
- Avoid in those with a history of prior gastrointestinal surgery
- The balloons are filled with saline and help increase satiety leading to smaller portions.

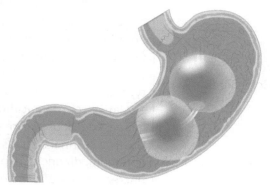

Image citation: Image created by Charu G. Copyright owned by Kevin Smith, DO
Reference: Up to Date: "Intragastric balloon therapy for weight loss"
Reference: Reshapelifesciences.com and Obera.com

177. (Content: III-D-1) A 61-year-old male presents to his primary care office with a desire to start a newer medication to treat his diabetes and help with weight loss. The medication discussed has two mechanisms of action. Which of the following is a contraindication to this medication?

    A. History of prior alcohol-induced pancreatitis
    B. End-stage renal disease
    C. Suicidal ideation
    D. Family history of medullary thyroid carcinoma
    E. History of nephrolithiasis

(D) The medication most likely discussed is tirzepatide, a dual incretin with both gastric inhibitory peptide (GIP) and a glucagon-like peptide 1 receptor agonist (GLP-1 RA) activity, which is currently FDA-approved to treat diabetes. It provides significant weight loss and is expected to soon acquire an FDA indication for weight loss. This medication, along with all GLP-1 RA, is contraindicated in those with a personal history or **family history of medullary thyroid carcinoma.**

Tirzepatide (Mounjaro®)	
Dose	Inject 2.5 mg subcutaneously weekly for one month. Increase the dose to 5 mg, 7.5 mg, 10 mg, 12.5 mg, and 15 mg weekly at one-month intervals.
Mechanism	Dual incretin (GLP-1 RA and GIP). GLP-1 RA activates the hypothalamus, reducing food intake, increasing satiety, decreasing caloric intake, and improving glucose metabolism (incretin). GIP also has an insulin incretin effect and slows gastric emptying.
Contraindications	Prior hypersensitivity to GLP-1 agonists, history of or family history of medullary thyroid carcinoma (black box warning), patients with multiple endocrine neoplasia type 2, and pregnancy (or pregnancy risk). *Relative contraindication: Severe gastroparesis and increased risk of pancreatitis[1]
Side Effects	Gastrointestinal distress (abdominal pain, nausea, vomiting), dizziness, hypoglycemia, increased lipase (increased risk of pancreatitis[1])

[1]Meta-analysis has shown no increased risk of pancreatitis or pancreatic cancer with GLP-1 use.

Reference: Tirzepatide package insert.

178. (Content: III-F-4) A 26-year-old female with severe obesity presents to a bariatric surgery consultation. Her prior medical history includes gastroesophageal reflux and obstructive sleep apnea. She takes prenatal vitamins and famotidine and admits adherence regarding her continuous positive airway pressure machine. Physical examination reveals acanthosis nigricans on the back of her neck and narrow striae on her abdomen. A recent complete metabolic panel and thyroid-stimulating hormone level were normal. Which of the following must be completed before this patient undergoes bariatric surgery?

A. Preoperative *Helicobacter pylori* testing
B. Right upper quadrant ultrasound
C. Serum dehydroepiandrosterone-sulfate (DHEA-S)
D. **Psychosocial-behavioral evaluation**
E. 5% mandatory weight loss preoperatively

(D) A formal **psychosocial-behavior evaluation** should be performed by a licensed behavioral health specialist with specialized knowledge and training regarding bariatric assessments on all patients before undergoing bariatric surgery. The areas of evaluation should focus on screening for eating disorders, motivation and understanding of the procedure, and environment and behavior factors. Also, screening for any unaddressed psychiatric illnesses or substance use is imperative.

Other mentioned screenings that should be performed preoperatively include:

- *H. pylori* screening in areas of high prevalence
- Right upper quadrant ultrasound if there are abnormal liver enzymes, to evaluate for metabolic-associated (nonalcoholic) fatty liver disease
- Total/bioavailable testosterone, DHEA-S, 4-androstenedione if there is a suspicion for polycystic ovarian syndrome

Note: There is no absolute weight loss requirement preoperatively. In addition, completing an extended weight loss program (i.e., 6 months) is not evidence-based in adults and often delays or creates barriers to surgical treatments.

Reference: AACE/TOS/ASMBS/OMA/ASA 2019 Guidelines: CLINICAL PRACTICE GUIDELINES FOR THE PERIOPERATIVE NUTRITION, METABOLIC, AND NONSURGICAL SUPPORT OF PATIENTS UNDERGOING BARIATRIC PROCEDURES – 2019 UPDATE. Table 7. Recommendations 13, 26, 27, 30, 31

179. (Content: III-D-2) A 29-year-old female who is one month postpartum is being evaluated for weight management. She is currently breastfeeding, and her BMI is 36 kg/m^2. She states her BMI has never been below 30 kg/m^2 during her adult life. She would like to start treatment to help with returning to her pre-conception weight. Which option would be most appropriate to initiate at this time?

A. Semaglutide
B. Phentermine/topiramate ER
C. Naltrexone/bupropion ER
D. Cellulose and citric acid hydrogel
E. Metformin

(D) Although most anti-obesity treatments should be avoided during pregnancy and while breastfeeding, cellulose and citric acid hydrogel is not systemically absorbed and would be the best choice in this patient currently breastfeeding.

Note: Cellulose and citric acid hydrogel is technically considered an FDA-cleared medical device, not a medication.

Cellulose and citric acid hydrogel (brand name Plenity®) is a volume-occupying treatment for those with a BMI of 25-40kg/m^2. It is taken before meals to decrease satiety. The capsule expands when taken with water, becoming the consistency of chewed vegetables. The particles eventually degrade in the colon, where the water is released and reabsorbed.

The characteristics of this device are discussed in the table below.

Cellulose and Citric Acid Hydrogel (Plenity®)	
Dose	Oral 2.25 g (3 capsules) twice daily (20-30 minutes before lunch and dinner meals) with 16 oz of water.
Mechanism	Contents form a three-dimensional matrix within the stomach and small intestines that occupies volume, providing a sensation of fullness and satiety.
Contraindications	Hypersensitivity to components and pregnancy.
Side Effects	-Abdominal pain and diarrhea. Avoid in those with dysphagia or active gastrointestinal disease. -May alter the absorption of other medications.

Reference: Cellulose and Citric Acid Hydrogel package insert

180. (Content: III-G-2) A 39-year-old female is presenting to her general surgeon, who performed her gastric bypass four months prior. She is having vague episodes of sharp mid- to upper abdominal pain that lasts 2-3 hours and then resolves. During these episodes, she feels nauseated but denies emesis. These occur 2 hours after eating, but she is unsure of the correlation to certain foods. She does admit to taking naproxen occasionally for a headache but is on concurrent omeprazole. A right upper quadrant ultrasound reveals cholelithiasis without cholecystitis. In working up her abdominal pain, which of the following statements is true?

A. She should be given a trial of rifaximin
B. NSAIDs should never be used after bariatric surgery
C. Endoscopic evaluation is high-risk after bariatric surgery
D. Traditional ERCP is preferred for choledocholithiasis evaluation
E. **Ursodeoxycholic acid may have prevented her symptoms**

(E) This patient presents with concerns of biliary colic, also known as symptomatic cholelithiasis. Cholelithiasis can occur from rapid weight loss after bariatric surgery, and **ursodeoxycholic acid may prevent** this complication.

Note: Endoscopy is safe after surgery and can be used to evaluate stricture, *H. pylori* testing, and celiac disease.

Important considerations of gastrointestinal complications after bariatric surgery are discussed below:

- Traditional ERCP is not possible after Roux-en-Y
- Although NSAIDs should be avoided, if unavoidable, the use of proton pump inhibitors should be used concurrently
- After sleeve gastrectomy, if patients develop severe GERD which is recalcitrant to medical therapy, conversion to Roux-en-Y should be considered

Reference: AACE/TOS/ASMBS/OMA/ASA 2019 Guidelines: CLINICAL PRACTICE GUIDELINES FOR THE PERIOPERATIVE NUTRITION, METABOLIC, AND NONSURGICAL SUPPORT OF PATIENTS UNDERGOING BARIATRIC PROCEDURES – 2019 UPDATE. Recommendation 72-75
Reference: Ursodeoxycholic acid for the prevention of symptomatic gallstone disease after bariatric surgery (UPGRADE): a multicentre, double-blind, randomised, placebo-controlled superiority trial. Lancet gastroenterol Hepatol. 2021 Dec;6(12):993-1001. doi: 10.1016/S2468-1253(21)00301-0. Epub 2021 Oct 27. PMID: 34715031.

181. (Content: III-D-3) A 22-year-old female is presenting to the weight-loss clinic to discuss the FDA-approved, long-term use anti-obesity medications. She denies any prior eating disorders, including bulimia and anorexia nervosa, which you state are contraindications to the combination oral medication that you want to prescribe. In addition, this medication carries a black box warning for which of the following conditions?

A. Congenital defects
B. **Suicidal ideation**
C. Medullary thyroid carcinoma
D. Pancreatitis
E. Ventricular arrhythmia

(B) Naltrexone/bupropion ER is the only long-term, anti-obesity medication contraindicated in patients with eating disorders such as bulimia or anorexia nervosa due to the increased seizure risk. In addition, this medication carries a black box warning for **increased suicide risk in young adults.**

Naltrexone/Bupropion ER (Contrave®)	
Dose	8 mg naltrexone/90 mg bupropion Tablet Week 1: Take one tablet daily in AM Week 2: Take one tablet twice daily Week 3: Take 2 tablets in AM, 1 tablet in PM Week 4: Take 2 tablets twice daily
Mechanism	Weak inhibitor of neuronal reuptake of dopamine and norepinephrine (not fully understood), affecting the hypothalamus (appetite) and reward system.
Contraindications	Hypersensitivity to bupropion or naltrexone, uncontrolled hypertension, seizure disorder, history of seizures, risk of seizures (bulimia, anorexia nervosa, alcohol or benzo withdrawal, etc.), chronic opioid use, pregnancy, concurrent use of MAO-I *Risk of suicide in young adults (black box warning)
Side Effects	Headache, nausea/vomiting, constipation, sleep disorder, dizziness

Reference: Naltrexone/bupropion ER package insert

182. (Content: III-F-4) A female patient meets with her dietician one final time before undergoing a Roux-en-Y gastric bypass. The dietician discusses starting a high-protein, liquid diet 2 weeks before the surgery. What is the reasoning behind this?

A. Develop good dietary habits for the post-operative period
B. **To prevent surgical complications from organ injury**
C. Reduce inflammation in the stomach and proximal intestines
D. Decrease colonic stool burden and risk of an intestinal leak
E. Increase the total percentage of post-operative weight loss

(B) Most patients are advised to initiate a low-calorie (<1200 kcal/day) diet that is high in protein and low in carbohydrates a few weeks prior to bariatric and metabolic surgery to promote a reduction in liver size. Studies have shown a 15-30% reduction in liver size if initiated 2 to 12 weeks before surgery, with 80% of this reduction occurring within the first two weeks. This decrease in liver sizes improves intraoperative laparoscopic visualization of vital structures and **decreases mechanical injury to the liver.**

A number of recommendations to reduce intraoperative and post-operate risks after bariatric surgery are made by the American Society for Metabolic and Bariatric Surgery (ASMBS), with some highlights including:

- Smoking cessation is completed at least 6 weeks before surgery
- Avoid post-operative hyperglycemia, although a specific hemoglobin A1c target pre-operatively should not delay surgery.
- Pre-operative nutrition should be optimized with the use of a dietician
- Insurance-mandated weight loss requirements or arbitrary time-based approaches (e.g., 6 months of dieting) pre-operatively is not beneficial.
- Pre-operative weight loss and adherence do not necessarily correlate with postoperative weight loss in the long-term.
- Patients are encouraged to have pre-operative age-appropriate cancer screenings completed before surgery.
- A TSH for screening is not recommended devoid of symptoms.
- Estrogen-containing birth control should be held for one month and hormone replacement therapy three weeks before surgery.

Reference: "ASMBS position statement on preoperative patient optimization before metabolic and bariatric surgery" Jonathan Carter, M.D., Julietta Chang, M.D., T. Javier Birriel, M.D., Fady Moustarah, M.D., et Al. Received 4 May 2021; accepted 27 August 2021

183. (Content: III-G-6) A 47-year-old female presents for a comprehensive metabolic and bariatric surgery consultation. Her BMI has consistently been over 50 kg/m² for the past ten years, which she attributes to pregnancies and genetics. She has a family history of endometrial cancer in her mother and prostate cancer in her father. Per the Centers for Disease Control and Prevention (CDC), aggressive weight loss will likely reduce the risk of malignancy affecting which of the following areas?

    A. Thyroid
    B. Lymph nodes
    C. Lung
    D. Skin
    E. Oral

(A) The CDC recognizes 13 malignancies that are increased in the setting of having excess weight (BMI ≥ 25kg/m²). This is thought to be from the increased inflammatory cytokines, sex hormones, and insulin resistance associated with excess adipose tissue. Of the options, only **thyroid cancer** is listed by the CDC.

The 13 types of cancers listed by the CDC make up 40% of cancers in the United States, with more likely being added to the list following ongoing research. It is estimated that excess weight accounts for 11% of cancers in females, 5% in males, and contributes to 7% of cancer-related deaths.

Interestingly, from 2005-2014 cancers not associated with obesity decreased (by 13%), whereas those found to have an association with excess weight increased by 7% (excluding colorectal cancer). This is consistent with an overall elevation in BMI in the United States during this period.

Malignancies Associated with an Elevated BMI	
Breast (post-menopausal)	Pancreas
Colorectal	Ovaries
Esophageal (adenocarcinoma)	Multiple myeloma
Gallbladder	Meningioma
Stomach (upper)	Uterus[1]
Kidneys	Thyroid
Liver	

[1]Endometrial cancer has a 7x relative risk (highest) in those with obesity compared to normal weight

Reference: CDC: Obesity and Cancer.
Reference: American Cancer Society: Does Body Weight Affect Cancer Risk?

184. (Content: III-D-2 and 9) A 6-year-old male presents to a geneticist after he is found to have hyperphagia. Testing reveals that pro-insulin levels are increased. The child's BMI is 150% of the 95th percentile. Genetic testing returns positive for a variant of the proprotein convertase subtilisin/Kexin type 1 (PCSK1) gene. Which of the following should be administered to this child?

    A. Amylin analogs
    B. Metreleptin
    C. Semaglutide
    D. Setmelanotide
    E. Gastric inhibitory polypeptide

(D) This patient has an abnormal PCSK1 gene that is likely contributing to his severely increased BMI and hyperphagia. **Setmelanotide** is approved for patients ≥ 6 years old with pathogenic POMC, PCSK1, or LEPR genetic defects and, as of 2022, Bardet-Biedl syndrome (BBS).

Note: Genetic testing for obesity should be considered in those with early-onset hyperphagia and obesity with or without intellectual disability.

The PCSK1 gene encodes for a convertase that cleaves many active peptide hormones involved in regulating energy, hunger, and energy homeostasis. Variants or deficiencies of this gene can lead to a variety of endocrinopathies. Initially, this presents as an infant with intestinal malabsorption (1st year of life) followed by hyperphagia and obesity.

Setmelanotide (Imcivree®)	
Indications	Chronic weight management in those with genetically confirmed pathogenic proopiomelanocortin (POMC), proprotein convertase subtilisin/kexin type 1 (PCSK1) genes or leptin receptor (LEPR) deficiency, and BBS.
Mechanism	Melanocortin 4 (MC4) receptor agonist
Contraindications	None currently listed
Significant Adverse Effects	New or worsening depression or suicidal ideation, increased sexual arousal (labial hypersensitivity and priapism), and skin hyperpigmentation

Reference: Setmelanotide package inserts.
Reference: Ramos-Molina B, Martin MG, Lindberg I. PCSK1 Variants and Human Obesity. Prog Mol Biol Transl Sci. 2016;140:47-74. doi:10.1016/bs.pmbts.2015.12.001

185. (Content: III-G-5) A 33-year-old female presents for a pre-operative consultation with a desire to undergo a Roux-en-Y gastric bypass. She is concerned as she states that she has been on buprenorphine-naloxone for the past five years due to a history of intravenous heroin use. Since stopping heroin, she has had a steady increase in weight, and her current BMI is 41 kg/m². She has an accountability partner, has been sober for the past 5 years, and is now counseling others on the effects of substance use. Which of the following statements is accurate to present?

A. A history of substance use is a contraindication to surgery
B. Buprenorphine-naloxone must be stopped prior to surgery
C. **The risk of alcohol use disorder is increased after surgery**
D. An underlying eating disorder will improve after surgery
E. Weekly urine drug screens will ensure adherence after surgery

(C) Patients undergoing bariatric and metabolic surgery should be thoroughly screened for underlying eating disorders, maladaptive eating patterns, substance use, and alcohol use disorder. After surgery, patients **are at an increased risk of alcohol use disorder,** likely due to rapid absorption of alcohol leading to immediate gratification and transference addiction. Active substance use is a contraindication for surgery. Those with risk factors or a history of should be managed/monitored by addiction specialists. Also, those with maladaptive eating disorders are likely to have less success unless treatment is initiated pre-operatively. A psychosocial evaluation for substance use, maladaptive eating patterns, and alcohol use is vital prior to surgery.

Note: In patients taking buprenorphine-naloxone, the naloxone portion is not orally bioavailable nor absorbed through the skin (transdermal patches). Thus, it is only added as a deterrent to injecting the medication by blocking the partial agonist effects of buprenorphine and preventing any euphoric effects. Therefore, it would not be contraindicated in the setting of surgery.

Reference: "ASMBS position statement on preoperative patient optimization before metabolic and bariatric surgery" Jonathan Carter, M.D., Julietta Chang, M.D., T. Javier Birriel, M.D., Fady Moustarah, M.D., et Al. Received 4 May 2021; accepted 27 August 2021
Reference: Buprenorphine-naloxone Package insert

186. (Content: III-A-1) A 32-year-old female is being evaluated by psychiatry before bariatric surgery. During the interview, the patient understands the risks and benefits of the planned gastric sleeve but shows a lack of motivation to maintain the dietary and exercise changes. The patient is asked to write a list of potential pitfalls or concerns the patient has regarding maintaining weight postoperatively. What key process of motivational interviewing is being displayed?

A. Engagement
B. Focusing
C. Evoking
D. Planning

(B) The psychiatrist is using the key process of motivational interviewing of **focusing,** in which the physician helps the patient identify their areas of ambivalence or potential struggles to begin setting goals accordingly. In addition to focusing, the other key processes include:

- **Engagement:** Establishing a therapeutic relationship (displaying empathy, acceptance, etc.) and utilizing OARS[1].
- **Evoking:** Discovering the patient's interest and motivation to change and being able to use these to reach their goals. Listening for words (DARN[2]) to cue you in that the patient is ready for changes
- **Planning:** Assisting the patient in making short and long-term goals and providing appropriate follow-up and guidance.

Motivational interviewing is a patient-centered technique that promotes change talk, which focuses on changing the patient's speech and actions from maintaining the status quo (sustain talk) to a direction of change.

One technique to incorporate change talk (and avoid sustain talk) is utilizing the importance ruler or readiness scale:

- On a scale of 1-10, how ready are you to _____?
    - Followed by: Why not a lower number?
    - Avoid asking why it is not a higher number

[1]**OARS:** **O**pen-ended questions, **A**ffirmation, **R**eflection, and **S**ummarize
[2]**DARN:** **D**esire, **A**bility, **R**easons, and **N**eed to change

Reference: Obesity medicine association: Obesity Algorithm (2021)

187. (Content: III-F-1 and 2) A multi-disciplinary weight management center has recently added the TransPyloric Shuttle (TPS)® to its list of options for weight loss. What is true regarding this device?

A. It is best for those with significant BMI levels as a bridge to surgery
B. It can only be kept in place for six months maximum
C. It is safe in pregnancy, although it must be removed before birth
D. **Patients must be on chronic acid suppression while device is in place**
E. Bowel obstruction is the most common adverse side effect

(D) TPS® is an endoscopically placed weight loss device that was FDA-approved in 2019. It uses a removable gastric bulb to affect the flow of food content through the stomach. Patients should be started on a **proton pump inhibitor** to reduce the risk of gastroesophageal tissue injuries.

- **Indications:** Adults with class I obesity with ≥ 1 obesity comorbidity or class II obesity, in conjunction with lifestyle modifications.
- **Contraindications:** Altered upper gastrointestinal anatomy such as a stricture or prior surgery, esophageal varices, erosions, ulcerations, untreated *H. pylori* infections, gastritis, pregnancy, and coagulopathy.
- **Duration:** The device must be removed after 12 months.
- **Effectiveness:** In the trial, 66% (vs 30% placebo) lost 5% of their weight, with an average of 9.3% total body weight loss (vs 2.8% placebo).

The larger smooth bulb ❶ of the TPS® sits in the stomach, while the small bulb ❷ is free to move into the proximal duodenum. This results in slowed gastric transit of food content ❸.

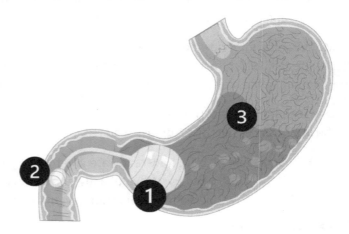

188. (Content: III-D-1) A 29-year-old female presents for a two-month follow-up appointment after her initial obesity medicine consultation. At the prior appointment, her medroxyprogesterone injection was discussed as being weight positive. She was started on tirzepatide to assist in weight loss and treat her diabetes mellitus type 2. She has since changed to an oral estrogen-progesterone contraceptive pill and is tolerating the tirzepatide well. Which lab finding may occur within the next year if her current medications are not addressed?

    A. Increased renin levels
    B. Hypokalemia
    C. Increased urine anion gap
    D. Hypoglycemia
    E. Positive urine HCG

(E) Tirzepatide is a dual incretin with both gastric inhibitory peptide and glucagon-like peptide-1 receptor agonist mechanisms. Both of these medications decrease the transit time of the stomach and intestines and therefore, can affect the efficacy of oral contraceptives. Thus, the manufacturer recommends adding barrier protection within four weeks of any increased dose of tirzepatide to prevent pregnancy **(positive urine HCG)**. Non-oral routes of birth control are not affected.

Tirzepatide has also been associated with an increased risk of fetal and maternal harm. Not only does oral birth control becomes less effective, but patients who lose weight have a higher chance of becoming pregnant. Therefore, recommendations when using tirzepatide in women of child-bearing age include:

- Using barrier protection if on oral contraceptives within four weeks of any increased dose of tirzepatide.
- Switching to non-oral options, including intra-uterine devices or progestin implants
- Although medroxyprogesterone injections are not affected by tirzepatide, they can cause significant weight increases.

Reference: Tirzepatide package insert

189. (Content: III-G-7) A 21-year-old female is having frequent migraines leading to missed days of work. Most headaches last up to two days and she has approximately eight debilitating headaches per month. She has tried NSAIDs and sumatriptan for abortive therapy and topiramate and propranolol for prevention. None of these have been effective. Recent head imaging was normal. She does not want to start on medications that will cause weight gain. Which is the best pharmacologic treatment for this patient?

A. Atenolol
B. Amitriptyline
C. Acetazolamide
D. **Erenumab**
E. Valproic acid

(D) Being aware of newer therapies for comorbidities that do not cause weight gain can improve the quality of our patient's lives and prevent complications (first, do no harm). Many migraine medications cause weight gain, but the newer monoclonal antibodies, such as **erenumab** that antagonize calcitonin gene-related peptide (CGRP) receptor function are very effective and weight neutral.

Erenumab is a once-monthly subcutaneous injection used for the prevention of migraines. Another CGRP antagonist, Rimegepant is used for both prevention and acute abortive migraine therapy, whereas Ubrogepant is currently only approved for abortive therapy.

Migraine Medications		
Weight Positive	**Weight Neutral**	**Weight Negative**
-Valproic acid	-NSAIDs	-Topiramate
-Propranolol and atenolol	-Triptans	-Zonisamide
-Amitriptyline	-CGRP antagonists	
	-Botox injections	

Weight effects are generalizations and may be based solely on observational trials and vary depending on dosing, treatment duration, and medication indications. Weight variability may be seen.
Note: Children/adolescents have more significant weight gain than adults with obesogenic medications

Reference: Obesity medicine association: Obesity Algorithm (2021)
Reference: Erenumab package insert

190. (Content: III-G-3) A 34-year-old male with a past medical history of anxiety and diabetes presents to his primary care physician two years after undergoing a sleeve gastrectomy. He initially lost 60 lbs (27.2 kg) within the first year, but then over this past year, he has slowly regained approximately 30 lbs (13.6 kg). Medications include metformin, detemir, and fluoxetine. He does admit nonadherence with his recommended daily vitamins but continues to exercise three times weekly. Given these findings, which of the following most likely explains his postoperative weight regain?

    A. Dilated gastric pouch
    B. Excess insulin administration
    C. Dietary indiscretion
    D. Psychologic issues
    E. Vitamin deficiencies

(C) Insufficient weight loss or weight regain after bariatric surgery is not uncommon. There can be many etiologies (some listed above). By far, the most common cause is behavioral-mediated and not surgical-related. Behavioral reasons for weight gain **include lack of dietary control** (i.e., snacking), nonadherence with calorie-restriction recommendations, lack of exercise, or increased psychosocial stressors. Also, undiagnosed eating disorders can play a role.

Note: Patients that are aware that behavioral modifications are just as crucial after surgery as they were before surgery often have improved success.

Important post-surgical lifestyle modifications include the following:

- Frequent follow-up with an obesity medicine specialist, dietician, and surgeon
- Support groups
- Continued physical activity
- Calorie monitoring and vitamin supplementation

Reference: Up to Date: "Bariatric surgery: Postoperative and long-term management of the uncomplicated patient"

191. (Content: III-G-6) A 49-year-old female who was recently widowed after her husband had complications from obesity presents to her family medicine physician for weight loss counseling. Her BMI is 42 kg/m², and she has a past medical history of hypertension, diabetes, and asthma. Comprehensive lifestyle changes are discussed. What is a reasonable weight loss goal, in terms of total body loss, for this patient within the next six months, according to the "2013 ACC/AHA/TOS Guidelines for the Management of Overweight and Obesity in Adults"?

    A. 0-5%
    B. 5-10%
    C. 10-15%
    D. 15-20%

(B) Although weight loss of 3-5% leads to some clinically meaningful reduction in cardiovascular risk factors, the expert panel recommends an initial weight loss goal **of 5-10% of baseline weight** within six months, as these more substantial weight losses produce more significant benefits.

Weight loss (WL) goals, in which improvements in obesity-related conditions are seen, according to the 2016 AACE/ACE guidelines, are summarized below.

Condition	% WL Goals
-Type 2 diabetes -Dyslipidemia -Polycystic ovarian syndrome (PCOS)	5% - ≥ 15%
-Metabolic syndrome -Prediabetes -Female infertility -Osteoarthritis -Gastroesophageal reflux	≥ 10%
Metabolic-associated fatty liver disease: -Steatosis -Steatohepatitis	5% or more 10%-40%
Male hypogonadism Urinary stress incontinence	5% - ≥ 10%
Asthma	7-8%

Reference: 2013 AHA/ACC/TOS Guideline for the Management of Overweight and Obesity in Adults. A Report of the American College of Cardiology/American Heart Association Task Force on Practice Guidelines and The Obesity Society. Box 9.
Reference: AACE/ACE Guidelines (2016). Table 8

192. (Content: III-F-4) A 33-year-old female with a past medical history of class III obesity, diabetes type 2, tobacco abuse, and polycystic ovarian syndrome presents for a bariatric evaluation. She is interested in a "gastric bypass." Her medications include metformin, oral contraceptive birth control, and a prenatal vitamin. After a thorough history and physical examination, you discuss preoperative recommendations, including a physical activity plan and healthy dietary patterns. What other perioperative education would be necessary for this patient?

A. Avoid becoming pregnant for at least 6 months after surgery
B. Birth control must be discontinued 1 week before surgery
C. Her hemoglobin A1c should be less than 9% preoperatively
D. Metformin is contraindicated after Roux-en-Y gastric bypass
E. Tobacco products must be stopped 6 weeks before surgery

(E) Tobacco use should be stopped as soon as possible, preferably one year preoperatively, but at a **minimum of six weeks before surgery**, due to the increased risk of poor wound healing and anastomotic ulcers.

Note: In women, pregnancy should be avoided preoperatively and 12-18 months postoperatively. Estrogen birth control should be stopped 1 cycle before surgery to prevent deep venous thrombosis (pre-menopausal).

Reasonable preoperative glycemic targets, which are associated with shorter hospital stays and improved bariatric procedure outcomes, include:

- HbA1c goal of 6.5-7% and peri-procedure glucose 80-180 mg/dL
- HbA1c goal of 7-8% is recommended in those with advanced micro/macrovascular complications, those with many comorbid conditions, or long-standing/difficult-to-control diabetes.
- Clinical judgment must be used if A1c is > 8%

*Metformin can be used postoperatively but should be converted to immediate release to improve absorption.

Reference: AACE/TOS/ASMBS/OMA/ASA 2019 Guidelines: CLINICAL PRACTICE GUIDELINES FOR THE PERIOPERATIVE NUTRITION, METABOLIC, AND NONSURGICAL SUPPORT OF PATIENTS UNDERGOING BARIATRIC PROCEDURES – 2019 UPDATE. Recommendation 14, 17, 18, 23

193. (Content: III-D-8) A 24-year-old female presents to her primary care physician's office for an evaluation regarding weight gain. She states she has been exercising five times weekly for approximately 30 minutes during her sessions. She has decreased her calories to 1200 kcal daily, focusing on a low-fat diet, but still has noticed a 10 lb (4.5 kg) weight gain in the past year. Medical history includes bipolar disease, which is well-controlled on aripiprazole. Previous laboratory work was within normal limits, including HbA1c, TSH, and CMP. Which would be the most effective in treating her weight gain?

A. **Prescribe metformin**
B. Prescribe orlistat
C. Intensify calorie restrictions
D. Change aripiprazole to olanzapine
E. Intensify exercise regimen

(A) This patient is experiencing antipsychotic-related weight gain, of which **metformin** is proven effective (off-label), with lots of supporting data. Metformin is commonly used (often off-label) in settings of insulin resistance, including polycystic ovarian syndrome, fatty liver disease, HIV protease inhibitor-associated lipodystrophy, and pre-diabetes.

Metformin	
Dose	Increase gradually. Maximum dose 1000 mg BID
Mechanism	-Decreases hepatic glucose production -Reduces intestinal absorption of glucose -Improves insulin sensitivity (peripheral utilization)
Contraindications	Hypersensitivity to metformin, eGFR < 30 mL/min, acute or chronic metabolic acidosis *Black box warning: Lactic acidosis (risk factors include age > 65 years old, contrasted studies, renal failure, hypoxia, significant alcohol use, etc.)
Side effects	Gastrointestinal distress: abdominal pain, nausea, vomiting, and diarrhea

Reference: Metformin package insert.
Reference: Baptista 2007; Chen 2013; Das 2012; de Silva 2016; Jarskog 2013; Wang 2012; Zheng 2015

194. (Content: III-H-3) A 12-year-old female who has struggled with obesity for the past five years is presenting to a bariatric tertiary center for a vertical sleeve gastrectomy evaluation. She has hypertension and severe obstructive sleep apnea that did not respond to tonsillectomy. She is sexually active and developmentally is at a Tanner Stage 3. Her BMI is currently 37 kg/m². Psychiatry evaluation reveals mild depression and a lack of understanding of the risks regarding the surgical procedure. Which of the following is a contraindication for this adolescent to undergo bariatric surgery?

A. Tanner Stage 3
B. Body mass index
C. Sexual activity
D. Depression
E. **Risk appreciation**

(E) This adolescent who has decision-making capacity may be a candidate for bariatric surgery if she fully understands and **acknowledges the risks** associated with surgery. Any lack of insight or motivation that would interfere with the postoperative treatment is a contraindication to pediatric bariatric surgery.

Surgery indications, contraindications, and complications in adolescents largely mirror those of adults desiring to undergo surgery. Contraindications include ongoing substance use or a recent history of use (within 1 year), medically correctable causes of obesity, current or planned pregnancy within 12-18 months of surgery, any condition (medical, psychiatric, psychosocial, or cognitive) that prevents adherence to the post-operative regimen.

Note: Pubertal status or physical maturity (Tanner Stage or bone age) are no longer included in determining surgery candidacy. The initial theory that rapid weight loss after surgery would inhibit linear bone growth has not been proven.

Reference: Obesity medicine association: Pediatric Obesity Algorithm (2020-2022)
Reference: Pratt JSA, Browne A, Browne NT, et al. ASMBS pediatric metabolic and bariatric surgery guidelines, 2018. Surg Obes Relat Dis. 2018;14(7):882-901. doi:10.1016/j.soard.2018.03.019

195. (Content: III-F-5b) A 28-year-old female is presenting to her primary care physician's office six months after undergoing a laparoscopic adjustable gastric banding (LAGB). She states two weeks ago, she had eaten too quickly, with subsequent nausea and vomiting. Since then, she has been unable to keep solids down and will regurgitate undigested food after small meals. In addition, her acid reflux has significantly worsened during this time. Which of the following is the next best step in management?

    A. CT of the abdomen
    B. Remove fluid from the band
    C. Surgical revision
    D. Diet changes
    E. Start omeprazole

(B) This patient's findings of nausea, vomiting, inability to tolerate solids, and worsening acid reflux is most consistent with the diagnosis of band slippage. This complication occurs in up to 5% of LABG. It may present with either loss of food restriction or an inability to pass food. The **initial step is to completely remove the fluid through the port,** thereby eliminating the restriction. Surgery may be indicated if this fails to relieve symptoms.

Note: Another potential complication after LABG that must be considered is an erosion, which may be asymptomatic and present as a loss of food restriction or present with findings of pain or infection at the port site.

Other complications of LAGB are discussed in the table below.

Complications of Laparoscopic Adjustable Gastric Banding	
Short-Term (30 Days)	**Long-Term**
-Death (1:1000)	-Band slippage (3-5%)
-Anastomotic leak (0.2%)	-Gastric pouch dilation (3-5%)
-Infection (1%)	-Erosion (1%)
-DVT/PE (1%)	-Port issue (2-5%)
-Dehydration (1%)	-Need for revision/removal (25%)

DVT: Deep venous thrombosis; **PE:** Pulmonary embolism

Reference: AACE/TOS/ASMBS/OMA/ASA 2019 Guidelines: CLINICAL PRACTICE GUIDELINES FOR THE PERIOPERATIVE NUTRITION, METABOLIC, AND NONSURGICAL SUPPORT OF PATIENTS UNDERGOING BARIATRIC PROCEDURES – 2019 UPDATE. Recommendation 78
Reference: Obesity medicine association: Obesity Algorithm (2021)

196. (Content: III-D-7 and III-G-3) A 35-year-old female presents as a follow-up three years after undergoing a sleeve gastrectomy. She states she had significant weight loss within the first year post-operatively but has since plateaued in her weight, approximately 30 lbs (13.6 kg) short of her goal. She has followed all recommendations but admits to an increased appetite. She would like to discuss anti-obesity medications to assist in helping with reaching her goals. Which of the following is the most appropriate recommendation to provide?

A. Weight-loss medications are contraindicated after bariatric surgery
B. Cellulose and citric acid hydrogel is preferred post-operatively
C. Revision surgery is most appropriate to reach your target weight
D. Body contouring surgery will likely allow you to reach your goal
E. **Starting semaglutide and phentermine will reduce weight**

(E) This patient has undergone successful bariatric and metabolic surgery but has plateaued prior to her weight-loss goals. Anti-obesity medications are an appropriate option to discuss at this visit. Most patients will plateau by the first year, and additional weight loss requires intensifying lifestyle modifications and/or the addition of weight loss medications. In this patient, **starting semaglutide and phentermine** will likely help reduce appetite and increase POMC/CART pathway activation, assisting in meeting her goals.

Anti-obesity medications are not only safe after bariatric surgery but are effective. These options should be considered for those who do not meet goals or have weight regain after surgery. Other options include:

- Surgical revisions, such as converting to another metabolic surgery (e.g., Single anastomosis duodeno–ileal bypass with sleeve gastrectomy) can be considered depending on desired and starting weight.
- A close review of dietary habits and physical activity is important
- Psychiatric evaluation should be considered to ensure any underlying eating disorders did not become uncovered or developed.

Finally, cellulose and citric acid hydrogel should be avoided in those with altered gastrointestinal anatomy due to the increased risk of obstruction.

Reference: Redmond IP, Shukla AP, Aronne LJ. Use of Weight Loss Medications in Patients after Bariatric Surgery. Curr Obes Rep. 2021 Jun;10(2):81-89. doi: 10.1007/s13679-021-00425-1. Epub 2021 Jan 25. PMID: 33492629.

197. (Content: III-H-3 and III-F-6) A 14-year-old female is being evaluated for a sleeve gastrectomy given her body mass index and comorbidities. Where should this evaluation be completed?

    A. Primary care physician's office
    B. Pediatric weight management center
    C. Tertiary care center
    D. Pediatric general surgery office

(C) Stage 4 of the four-tiered approach to managing obesity involves **a tertiary weight-loss center,** and includes interventions such as a very low-calorie diet, anti-obesity medications, and metabolic weight-loss surgery.

The 4-Tiered system was initiated in 2007. If no improvements are seen after 3-6 months, you progress to the next stage (varies by patient).

4-Tiered Approach for Management of Pediatric Obesity		
Stage and Name	**Location of Intervention**	**Follow-up**
1: Prevention plus	Primary care office	Monthly visits with similar interventions as in prevention[1], but with a goal of improved BMI
2: Structured weight management	Primary care office with support	Monthly visits with motivational interviewing, dieticians, and +/- physical therapists to create a targeted treatment plan
3: Comprehensive multidisciplinary intervention	Pediatric weight management center	Weekly visits targeting behavioral modification, negative energy balance, and stricter dietary and activity plans with monitoring
4: Tertiary care intervention	Tertiary care center	Weekly follow-up. High acuity care with additions of anti-obesity medications and preparation for possible metabolic surgical options

[1]**Prevention:** Limit screen time to 2 hours daily, encourage sleeping ≥ 9 hours nightly, ≥ 5 servings of fruits and vegetables daily, eliminate sugar-sweetened beverages, prepare meals at home when possible, eat at the table with family ≥ 5 times weekly, consume a healthy breakfast every morning, and perform at least 60 minutes of physical activity daily.

Reference: Expert Committee Recommendations Regarding the Prevention, Assessment, and Treatment of Child and Adolescent Overweight and Obesity: Summary Report. Sarah E. Barlow. Pediatrics Dec 2007, 120 (Supplement 4) S164-S192; DOI: 10.1542/peds.2007-2329C

198. (Content: III-B-1) A 59-year-old male is interested in initiating the exchange diet into his daily routine. He is currently planning on eliminating one of his snacks daily and substituting two servings of vegetables for his 2 starches.

American Diabetes Association Exchange Servings				
1 Serving	Protein	Carbohydrate	Fat	Calories
Starches	3 g	15 g	<1 g	80 kcal
Vegetables	2 g	5 g	0 g	25 kcal
Fat	0 g	0 g	0 g	45 kcal
Fruit	0 g	15 g	0 g	60 kcal
Dairy	8 g	15 g	0-8 g	90-150 kcal
Protein	7 g	0 g	2-5 g	55-75 kcal
Snacks	3 g	15 g	0-1 g	80 kcal

How many daily calories will he reduce by making these changes?

A. 80 kcal/day
B. 130 kcal/day
C. 190 kcal/day
D. 240 kcal/day
E. 270 kcal/day

(C) The American Diabetes Association created the exchange diet as a way for a patient to reduce their carbohydrate intake by exchanging one food for another. In this example, the patient is eliminating 1 snack (80 kcal and 15 g of carbohydrates) and exchanging 2 starches (80 kcal and 15g of carbohydrate each) for 2 vegetables (25 kcal and 5g of carbohydrates each). Thus, every day he is eliminating 80 kcal (snack) + {160 kcal (2 starches) – 50 kcal (2 vegetables)} = **190 kcal/day and 35 g of carbohydrates.**

Note: You will not be required to memorize these values, although you should know 1 serving of fruit is 60 kcal.

The idea of an exchange diet is to group foods together according to their nutritional value. A list of foods that constitute a serving is available and is useful for those who desire to substitute a food choice that may be higher in carbohydrates and calories for one that is lower.

Reference: Gray A, Threlkeld RJ. Nutritional Recommendations for Individuals with Diabetes. [Updated 2019 Oct 13]. In: Feingold KR, Anawalt B, Boyce A, et al., editors. Endotext [Internet]. South Dartmouth (MA): MDText.com, Inc.; 2000-. Available from: https://www.ncbi.nlm.nih.gov/books/NBK279012/

199. (Content: III-G-7) A 19-year-old female presents to her obstetrician to discuss options for birth control. She wants to maintain a healthy weight, given her family history of diabetes and early-onset coronary artery disease. She is sexually active and does not want to become pregnant. Which of the following is associated with the most weight gain?

A. Intrauterine device
B. Barrier method
C. Progesterone-only pill
D. Etonogestrel implant
E. Progesterone depo injections

(E) Many birth control options are considered weight-neutral, including most options above, except for **medroxyprogesterone.** This quarterly intramuscular progesterone-only injection is great for preventing pregnancy but notorious for causing weight gain.

Weight gain for medroxyprogesterone is reported to occur in up to 38% of females and is the most common cause of discontinuation. Approximately 2 kg (4.4 lbs) was gained within the first year, and nearly double that was seen in subsequent years. Not everyone will experience this weight gain, but it is important to discuss this possibility with patients and provide alternative options if there are no contraindications.

Birth Control Options	
Weight Positive	**Weight Neutral**
-Medroxyprogesterone (Depo-Provera®)	-Intrauterine devices -Barrier methods -Long-acting reversible contraceptives -Progesterone-only pills

Weight effects are generalizations and may be based solely on observational trials and vary depending on dosing, treatment duration, and medication indications. Weight variability may be seen.
Note: Children/adolescents have more significant weight gain than adults with obesogenic medications

Reference: Obesity medicine association: Obesity Algorithm (2021)
Reference: Medroxyprogesterone acetate package insert

200. (Content: III-D-5) A 32-year-old male presents to his primary care physician for yellowing of his eyes and noticing increased fatigue. He takes no prescribed medication but does admit to taking a combination herbal supplement for weight loss. Although it is recommended to take twice daily, he has been taking approximately ten daily, and has noticed a 14 lb (6.4 kg) weight loss. AST, ALT, bilirubin, and INR are markedly elevated. Which of the following ingredients in his supplement is most likely contributing to his current condition?

A. Chitosan
B. Ephedra
C. Glucosinolates
D. Green tea extract
E. Raspberry ketone

(D) **Green tea extract** is an important and well-known cause of hepatic injury, along with the more common side effects similar to caffeine excess. In general, increased herbal and dietary supplement use is directly proportional to increased hepatotoxicity rates, accounting for nearly 20% of cases within the United States. Anabolic steroids and green tea extract are the most commonly implicated agents.

The other supplements listed above have side effects that include:

- **Chitosan:** Indigestion, bloating, and constipation
- **Glucosinolates:** Goiter and hypothyroidism
- **Raspberry extract:** Significant burping

In addition, the FDA has banned certain supplements, as listed below:

- **Ephedra (mu Huang):** Used to reduce appetite; this is associated with palpitations, myocardial infarctions, stroke, and sudden death.
- **Human chorionic gonadotropin (HCG):** In 2016, the AMA passed a policy that HCG for weight loss is inappropriate. The FDA has mandated a disclaimer describing its lack of efficacy.

Reference: Obesity medicine association: Obesity Algorithm (2021)

201. (Content: III-B-2 and III-G-2) A 29-year-old male presents to his dietician after starting a very low-calorie diet. He has done some research and determined that he would like to maintain less than 800 kcal/day and eliminate all fat from his diet. Currently, he is consuming 1300 kcal/day without significant weight loss. The dietician discusses the importance of close monitoring and recommends adding some fat to his diet instead of eliminating it altogether. Without this recommendation, what possible complications could arise?

A. Electrolyte imbalance
B. Gout flares
C. **Cholelithiasis**
D. Electrolyte derangements
E. Cold intolerance

(C) A very low-calorie diet (VLCD) is any diet under 800 kcal/day which requires close monitoring to prevent complications. One complication that may arise with eliminating fat from the diet, instead of taking in small amounts (10-20 g) including essential fatty acids, **is gallstones.**

In VLCD, the typical diet consists of a predominance of protein (suppresses hunger), with a target of 1.5 g/kg and 1.2 g/kg ideal body weight in men and women, respectively (average 75-110 g/day). Carbohydrates are usually restricted to 50-100 grams daily, and a fat intake of at least 10-20 g is preferred.

There is little evidence to support that a VLCD is superior to a low-calorie diet (800 -1500 kcal/day), and there is no long-term weight benefits between the two approaches. In fact, there are a number of potential complications of VLCD:

- Electrolyte disturbances, especially sodium and potassium, which require carbohydrates as a cofactor for absorption
- Essential fatty acid deficiency and gallstones
- Gout (often pre-treated with allopurinol)
- Cardiac arrhythmias
- Irritability, depression, apathy, insomnia, and anxiety

Reference: Up to Date: "Obesity in adults: Dietary therapy"
Reference: Weinsier RL, Ullmann DO. Gallstone formation and weight loss. Obes Res. 1993;1(1):51-56. doi:10.1002/j.1550-8528.1993.tb00008.x

202. (Content: III-F-3) A 26-year-old female underwent a one-anastomosis gastric bypass and has since had a persistent burning sensation in her mid-epigastric region. She states that proton pump inhibitors have not helped and sucralfate provided no relief. She denies any other symptoms, including fever, nausea, or vomiting. Endoscopic evaluation reveals no strictures or anastomotic ulcers, and a histologic sample shows mild stomach inflammation. A CT of the abdomen is unremarkable. Which of the following is the most likely cause of her symptoms?

A. Cardiac ischemia
B. Bile acid gastritis
C. *H. pylori* infection
D. Recalcitrant acid reflux
E. Esophageal spasm

(B) This patient who underwent a mini-gastric bypass or one-anastomosis gastric bypass, despite a negative endoscopic and CT image evaluation, is most likely experiencing bile acid gastritis. Bile reflux occurs near the anastomotic site in approximately 4% of patients undergoing this procedure, with endoscopic (and histologic) findings non-specific, thus making it a diagnosis of exclusion. Treatment often requires conversion to a Roux-en-Y gastric bypass (RYGB).

The one-anastomosis gastric bypass is one of the newer ASMBS-endorsed bariatric and metabolic surgeries (2022), which involves creating a gastric pouch ❶ and anastomosing a loop of the bowel to this pouch ❷. It is considered more malabsorptive than a RYGB, but with similar weight loss and comorbidity improvements.

Image citation: Image created by Charu G. Copyright owned by Kevin Smith, DO
Reference: Chaim EA, Ramos AC, Cazzo E. MINI-GASTRIC BYPASS: DESCRIPTION OF THE TECHNIQUE AND PRELIMINARY RESULTS. Arq Bras Cir Dig. 2017 Oct-Dec;30(4):264-266. doi: 10.1590/0102-6720201700040009. PMID: 29340551; PMCID: PMC5793145.

203. (Content: III-D-3) A 44-year-old male presents to his primary care clinician for a three-month follow-up appointment. He has a history of obesity class II, hypertension, obstructive sleep apnea, and hyperlipidemia. He started an off-label medication for weight loss at his prior appointment and is tolerating it well. His lab work before and after initiating the anti-obesity medication, is shown below. Which of the following medications was likely started?

Test	Initial	Today	Reference Range
Sodium	138 mEq/L	136 mEq/L	136–145 mEq/L
Potassium	3.8 mEq/L	4.1 mEq/L	3.5-5.0 mEq/L
Chloride	99 mEq/L	107 mEq/L	95-105 mEq/L
Bicarbonate (HCO_3)	24 mEq/L	18 mEq/L	22–28 mEq/L
BUN	16 mg/dL	18 mg/dL	6-20 mg/dL
Creatinine	0.8 mg/dL	0.9 mg/dL	0.6–1.2 mg/dL
Glucose	88 mg/dL	83 mg/dL	70–110 mg/dL

A. Phentermine
B. Metformin
C. Bupropion
D. Topiramate
E. Tirzepatide

(D) This patient presents with hyperchloremic metabolic acidosis (non-anion gap metabolic acidosis) after starting a new medication. Of the options, only **topiramate** has this quality, given its carbonic anhydrase inhibition. Acidosis also predisposes to nephrolithiasis formation.

Note: Anion gap is measured by taking sodium – (chloride + bicarbonate). If this value is less than 12, it is considered a non-anion gap metabolic acidosis. Although it is unlikely to be required to calculate this on the ABOM examination, recognizing hyperchloremia and acidosis will be important.

Topiramate is used for several conditions, including off-label uses:

- Migraine headache prevention
- Weight-loss (off-label if used as monotherapy)
- Seizures
- Binge-eating disorder (off-label)

Reference: Topiramate package insert

204. (Content: III-D-8) A 31-year-old female presents to her primary care physician's office with complaints of significant anxiety. She has tried counseling and has noted slight improvements, but the anxiety still interferes with her life. She denies depression. She is concerned that initiating pharmacotherapy for anxiety could cause her to gain weight. Vital signs are normal. BMI is 32 kg/m². If pharmacotherapy is started, which would be the most appropriate?

A. Bupropion
B. Fluoxetine
C. Duloxetine
D. Aripiprazole
E. Propranolol

(B) This patient, who is struggling with anxiety and is concerned about weight gain, should be placed on a selective serotonin reuptake inhibitor (SSRI). Of the SSRIs, **fluoxetine** is considered to be the most weight neutral. Beta-blockers, antipsychotics, and SNRIs tend to cause slight weight gain. Finally, although weight-negative, bupropion is not approved for anxiety and can worsen anxiety symptoms.

Psychiatric Medication Considerations in Obesity Medicine		
Condition	**Weight Positive**	**Weight Neutral/Variable**
Depression	-TCA: Amitriptyline, doxepin, imipramine -SSRI/SNRI: Paroxetine, citalopram, venlafaxine -Mirtazapine -Trazodone	-TCA: Desipramine, nortriptyline -SSRIs: Fluoxetine, sertraline -SNRI: Desvenlafaxine, duloxetine -Bupropion[1]
Anxiety	Propranolol	Fluoxetine
Mood Stabilizers	Divalproex, lithium, carbamazepine	Lamotrigine, oxcarbazepine
Antipsychotics	Olanzapine, lithium, quetiapine, clozapine, risperidone	Aripiprazole, ziprasidone, haloperidol

Weight effects are generalizations and may be based solely on observational trials and vary depending on dosing, duration of treatment, and indications of medication. Weight variability may be seen.
Note: Children/adolescents have more significant weight gain than adults with obesogenic medications
[1]Weight negative

Reference: Obesity medicine association: Obesity Algorithm (2021)

205. (Content: III-G-7) A 38-year-old male with a history of obesity presents to his internist's office for an annual exam. The patient denies any new symptoms since his last appointment but has noticed some weight gain, especially around his waist. His current weight is 241 lbs (109.3 kg), which is an increase of 14 lbs (6.4 kg) since last year, placing his BMI at 39 kg/m^2. His lipid panel is within normal limits, however, his HbA1c is currently 5.9% (reference range: < 5.7%), and his fasting glucose level is 119 mg/dL (reference range: < 100 mg/dL). Which of the following would be the most appropriate recommendation at this time?

A. **Initiate metformin therapy**
B. Obtain C-peptide levels
C. Recheck HbA1c levels in 3 months
D. Recommend resistance training
E. Initiate an SGLT-2 inhibitor

(A) Prevention of prediabetes to type 2 diabetes includes multiple interventions. **Pharmacotherapy with metformin should be considered in those with prediabetes** (HbA1c 5.7%- 6.4%), especially if the patient is < 60 years old, has a BMI ≥ 35 kg/m^2, or in females with a history of gestational diabetes. Metformin reduces the risk of progression to diabetes by 31%.

Diabetes affects 30 million people in the United States, with another 84 million having pre-diabetes. Therefore interventions that prevent the progression to diabetes is vital and may include the following:

- Weight loss: A 6% weight loss leads to a relative risk reduction of 58%.
- Nutrition: Macronutrient diets should be individualized.
- Physical activity: Recommendations are similar to the general population; encourage moderate-intensity activity for a minimum of 150 minutes/week.

Reference: American Diabetes Association: Standards of Medical Care in Diabetes—2020 Abridged for Primary Care Providers; Clinical Diabetes 2020 Jan; 38(1): 10-38. https://doi.org/10.2337/cd20-as01
Reference: Knowler WC, Barrett-Connor E, Fowler SE, et al. Reduction in the incidence of type 2 diabetes with lifestyle intervention or metformin. N Engl J Med. 2002;346(6):393-403. doi:10.1056/NEJMoa012512

206. (Content: III-D-2) A 52-year-old male presents for a follow-up for weight loss. He was started on phentermine 15 mg in the morning and states it works well, but he notices the effects wear off by midafternoon. He wants to avoid increasing the morning dose of phentermine due to some tremors he noticed on the higher dose. He has a history of nephrolithiasis and cannot afford GLP-1 medications due to a lack of insurance coverage. Which of the following would be a potential treatment option?

A. Initiate tirzepatide
B. **Add diethylpropion in the afternoon**
C. Add topiramate
D. Continue current regimen
E. Add metformin

(B) This patient is presenting with increased appetite in the afternoon, although his phentermine works well in the morning. Given his history of nephrolithiasis, he should not start topiramate. If insurance does not cover GLP-1 medications, they will not cover tirzepatide (GLP-1/GIP) off-label. Of the options, adding a shorter-acting sympathetic amine **(diethylpropion)** to cover his afternoon appetite is appropriate. This medication has a half-life elimination of only 4-6 hours, compared to phentermine (DEA schedule IV) with a half-life elimination of 20 hours, so it is less likely to cause insomnia.

Short-Acting Sympathetic Amines for Weight Loss	
Options (DEA schedule) *Half-life*	-Diethylpropion (Class IV): *4-6 hours* -Benzphetamine (Class III): *4-6 hours* -Phendimetrazine (Class III): *3-7 hours*
Mechanism	Sympathomimetic amines stimulate the hypothalamus to release norepinephrine, resulting in decreased appetite and increased energy expenditure.
Contraindications	Hypersensitivity to phentermine or other formulary components, concurrent MAOI use, hyperthyroidism, glaucoma, and pregnancy. Avoid in those with coronary artery disease and severe anxiety
Side Effects	Insomnia, constipation, xerostomia, tachycardia

Reference: Package insert for phentermine, diethylpropion, benzphetamine, and phendimetrazine

207. (Content: III-D-1) A previously healthy 28-year-old female with a current BMI of 28 kg/m² presents for a follow-up appointment with her primary care. Over the past six months, she has intensified her exercise regimen to 200 minutes/week, restricted her diet to 1300 kcal/day, and eliminated fast food and soda. However, she is frustrated that she has not met her weight loss goals and is interested in pharmacotherapy. If prescribed, which would most likely help her accomplish her 10% weight loss goal if titrated to maximum recommended strength?

    A. **Phentermine/topiramate ER**
    B. Phentermine monotherapy
    C. Liraglutide
    D. Naltrexone/bupropion ER

(A) Of the options listed, the combination weight-loss drug **Phentermine/topiramate ER** had the highest percentage of participants achieving a 10% weight loss (48%) compared to placebo.

The table below summarizes the number of patients who achieved weight loss targets of 5% and 10%, respectively, in large, randomized control trials. Those who received recommended doses of anti-obesity medications are compared to those who received the placebo (in parenthesis).

Those Achieving 5% and 10% Weight Loss (WL) at Max Dose vs. (Placebo)					
% WL	Naltrexone/ Bupropion ER	Liraglutide 3 mg	Semaglutide 2.4 mg	Orlistat	Phentermine/ Topiramate ER
5%	48 (16)	63.2 (27.1)	86.4 (31.5)	50.5 (30.7)	70 (21)
10%	25 (7)	33.1 (10.6)	69.1 (12.0)	28.6 (11.3)	48 (7)

Note: Tirzepatide (Mounjaro®) is currently FDA approved for diabetes, with an expected indication for weight loss soon. Data shows that 91% of participants had a weight reduction of 5% or more (35% for placebo), but 57% had a weight reduction of 20% or more (compared to 3% in placebo arm) at the 15 mg dose in the SURMOUNT-1 trial.

Reference: AACE/ACE Guidelines: AMERICAN ASSOCIATION OF CLINICAL ENDOCRINOLOGISTS AND AMERICAN COLLEGE OF ENDOCRINOLOGY COMPREHENSIVE CLINICAL PRACTICE GUIDELINES FOR MEDICAL CARE OF PATIENTS WITH OBESITY (2016). Table 10.

208. (Content: III-B-1) A 17-year-old female who has struggled with the disease of obesity since childhood is meeting with a dietician to discuss weight loss goals. In addition to keeping a food diary, the patient downloads an application on her smartphone that keeps track of calories. Upon a follow-up visit, she is averaging 1900 kcal/day. She should be counseled to reduce her calories by a minimum of what additional amount?

A. 300 kcal/d
B. 600 kcal/d
C. 900 kcal/d
D. 1200 kcal/d

(B) Weight loss requires sustaining a calorie deficit through both total calorie restriction and increased physical exercise. An energy deficit of ≥ 500 kcal/day is recommended and may be achieved with a daily caloric intake as below:

- Male: 1500-1800 kcal/d
- Female: 1200-1500 kcal/d

Therefore, this patient needs to reduce her calorie count **by at least 600 kcal/day** to meet this goal (making it 1300 kcal/d).

Note: Only in limited circumstances is a restricted caloric intake of < 800 kcal/d recommended, of which close medical supervision is necessary.

Reference: 2013 AHA/ACC/TOS Guideline for the Management of Overweight and Obesity in Adults. A Report of the American College of Cardiology/American Heart Association Task Force on Practice Guidelines and The Obesity Society. Box 9.

209. (Content: III-D-9) A 67-year-old male presents with concerns of uncontrolled diabetes and increased weight gain. He is petrified of needles and refuses medications that require administration through needles, including insulin. Medications include metformin ER and dapagliflozin. He exercises 30 minutes daily and follows recommendations from his dietician. Which of the following is the next best step in management?

    A. **Initiate oral semaglutide**
    B. Discuss tirzepatide
    C. Start pioglitazone
    D. Intensify exercise routine
    E. Prescribe continuous glucose monitoring

(A) Semaglutide is approved for diabetes in an **oral form (Rybelsus®).** This medication is taken daily, with the initial dose (3 mg) being used only to improve gastrointestinal tolerance but provides no significant glucose control. Therefore, up-titration to 7 mg or 14 mg is important.

Semaglutide (Ozempic®, Rybelsus®)	
Dose	**Ozempic®:** Inject 0.25 mg subcutaneously weekly for one month. Increase the dose to 0.5 mg, 1.0 mg, and 2.0 mg weekly at one-month intervals, as needed **Rybelsus®:** Oral 3 mg daily (≥ 30 minutes before first meal). Increase to 7 mg then 14 mg monthly.
Mechanism	Glucagon-like peptide 1 receptor agonists activate the hypothalamus, reducing food intake, increasing satiety, decreasing caloric intake and improving glucose metabolism (incretin).
Contraindications	Prior hypersensitivity to GLP-1 agonists, history of or family history of medullary thyroid carcinoma (black box warning), patients with multiple endocrine neoplasia type 2, and pregnancy. *Relative contraindication: Severe gastroparesis and increased risk of pancreatitis
Side Effects	Gastrointestinal distress (abdominal pain, nausea, vomiting), dizziness, hypoglycemia, increased lipase (increased risk of pancreatitis)

[1]Meta-analysis has shown no increased risk of pancreatitis or pancreatic cancer with GLP-1 use.

Reference: Semaglutide package inserts.

210. (Content: III-F-7) A 59-year-old female presents to her bariatric surgeon's office one week before undergoing a Roux-en-Y gastric bypass. Her current comorbidities include hyperlipidemia, hypothyroidism, obstructive sleep apnea, osteoarthritis, hypertension, and type 2 diabetes. She is hopeful of decreasing or discontinuing some of her medications after surgery. Despite improvements in many obesity-related comorbidities, which of the following conditions may likely need to have medications increased after her bariatric surgery?

A. Hyperlipidemia
B. Diabetes
C. Hypertension
D. Hypothyroidism
E. Osteoarthritis

(D) Many medical conditions related to obesity improve after bariatric surgery, including many of the above, requiring monitoring and dose adjustment with progressive weight loss. Although some patients may be able to decrease their **levothyroxine** dose with weight loss (especially after a sleeve gastrectomy), the dose may need to be increased in the setting of malabsorption.

After a malabsorptive surgery, liquid or soft gel formulations are preferred if TSH suppression is difficult to achieve.

The table below shows comorbidity improvements after bariatric surgery:

Medical Outcomes after Bariatric Surgery	
Disease	% Resolved or Improved
Type 2 Diabetes Mellitus	86
Hypertension	78.5
Obstructive Sleep Apnea	85.7
Hyperlipidemia	78.5

[1]In addition, a reduction of up to 60% in mortality from cancers (especially colon and breast) is seen.

Reference: AACE/TOS/ASMBS/OMA/ASA 2019 Guidelines: CLINICAL PRACTICE GUIDELINES FOR THE PERIOPERATIVE NUTRITION, METABOLIC, AND NONSURGICAL SUPPORT OF PATIENTS UNDERGOING BARIATRIC PROCEDURES – 2019 UPDATE. Recommendation 68- 71
Reference: Buchwald H, Avidor Y, Braunwald E, et al. Bariatric Surgery: A Systematic Review and Meta-analysis. JAMA. 2004;292(14):1724–1737. doi:10.1001/jama.292.14.1724

211. (Content: III-F-3) A medical student is rotating with a surgeon who is about to perform a Roux-en-Y gastric bypass. He describes the procedure as one in which he will create a gastric pouch, then connect this new pouch to the jejunum, bypassing the duodenum. He describes a potentially severe complication that may follow the procedure, associated with high morbidity and prolonged hospital stays. What is true of this potential complication?

    A. Barium studies are the preferred imaging
    B. Failure to extubate may be the presenting sign
    C. Procalcitonin has no role in evaluation
    D. It is more frequently seen in a sleeve gastrectomy

(B) Failure to extubate should prompt an evaluation for a pulmonary embolism or **an anastomotic leak**, which is best evaluated by computed tomography. C-reactive protein and procalcitonin can assist in diagnosis. Given the multiple anastomosis sites, this complication is more commonly seen in Roux-en-Y gastric bypass (RYGB) and biliopancreatic diversion with a duodenal switch.

During a RYGB, a stomach pouch is created **1**. A portion of the small intestines (jejunum) is cut and anastomosed **2** to the stomach pouch. The portion of the intestine that was cut is then anastomosed to the alimentary tract **3**. This is where the food contents and the digestive enzymes will meet for the first time. This procedure is considered reversible, as no sleeve gastrectomy is performed.

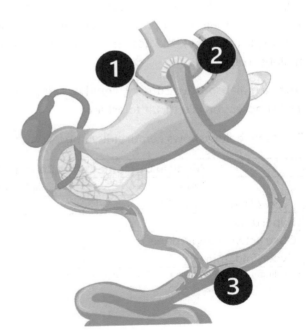

Reference: AACE/TOS/ASMBS/OMA/ASA 2019 Guidelines: CLINICAL PRACTICE GUIDELINES FOR THE PERIOPERATIVE NUTRITION, METABOLIC, AND NONSURGICAL SUPPORT OF PATIENTS UNDERGOING BARIATRIC PROCEDURES – 2019 UPDATE. Recommendation 47

212. (Content: III-D-8) A patient with type 1 diabetes and obesity class I presents to the clinic to discuss an indicated medication to help reduce appetite and insulin intake. A subcutaneous medication is initiated after a thorough discussion, including hypoglycemia symptoms. Which mechanism or class of medication is associated with the initiated medication?

A. **Amylin analog**
B. Biguinide
C. GLP-1 receptor agonist
D. GLP-1 and GIP agonist
E. Sympathetic amine

(A) An **amylin analog,** such as pramlintide, can be utilized in type 1 and type 2 diabetes to reduce mealtime insulin intake and reduce caloric intake via centrally-mediated POMC/CART activation, leading to weight loss and improved hemoglobin A1c levels.

Importantly, amylin can cause hypoglycemia and a discussion with the patient about the associated symptoms, including tremors, headaches, and diaphoresis, should be initiated.

Pramlintide (SymlinPen ®)	
Indication	Type 1 diabetes or insulin-dependent type 2 diabetes. Adjuvant treatment for mealtime insulin in those who have not achieved glucose control despite optimal insulin therapy[1]
Dose	**Type 1 diabetes:** 15 mcg subQ before major meals to a target dose of 30-60 mcg before meals **Type 2 diabetes:** 60 mcg subQ before major meals to a target dose of 120 mcg before meals
Mechanism	Amylin synthetic analog which reduces postprandial glucose via prolonged gastric emptying time, decreased glucagon secretion, and centrally-mediated caloric reduction.
Contraindications	Gastroparesis or hypoglycemic unawareness.
Side Effects	Headaches, severe hypoglycemia, nausea, anorexia, or vomiting.

[1]Patients should reduce mealtime insulin dose by 50% with pramlinatide

Reference: Pramlintide package insert

213. (Content: III-D-9) A 37-year-old male with a past medical history of chronic migraines and well-controlled hypertension is presenting to his primary care physician for evaluation of weight management. He has lost 9 lbs (4 kg) with lifestyle modifications but has plateaued and wants to start pharmacotherapy. His current BMI is 32 kg/m². Insurance denies the use of combination weight loss pills. Which of the following, if used off-label, would be the most appropriate medication to start now?

A. **Topiramate**
B. Phentermine
C. Bupropion
D. Naltrexone
E. Metformin

(A) This patient with a concurrent history of chronic migraines would benefit from being prescribed **topiramate**, a medication FDA-approved for chronic migraines. Although it is considered off-label for obesity, it is commonly prescribed for this reason, with many studies backing its efficacy.

Note: A patient affected by obesity, who frequently awakens with morning headaches, should be screened for obstructive sleep apnea.

When possible, a patient's comorbidities should be considered when prescribing anti-obesity medications, as there may be dual indications.

- **Bupropion:** Smoking cessation, major depression disorder, seasonal affective disorder
- **Topiramate:** Migraine prevention, epilepsy, binge eating disorder
- **Metformin:** Insulin resistance, PCOS, anti-psychotic induced weight gain, diabetes type II, and pre-diabetes

Interestingly, topiramate also can make soda undesirable due to its carbonic anhydrase inhibition and may be beneficial for obesity management in those having difficulty discontinuing soda.

Reference: Topiramate package insert.
Reference: Up to Date: "Obesity in adults: Drug therapy"

214. (Content: III-A-2) A 29-year-old female, two months post-partum who is currently breastfeeding, presents to her family practitioner to jump-start weight-loss. She states her goals are to lose weight healthily and not disrupt milk production. She is up multiple times nightly with her infant and always feels tired. She walks for 15 minutes daily and drinks 1-2 sodas daily. Her pre-pregnancy weight was 178 lbs (80.7 kg). Currently, she is at 212 lbs (96.2 kg). Which of the following would be an example of a SMART goal to set for this patient while utilizing shared-decision making?

A. Decrease calories to < 1000 kcal/day
B. Increase exercise as much as tolerated
C. Lose 5 lbs (2.3 kg) weekly until at pre-pregnancy weight
D. Decrease soda intake by 3 cans weekly until discontinued
E. Start and titrate liraglutide to a goal of 3 mg daily

(D) This post-partum female who is breastfeeding aims to lose weight but desires to do so in a manner that does not disrupt milk production. Therefore, a rapid decrease in calories would be detrimental to one of her main goals. Hence, an ideal SMART goal will **decrease her soda intake,** thereby improving her weight and fatigue while not reducing milk production.

Note: All FDA-approved anti-obesity medications are contraindicated in pregnancy, and most should be avoided while breast-feeding.

A SMART goal refers to an acronym for setting a quality and challenging goal. The abbreviation and corresponding examples are shown below.

- **S**pecific: Losing 10% body weight or eliminating sugary drinks
- **M**easurable: Pounds, calories, minutes, sodas
- **A**chievable: (Must be realistic!) 5% weight loss in 4 months
- **R**elevant: (Important to the patient) goals may be related to improving blood pressure, fitting into jeans, being able to swim with kids, etc.
- **T**imed: Per week, by three months, by the patient's birthday

Reference: Bovend'Eerdt TJ, Botell RE, Wade DT. Writing SMART rehabilitation goals and achieving goal attainment scaling: a practical guide [published correction appears in Clin Rehabil. 2010 Apr;24(4):382]. Clin Rehabil. 2009;23(4):352-361. doi:10.1177/0269215508101741

215. (Content: III-G-7) A neurologist calls to discuss a mutual patient who needs treatments for partial seizures. The neurologist offers a few options listed below but would like your feedback based on the patient's comorbidities. The patient has diabetes mellitus type II with retinopathy, obesity class I, and hypertension. Which of the following options is most appropriate to recommend?

A. Carbamazepine
B. Gabapentin
C. Valproate
D. Zonisamide
E. Pregabalin

(D) **Zonisamide** is FDA-indicated as an adjunctive treatment for focal-onset seizures and used off-label as an alternative in those that do not tolerate topiramate for binge-eating disorder and weight loss. Of the options, it is the only weight-negative medication listed.

Although pregabalin and gabapentin are commonly used for diabetic neuropathy, this patient has diabetes complicated by retinopathy, not neuropathy. All other listed options are weight-positive and should be avoided, if possible, in this patient with obesity class I.

Note: Similar to topiramate, zonisamide may increase the risk of nephrolithiasis and should be avoided in patients with a history or calcium renal stones.

Anti-Seizure Medications	
Weight Positive	**Weight Negative**
-Carbamazepine	-Lamotrigine
-Pregabalin	-Zonisamide
-Valproate	-Topiramate
-Gabapentin	

Weight effects are generalizations and may be based solely on observational trials and vary depending on dosing, treatment duration, and medication indications. Weight variability may be seen.
Note: Children/adolescents have more significant weight gain than adults with obesogenic medications

Reference: Obesity medicine association: Obesity Algorithm (2021)

216. (Content: III-F-1) A 45-year-old male with a past medical history of acid reflux, class III obesity, hypertension, and osteoarthritis presents for a bariatric surgery evaluation. He takes a proton pump inhibitor twice daily but admits that he still has gastroesophageal symptoms regularly. A barium swallow evaluation is performed, as shown below. If bariatric surgery is pursued, which of the following should be recommended?

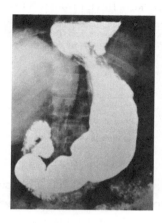

A. Sleeve gastrectomy
B. Biliopancreatic diversion with a duodenal switch
C. Adjustable gastric banding
D. Intra-gastric balloon
E. **Roux-en-Y gastric bypass**

(E) **Roux-en-Y gastric bypass** is the bariatric surgery of choice for patients with moderate-severe gastroesophageal reflux symptoms, hiatal hernia (as shown in the esophageal barium image), esophagitis, or Barrett's esophagus. An intra-gastric balloon may increase GERD symptoms and <u>should not</u> be used in this setting.

Reference: AACE/ACE Guidelines: AMERICAN ASSOCIATION OF CLINICAL ENDOCRINOLOGISTS AND AMERICAN COLLEGE OF ENDOCRINOLOGY COMPREHENSIVE CLINICAL PRACTICE GUIDELINES FOR MEDICAL CARE OF PATIENTS WITH OBESITY (2016): Recommendation 62.

217. (Content: IV-A-1) A 45-year-old male reluctantly presents to a bariatric seminar. He has wanted to attend for the past few years, but always cancels due to concerns of what others may think. In particular, his coworkers have already verbalized that he is less valuable compared to more active and fit employees. Thus, if he takes 2-3 weeks off from work for surgery, he feels this may exacerbate their views. What is the term that describes this labeling of decreased value that his coworkers have imparted on him?

A. Bias
B. Self-efficacy
C. Implicit bias
D. Prejudice
E. Stigma

(E) This patient is experiencing **stigma,** which is a physical or character trait that labels the bearer as having lower social value. His coworkers view him as less valuable simply based on his weight. In contrast, bias is when a victim becomes the target of prejudice or unfavorable treatment. Nothing in the question indicates he is treated any differently, but rather that their views of him are lesser.

Importantly, this same stigma can occur amongst physicians as well. Physicians self-report that they often view their patients with obesity as being non-adherent, dishonest, lazy, unsuccessful, and lacking self-control.

Note: Implicit bias occurs when the person is unaware of these deep-rooted views, often affecting how they act or treat an individual.

Bias, on the other hand, is the action that occurs when emotions result from stigma (disgust, anger, blame, etc.), leading to prejudice or unfavorable treatment.

Reference: Puhl RM, Heuer CA. Obesity stigma: important considerations for public health. Am J Public Health. 2010;100(6):1019-1028. doi:10.2105/AJPH.2009.159491

218. (Content: IV-B-2 and 4) A primary care physician is treating a patient who is interested in bariatric surgery. She wants to understand the potential mortality, morbidity, and predicted amount of weight loss she could experience, given her comorbidities. More specifically, she wants to compare and contrast these parameters between a sleeve gastrectomy and a Roux-en-Y gastric bypass to help her decide the best option for her. In addition to referring her to a bariatric surgeon, what resource will likely be able to assist in providing her with the information she is looking for?

    A. American College of Sports Medicine
    B. Metabolic and Bariatric Surgery Accreditation Quality Improvement
    C. Obesity Medicine Association
    D. The Obesity Society
    E. United States Preventive Services Task Force

(B) Although all of the above options are excellent resources and should be utilized to some capacity regarding patients undergoing bariatric surgery, the **Metabolic and Bariatric Surgery Accreditation and Quality Improvement Program (MBSAQIP)** provides a surgical risk/benefit calculator that compares different surgical options, including expected weight loss, complications, DVT risk, etc. This would be the best resource for what this patient is seeking.

Bariatric resources are vital for patient education. Some excellent resource options are listed below:

- **MBSAQIP Calculator**
  - https://riskcalculator.facs.org/
- **Obesity Medicine Association (OMA):** Obesity algorithm
  - https://obesitymedicine.org/obesity-algorithm
- **American Association of Clinical Endocrinologists (AACE)**
  - https://pro.aace.com/disease-state-resources/nutrition-and-obesity
- **American Heart Association/American College of Cardiology /The Obesity Society (AHA/ACC/TOS)**
  - https://www.ncbi.nlm.nih.gov/pmc/articles/PMC5819889/
- **American Society for Metabolic and Bariatric Surgery (ASMBS)**
  - https://asmbs.org/
- **American College of Sports Medicine**
  - http://www.acsm.org/

219. (Content: IV-C) A cardiologist is teaming up with a bariatric clinic to provide multidisciplinary expertise regarding exercise safety. They have created an algorithm to screen asymptomatic individuals who would benefit from performing an exercise electrocardiogram stress test before engaging in a robust exercise program. Which patient would most likely fall into a moderate-risk category for suffering a cardiac event during exercise and, therefore, should be recommended for an exercise stress test before beginning aerobic exercise?

    A. 52-year-old male starting moderate-intensity exercise
    B. 49-year-old female initiating vigorous-intensity exercise
    C. 61-year-old male starting water-walking
    D. 41-year-old male beginning vigorous-intensity workouts

(D) The United States Preventative Task Force does not support routine stress electrocardiograms (ECG) in asymptomatic, low cardiovascular-risk individuals and does not have sufficient evidence to say whether these are beneficial in higher-risk patients. However, the American College of Cardiology (ACC) has recommended performing stress electrocardiograms in high-risk individuals before starting exercise programs. Of these, a **male > 40 years old who is beginning vigorous-intensity workouts** meets the criteria, especially in a previously sedentary individual.

The ACC has a Class II, Level of Evidence B, recommendation in favor of performing a stress electrocardiogram in asymptomatic patients that meet one of the following criteria:

- Multiple cardiac risk factors
- Men > 40 years old who plan to start vigorous exercise
- Women > 50 years old who plan to start vigorous exercise

These recommendations are particularly important in those who are sedentary or involved in occupations in which impairment may impact public safety (i.e., pilots).

Reference: Screening for cardiovascular disease risk with electrocardiogram: USPTF Recommendation. https://www.acc.org/latest-in-cardiology/journal-scans/2018/06/14/14/41/screening-for-cardiovascular-disease-risk-with-ecg

220. (Content: IV-A-3) A mother of a 12-year-old son with cognitive delays and class III obesity has brought a formal complaint to the medical board regarding the denial of a metabolic bariatric surgery evaluation. The surgeon states that although the patient meets criteria for surgery based on body mass index and comorbidities, he is concerned that the cognitive disability would make post-operative follow-up more difficult. Thus, he denied the adolescent entrance into the comprehensive bariatric program. This physician may be found in violation of which of the following principles?

A. Respect for autonomy
B. Beneficence
C. Nonmaleficence
D. Justice
E. American disability act

(D) Although this physician had appropriate concern for post-operative care, denying an initial evaluation based on cognitive disability violates the principle of **fairness (justice).** This patient should be provided consultation, treatment options, and evaluation of adherence to a medical, dietary, and physical plan before determining surgical candidacy.

Note: Although any medical, psychiatric, psychosocial, or cognitive condition that prevents adherence to postoperative regimens is a contraindication to surgery, social and family support should be evaluated. A patient with a cognitive disability but great family support that can assist in post-operative adherence may be a better surgical candidate than someone with decision-making capacity with little motivation or appreciation of the surgery.

Ethical principles regarding patient care include:

- Autonomy: Respecting the patient's decision to refuse or accept treatments based on the patient's preferences
- Beneficence: Doing what is best for the patient
- Nonmaleficence: "First, do no harm"
- Justice: Treat and provide care fairly to all patients

Reference: Pratt JSA, Browne A, Browne NT, et al. ASMBS pediatric metabolic and bariatric surgery guidelines, 2018. Surg Obes Relat Dis. 2018;14(7):882-901. doi:10.1016/j.soard.2018.03.019

221. (Content: IV-A-1) A Master of Public Health candidate is interviewing clinicians for her dissertation focused on the biased treatment of those living with obesity. In particular, she wants to understand the clinician-patient relationship, including support staff, regarding the perception of those with obesity in the medical setting. Which of the following is the most accurate statement regarding this topic?

A. Patients with obesity seek out medical care as a safe haven for bias
B. The FDA treats medications for obesity similarly to other medications
C. **Clinicians with a normal BMI are more comfortable discussing weight**
D. Physicians self-report that obesity is a disease similar to diabetes
E. Patients with obesity tend to receive longer office visits

(C) Unfortunately, weight stigma and bias are rampant not only within the community but also within the medical environment. All of the above are false, except for **clinicians with a normal BMI are more comfortable discussing weight** and counseling patients on this disease.

Obesity is treated differently from other chronic diseases, likely because it is often a visual diagnosis. Clinicians with excess weight felt they were less trustworthy in providing obesity care because they felt like they were poor role models. This finding is not present with other less noticeable medical conditions.

Studies have shown many physicians associate obesity with laziness, lack of self-control, and lack of success or intelligence. In addition, a study showed that 31% of nurses would prefer to treat patients without obesity and 24% were repulsed by those with obesity. Even prescribing medications has additional barriers, including Risk Evaluation and Mitigation Strategies (REMS) safety program for prescribing topiramate (Qsymia®) for obesity, though not required for topiramate if used for an alternative diagnosis (i.e., migraines).

Reference: Obesity Action Coalition
Reference: Flint SW, Oliver EJ, Copeland RJ. Editorial: Obesity Stigma in Healthcare: Impacts on Policy, Practice, and Patients. Front Psychol. 2017 Dec 11;8:2149. doi: 10.3389/fpsyg.2017.02149. PMID: 29312036; PMCID: PMC5732360.
Reference: Puhl RM, Heuer CA. Obesity stigma: important considerations for public health. Am J Public Health. 2010 Jun;100(6):1019-28. doi: 10.2105/AJPH.2009.159491. Epub 2010 Jan 14. PMID: 20075322; PMCID: PMC2866597.

222. (Content: IV-E-2) An employer of a mid-level business is evaluating ways to improve productivity while decreasing costs. He would like to implement a physical activity initiative in which his employees would reap the cost-savings of an overall healthier workforce. Which of the following has the highest cost for an employer of workers affected by obesity compared to workers with a healthy weight?

A. Absenteeism
B. Health insurance premiums
C. **Presenteeism**
D. Retirement plans
E. Accidental death insurance

(C) **Presenteeism** is the opportunity cost (indirect cost) related to decreased productivity while the employee is at work. On average, workers with a body mass index ≥ 35 kg/m^2 experience a 4.2% (1.18% more than other employees) health-related loss in productivity, equating to $506 annually per worker in lost productivity.

Similarly, lost production due to the employee not being at work (hospitalized, doctor's appointments, injury, etc.) is termed absenteeism and costs approximately $79-132 per person in those with a BMI ≥ 35 kg/m^2.

Obesity healthcare costs in the United States range from $170-210 billion annually. Individually, annual costs are approximately $1800 more than healthy-weight individuals. This is related to the following:

- **Direct costs:** Hospitalizations, physician visits (preventative, diagnostic, and treatments), prescription drug use, and management of obesity-related comorbidities.
- **Indirect costs:** Absenteeism, presenteeism, and premature disability and mortality.

Reference: Obesity and Presenteeism: The Impact of Body Mass Index on Workplace Productivity. Journal of Occupational and Environmental Medicine: January 2008 - Volume 50 - Issue 1 - p 39-45;
Reference: Reference: Adult Obesity Prevalence Maps. Centers for Disease Control and Prevention. National Center for Chronic Disease Prevention and Health Promotion, Division of Nutrition, Physical Activity, and Obesity. 27 September 2022. https://www.cdc.gov/obesity/data/prevalence-maps.html

223. (Content: IV-E-3) A 19-year-old female presents to her primary care physician. She has a diagnosis of systemic lupus erythematosus with nephritis, and she has gained nearly 50 lbs (22.7 kg) since starting treatment. Her current BMI is 33 kg/m². Which of the following is the best primary diagnosis code used for billing in this patient?

    A. E66.01: Severe obesity due to excess calories
    B. E66.1: Drug-induced obesity
    C. E66.9: Obesity, unspecified
    D. Z68.33: Body mass index (BMI) 33.0-33.9, adult
    E. Z68.53: BMI pediatric, 85% to less than 95th percentile for age

(B) The best primary code (in the absence of pregnancy) is an E66 code, with the most specific explanation preferred. In this case, **drug-induced obesity (E66.1) is the most descriptive**, as her weight gain is likely from the initiation of glucocorticoids.

Billing for patients with the disease of obesity consists of identifying their severity (overweight, obesity, etc.), contributing factors (drug-induced or excessive calories), associations (pregnancy), and symptoms (BMI or alveolar hypoventilation). Use E66 codes for primary diagnosis and Z68 codes for secondary diagnosis.

- E66.01: Severe obesity due to excess calories
- E66.09: Other obesity due to excess calories
- E66.1: Drug-induced obesity
- E66.2: Severe obesity with alveolar hypoventilation
- E66.6: Overweight
- E66.8: Other obesity
- E66.9: Obesity, unspecified
- Secondary: Z68.1-Z68.44 index codes for BMI (Used for adults only)
  - Kids (age 2-20) based on percentile for age range (Z68.5-)

If the code for obesity complicating pregnancy, childbirth, or puerperium is used (O99.21), use an additional code to identify BMI (Z68).

Note: These unique codes do not need to be memorized for the board exam, but a basic understanding of how they are applied is necessary.

Reference: AAPC: Obesity: ICD-10-CM Code Assignment

224. (Content: IV-B-1) A primary care physician will start to see bariatric patients in his clinic as part of a multi-disciplinary approach to treating patients that are planning to undergo bariatric surgery. He plans to perform a preoperative screening, education, and postoperative follow-up visits. In preparing his office for this influx of patients with obesity, what would be recommended to make the patients feel more comfortable when presenting to his office?

A. Ensure his scales can weigh up to 300 lbs (136 kg)
B. Ensure standard chairs have handrails on either side
C. Order additional medium and large blood pressure cuffs
D. **Ensure reading material in the waiting room is obesity-sensitive**
E. Provide additional obesity-culture training only to the nursing staff

(D) A patient with obesity should feel comfortable in the setting in which they are being seen. Therefore, forethought should go into preparing your office in regards to equipment and staffing culture. One of the initial impressions your patient will experience is the waiting room. If there is not **obesity-sensitive reading materials available,** this can cause discomfort and potential shame. In addition, magazines that promote fad or unhealthy diets should be removed.

Other necessary preparations are discussed below:

- Furniture to accommodate > 300 lbs
- Wide chairs with handrails or standard chairs without side rails
- Exam tables with a capacity of up to 600 lbs
- Blood pressure cuffs and gowns in large and extra-large sizes
- Scales that weigh up to 350 lbs- 700 lbs (calibrated monthly and located in a private area) based on clientele (500 lbs or more preferred).

Also, all staff should be trained in appropriate first-person language, free of bias, stigma, shaming, or embarrassment.

Reference: Toward Sensitive Treatment of Obese Patients
Syed M. Ahmed, MD, MPH, DrPH, Jeanne Parr Lemkau, PhD, and Sandra Lee Birt

225. (Content: IV-E-1 and 2) A physician is meeting with a United States senator regarding reimbursement for obesity therapy, including pharmacotherapy. The senator discusses the cost burden associated with obesity and his concerns that additional finances for coverage of extra office visits, bariatric surgery, and pharmacotherapy would ultimately not be worth the extra cost. Which of the following statements is true regarding the value of obesity therapy?

A. A patient with a BMI of 35 kg/m^2 infers an additional annual average medical cost of $500 compared to someone with a BMI of 25 kg/m^2
B. Nationally, the burden of obesity accounts for $50 billion in additional healthcare costs
C. **Anti-obesity interventions cumulatively could generate $20 billion in savings for Medicare within ten years**
D. Although bariatric surgery provides decreased morbidity, no studies have confirmed improved mortality rates
E. Physicians should only use FDA-approved anti-obesity medications despite the cost, as off-label medications have little evidence.

(C) The astronomical cost of treating obesity and its related complications account for nearly $150 billion annually (approximately $1900 annually per individual with a BMI $\geq$ 30 kg/m^2). In contrast, anti-obesity interventions for eligible individuals could generate **Medicare budgetary savings of $20-$23 billion over 10 years,** justifying the upfront costs associated with appropriate treatment.

In conclusion, individually, the cost of obesity intervention would be approximately $1800, with individual savings of $7000 (over ten years) for intensive therapy.

Note: Off-label use of medications is commonly done in obesity medicine to help patients offset prescription costs. There is ample evidence to support this practice, with many medical societies supporting this practice and providing guidance.

Reference: Ten-year Medicare budget impact of increased coverage for anti-obesity intervention. Chen F, Su W, Ramasamy A, Zvenyach T, Kahan S, Kyle T, Ganguly R. J Med Econ. 2019 Oct;22(10):1096-1104. doi: 10.1080/13696998.2019.1652185. Epub 2019 Aug 19.

226. (Content: IV-A-1) A school counselor is evaluating a 9-year-old male. The child states that two other boys in his class relentlessly tease him about his weight during recess. This has caused the student to withdraw from friends and academically decline. He is very conscious of what he eats now and states, "I wish they would just leave me alone!" The counselor calls the parents to discuss the situation. Which of the following would be the most constructive advice to provide to the parents?

A. Encourage them to seek medical care for the child's weight
B. Reassure the parents this will likely resolve with disciplinary action against the students initiating the bullying
C. Recommend scheduled counseling for the child
D. Encourage parents to teach the child to stand up for himself
E. Inform the parents that ignoring bullying is an effective technique

(C) Bullying is a common stressor incurred by children, with teasing based on a child's weight being one of the most common causes of victimization. **Counseling** is beneficial to help with coping skills, screening for severe depression, and improving self-worth and self-esteem.

Note: Although encouraging the parents to seek help for the child's weight seems appropriate, it does not address the child's underlying coping skills or provide an evaluation for depression.

A child undergoing teasing due to increased weight leads to mental and emotional health consequences causing academic decline and social avoidance. These ultimately contribute to potential mental health disorders such as low self-esteem, depression, and suicide.

General recommendations include:

- Avoid encouraging children to fight back with physical aggression, as this often only worsens and encourages increased teasing.
- Ignoring the bullying by the child often does not improve, and may even escalate, teasing.
- Seek counseling or psychiatric evaluation, especially if the child has severe depression, suicidality, or daily activity withdrawal symptoms.

Reference: Obesity medicine association: Pediatric Obesity Algorithm (2020-2022)

227. (Content: III-H-4 and IV-A-3) A 14-year-old male with Down syndrome and class II obesity with obstructive sleep apnea, hyperlipidemia, and prediabetes presents for follow-up at a bariatric center. The patient has been evaluated for bariatric surgery and was started on lifestyle modifications. His mother states he eats what he is given and rarely snacks. The patient and his family have been walking together every night for 1 hour. However, he has not lost any weight despite these measures. When discussing the procedure, the patient does not show an understanding of the procedure but states, "I want to be skinny." What is the most appropriate surgical management?

A. **Obtain surgical consent from the parents**
B. Continue to educate the patient and only perform the surgery when he can understand and provide consent
C. Two physicians that agree that surgery is appropriate, along with the parent's consent, is sufficient for pre-operative consent
D. Do not perform surgery due to a lack of understanding
E. Intensify lifestyle modifications

(A) This patient has many obesity-related complications and meets the criteria for metabolic surgery. However, he cannot provide consent due to a lack of decision-making capacity. Despite this, he has shown a solid support system and adherence with lifestyle modifications. Therefore, **informed consent by the parents or guardian** is sufficient to pursue metabolic surgery.

If surgery is determined to be the only effective treatment in preventing long-term morbidity, intellectual disability should not exclude the patient. However, to meet the criteria for surgery, appropriate support and adherence with pre-operative eating and physical activity should be demonstrated to ensure that recommendations can be followed to improve the likelihood of sustainable and effective results post-operatively. If this standard is not met, surgery provides more short-term risks than long-term benefits.

Reference: Pratt JSA, Browne A, Browne NT, et al. ASMBS pediatric metabolic and bariatric surgery guidelines, 2018. Surg Obes Relat Dis. 2018;14(7):882-901. doi:10.1016/j.soard.2018.03.019

228. (Content: IV-A-2) An obesity clinic is trying to determine the best way to reach different ethnicities by utilizing cultural-specific resources effectively. Given the clinic's central location, its patient population consists of many minority groups. Generally speaking, which strategy would be the most effective therapeutic addition for a culturally tailored approach to weight-loss?

    A. Provide a heart disease class for American Indians
    B. Have Caucasians teach weight-loss strategies to Chinese Americans
    C. Discuss alcohol avoidance within the Muslim population
    D. Utilize a faith-based setting for African Americans

(D) Culturally tailored communication is an integral part of healthcare and can effectively improve obesity rates. Different studies have evaluated communication approaches within ethnicities to find more effective ways to reach minorities. In particular, **African Americans have improved retention when support/education groups are located in a faith-based setting.**

Other findings are discussed below:

- **Chinese Americans:** Incorporating cultural values and customs while providing bilingual staff (when appropriate) was shown to improve retention.
- **American Indians/Alaskan natives:** Due to the high levels of diabetes with diabetes-related complications, focusing on weight loss to prevent these complications is more effective than targeting obesity or weight loss alone.
- **Muslims:** Utilizing imams (Muslim religious leaders) in specific health education yielded more effective results. In addition, working with patients in the setting of Ramadan (prolonged fasting periods) to incorporate healthy practices (e.g., avoiding SGLT-2 inhibitors, modifying physical activity, etc.)

Reference: Wanda Martin Burton, Ashley N. White & Adam P. Knowlden (2017) A Systematic Review of Culturally Tailored Obesity Interventions among African American Adults, American Journal of Health Education, 48:3, 185-197, DOI: 10.1080/19325037.2017.1292876
Reference: Ya-Ching Huang & Alexandra A. Garcia (2020) Culturally-tailored interventions for chronic disease self-management among Chinese Americans: a systematic review, Ethnicity & Health, 25:3, 465-484, DOI: 10.1080/13557858.2018.1432752

229. (Content: IV-A-1) A 27-year-old male with a body mass index of 34 kg/m² presents to his primary care physician for follow-up from an emergency department visit for intractable nausea that has since resolved. He is very disappointed with his experience, as he requested hospital records and found in the emergency room notes that the physician used wording that he felt was hurtful and counterproductive. Which of the following statements would be an appropriate opening identifying statement regarding his weight?

A. A 27-year-old morbidly obese male
B. A 27-year-old individual affected by obesity
C. A 27-year-old obese patient
D. A class 1 obese 27-year-old male

(B) People-first language is a term that recognizes the importance of not labeling individuals by their disease, in order to prevent the potential hazards and adverse provider-patient relationships that may subsequently ensue. Therefore, **stating a patient is affected by obesity is preferred** over labeling the person as an "obese individual."

People-first language: Name the person first and the disease second.

People-first language should be incorporated not only in obesity medicine but in all areas of practice, as it replaces the feelings of assumptions or stereotypes with more positively associated terms.

The table below further provides some examples.

People-First Language and Avoiding Stigma	
Avoid	**Use Instead**
Obese/overweight patient	Patient with obesity/overweight[1]
Fat	Excess/unhealthy weight or adiposity
Morbidly obese	Severe or class III obesity
Diet	Healthy eating habits or patterns
Exercise	Physical activity or patterns
Large size/heaviness	High BMI

[1]Pre-obesity may be used with patients to describe overweight

Reference: Obesity medicine association: Obesity Algorithm (2021)
Reference: Obesity Action Coalition (http://www.obesityaction.org)

Test Content Outline and Answer List Summary

I. Basic Concepts – 25%

A. Determinants of Obesity
    1. Lifestyle/Behavioral
    2. Environmental/Cultural
    3. Genetic
    4. Secondary
    5. Epigenetics and Fetal Environment

B. Physiology/Pathophysiology
    1. Neurohormonal
    2. Enterohormonal/Microbiota
    3. Body Fat Distribution
    4. Pathophysiology of Obesity-Related Disorders/ Comorbidities
    5. Body Composition and Energy Expenditure
    6. Energy Balance and Hormonal Adaptation to Weight Loss
    7. Obesity Related Cell Physiology and Metabolism
    8. Brain, Gut, Adipocyte Interaction

C. Epidemiology
    1. Incidence and Prevalence, Demographic Distribution
    2. Across the Life Cycle

D. General Concepts of Nutrition
    1. Macro and Micronutrients
    2. Gastrointestinal Sites of Nutrient Absorption
    3. Obesity Related Vitamin and Mineral Metabolism
    4. Macronutrient Diet Composition and Effects on Body Weight and Metabolism

E. General Concepts of Physical Activity
    1. Biomechanics and kinesiology
    2. Cardiorespiratory Fitness and Body Composition

II. Diagnosis and Evaluation – 30%

A. History
  1. Medications
  2. Family History
  3. Comorbidities/Assessment and evaluation
  4. Sleep
B. Lifestyle/Behavior/Psychosocial
  1. Demographic/Socioeconomic/Cultural/Lifestyle/Occupational
  2. Physical Activity
  3. Nutrition/Diet
  4. Eating Disorders/Disordered Eating
  5. Body image disturbance
C. Physical Assessment
  1. BMI
  2. Waist Circumference
  3. Physical Findings of obesity and Comorbid Conditions
  4. Vital Signs
  5. Underlying Syndromes
  6. Signs of Nutritional Deficiency
  7. Growth indices
D. Procedures and Laboratory Testing
  1. Resting Metabolic Rate
  2. Body Composition Analysis
  3. Diagnostic Tests
      a. Comorbidities
      b. Secondary Obesity
E. Screening Questionnaires
F. Research Tools

III. Treatment – 40%

A. Behavior
    1. Behavioral Counseling Techniques/Therapies
    2. Self-Monitoring Techniques/Tools
B. Diet
    1. Calorie and Micro/Macronutrient
    2. Very Low Calorie Diet
    3. Meal Replacements
    4. Effect on Comorbid Conditions
C. Physical Activity
    1. Prescription
    2. Mechanisms of Action
    3. Effect on Comorbid Conditions
D. Pharmacotherapy, Pharmacology and Pharmacokinetics
    1. Risks, Benefits, and Adverse Effects
    2. Indications/Contraindications
    3. Monitoring and Follow Up
    4. Prescription Dose and Frequency
    5. Drug-Drug, Drug-Nutrient, Drug-Herbal Interactions
    6. Off Label Usage/Over-the-counter (OTC)
    7. Multi-drug/Combination Therapy
    8. Management of Drug-Induced Weight Gain
    9. Effect on Comorbid Conditions
E. Alternative, Emerging, and Investigational Therapies
F. Surgical Procedures
    1. Types, Risks, Benefits
    2. Indications and Contraindications
    3. Complications
    4. Pre-operative Assessment and Preparation
    5. Post-operative Management
        a. Medical Inpatient
        b. Medical Outpatient
        c. Nutritional
    6. Adolescent Surgery
    7. Effect on Comorbid Conditions

G. Strategies

    1. Age-Related Treatment

    2. Risks Associated with Excessive Weight Loss

    3. Management of Weight Plateau

    4. Prevention of Obesity and Weight Gain

    5. Management of Comorbid Conditions During Weight Loss

    6. Effect of Weight Loss on Comorbid Conditions

    7. Treatment of Comorbid Conditions

H. Pediatric obesity

    1. Treatment Guidelines

    2. Pharmacotherapy

    3. Bariatric Surgery

    4. Family Support and Participation

IV. Practice Management – 5%

A. Patient care Issues
    1. Weight Bias, Stigma/Discrimination
    2. Culturally Tailored Communication
    3. Ethics
B. Office Procedures
    1. Policies and Protocols
    2. Adult Obesity Management Guidelines and Recommendations
    3. Physician Personal Health Behaviors
    4. Online and remote management tools
C. Interdisciplinary Team
D. Advocacy/Public Health
E. Other
    1. Cost Effectiveness of Treatment Options
    2. Awareness of Societal Cost of Obesity
    3. Reimbursement and Coding

Content breakdown per life cycle:

- Pediatric and adolescent content: 15%
- Adult content: 20%
- Content relevant to all life cycles: 65%

Answers

1. C	31. D	61. D	91. E
2. A	32. E	62. C	92. B
3. D	33. B	63. C	93. D
4. A	34. A	64. A	94. E
5. B	35. D	65. D	95. A
6. E	36. B	66. C	96. A
7. C	37. B	67. A	97. A
8. A	38. D	68. B	98. B
9. C	39. A	69. C	99. B
10. D	40. B	70. C	100. C
11. B	41. D	71. D	101. C
12. D	42. A	72. A	102. A
13. A	43. E	73. D	103. C
14. C	44. B	74. B	104. E
15. D	45. B	75. A	105. C
16. A	46. A	76. B	106. D
17. A	47. D	77. B	107. B
18. D	48. E	78. C	108. C
19. B	49. C	79. A	109. E
20. E	50. B	80. E	110. A
21. E	51. C	81. C	111. A
22. D	52. A	82. C	112. E
23. E	53. E	83. D	113. D
24. B	54. B	84. C	114. B
25. D	55. E	85. E	115. A
26. B	56. C	86. D	116. B
27. A	57. D	87. B	117. B
28. B	58. E	88. C	118. D
29. C	59. C	89. B	119. D
30. C	60. D	90. A	120. D

121. A	151. E	181. B	211. B
122. B	152. C	182. B	212. A
123. A	153. B	183. A	213. A
124. B	154. E	184. D	214. D
125. B	155. D	185. C	215. D
126. B	156. A	186. B	216. E
127. A	157. A	187. D	217. E
128. B	158. D	188. E	218. B
129. E	159. C	189. D	219. D
130. A	160. B	190. C	220. D
131. C	161. C	191. B	221. C
132. B	162. D	192. E	222. C
133. C	163. B	193. A	223. B
134. E	164. D	194. E	224. D
135. D	165. A	195. B	225. C
136. D	166. A	196. E	226. C
137. B	167. C	197. C	227. A
138. C	168. A	198. C	228. D
139. B	169. D	199. E	229. B
140. D	170. B	200. D	
141. A	171. D	201. C	
142. D	172. A	202. B	
143. B	173. A	203. D	
144. B	174. E	204. B	
145. B	175. D	205. A	
146. D	176. C	206. B	
147. C	177. D	207. A	
148. C	178. D	208. B	
149. D	179. D	209. A	
150. D	180. E	210. D	

Provide Feedback After the Exam

Be entered to win a $100 Amazon gift card!

Drawing October 29th, 2023. Five winners will be chosen.
Constructive and detailed feedback appreciated.

Made in United States
Troutdale, OR
09/10/2023

12763490R00206